100 YEARS OF THE INTERNATIONAL CONFEDERATION OF MIDWIVES

First published 2022

Copyright © Joyce E Thompson, Joan Walker, Ann M Thomson & Margaret H Peters 2022

The right of Joyce E Thompson, Joan Walker, Ann M Thomson & Margaret H Peters to be identified as the authors of this work has been asserted in accordance with the Copyright, Designs & Patents Act 1988.

All rights reserved. No part of this book may be reproduced, stored in a retrieval system, or transmitted in any form or by any means, electronic, electrostatic, magnetic tape, mechanical, photocopying, recording or otherwise, without the written permission of the copyright holder.

Published under licence by Brown Dog Books and
The Self-Publishing Partnership Ltd, 10b Greenway Farm, Bath Rd,
Wick, nr. Bath BS30 5RL

www.selfpublishingpartnership.co.uk

ISBN printed book: 978-1-83952-529-2
ISBN e-book: 978-1-83952-530-8

Cover design by Kevin Rylands
Internal design by Andrew Easton

Printed and bound in the UK

This book is printed on FSC® certified paper

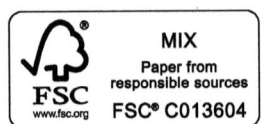

100 YEARS OF THE INTERNATIONAL CONFEDERATION OF MIDWIVES

EMPOWERING MIDWIVES AND EMPOWERING WOMEN

1922–2022

Joyce E Thompson
Joan Walker
Ann M Thomson
Margaret H Peters

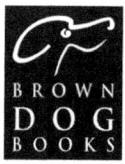

Dedication of the Book

This book is dedicated to the midwives and women of the world, the International Confederation of Midwives (ICM) and its member associations, the ICM's Partners, and others interested in global midwifery. It is also written In Memoriam to all those wise women and midwives on whose shoulders we, the authors, stand.

100 YEARS OF THE INTERNATIONAL CONFEDERATION OF MIDWIVES

EMPOWERING MIDWIVES AND EMPOWERING WOMEN

1922–2022

Joyce E Thompson
Regional Representative,
Deputy Director & Director 1990–2005
International Confederation of Midwives
International Midwifery Consultant
Michigan, USA

Joan Walker
Secretary General 1990–1998
International Confederation of Midwives
International Midwifery Consultant
Reading, UK

Ann M Thomson
Professor (Emerita) of Midwifery
University of Manchester
Former Editor Midwifery

Margaret H Peters
President,
Deputy Director & Director 1981–1999
International Confederation of Midwives
Melbourne, Australia

Contributing Authors

Franka Cadée
President 2017–2023
International Confederation of Midwives
The Netherlands
Chapter 18

Katherine A Dawley
Midwife Historian
Philadelphia,
PA, USA
Chapter 2

Karen Guilliland
Regional Representative
International Confederation of Midwives
Midwifery Consultant
New Zealand College of Midwives
Chapter 14

ACKNOWLEDGEMENTS

Librarians / Archivists
Archivists at the Royal College of Obstetricians & Gynaecologists
Gertrude M Ayerle: Assisted in locating paper about the 1900 conference
Jan Ayres, Librarian (retired), Photographer
British Library Staff
Jill Caughley, researching history ICN in 2007 who sent key WHO documents to JET
Mary Dharmachandran, Librarian at the Royal College of Midwives
Wellcome Collection Archivists and Library staff: Obtained ICM files from catalogued and uncatalogued sources and assisted Joan Walker whilst she worked in the library.

Interviewees / Contributors[1]
All the Midwives of the world who met with the Authors since 2014[2]
The ICM Headquarters' Staff
Roa Altaweli (Saudi Arabia): ICM Eastern Mediterranean Regional Representative
Sabaratnam Arulkumaran: FIGO
Ruth Ashton (UK): ICM Treasurer
Luc de Bernis: WHO, FIGO
Judith Marie Brown (Australia): ICM Deputy Director, Director Board of Management
Franka Cadée (The Netherlands): ICM President
Kim Campbell (British Columbia): ICM Treasurer, ICM Council member
Karin Christiani (Sweden): Director, ICM Board of Management
Alicia Cillo (Argentina): ICM Regional Representative
Dame Karlene Davis (UK): ICM Appointed President
Frances Day-Stirk (UK): ICM President
Jemima Dennis-Antwi (Ghana): ICM Anglophone Africa Regional Representative
Elizabeth Duff (UK): Editor of ICM newsletter

Vincent Fauveau: UNFPA
Judith Fullerton (USA): Consultant ICM Essential Competencies process
Frances Ganges (USA): ICM Secretary General/Executive Officer
German Midwives Association: Ingela Wiklund
Pandora Hartmann (USA): ICM Americas Regional Representative
Kathy Herschderfer (The Netherlands): ICM Secretary General
Petra ten Hoope-Bender (Netherlands): ICM Secretary General
Nicola King: Indexer
Ann Kinnear (Australia): Western Pacific Regional Representative
Anneka Knutsson: SIDA, UNFPA
Junko Kondo (Japan): ICM Asia-Pacific Regional Representative
Barbara E Kwast (Netherlands): WHO staff and ICM Liaison
Jerker Liljestrand: FIGO
Bridget Lynch (Ontario): ICM President
Nester T Moyo (Zimbabwe): ICM Programme Manager
Sandra Oyarzo (Chile): ICM Americas Regional Representative, ICM Vice President
Judith Oulton (Geneva): Executive Director, International Council of Nurses
Sally Pairman (New Zealand): ICM Chief Executive
Anja Peters (Germany): Author of IMU President Nanna Conti's biography
Leah Phillips (UK): Timeline graphic
Julie Berry Foster (USA) Graphic Designer at Printex printing and graphics
Frances Prior-Reeves: Brown Dog Books Managing editor
Khama Rogo: World Bank; Co-Chair PSMNH
Anita Román (Chile): Latin American midwifery perspective
Kerri Schuiling (USA): Story of International Journal of Childbirth
Gloria Seguranyes (Spain): ICM European Regional Representative
Della Sherratt (UK): WHO staff and ICM liaison; Interim ICM Secretary General Ann Starrs: Family Care International
Sister Anne Thompson (UK): ICM Treasurer, provided 75th ICM anniversary documents
Kim Updegrove (USA): Story of first ICM website
Paul Van Look: WHO
Caroline Weaver (Australia): ICM Appointed President

Reviewers
Roa Altaweli
Ruth Ashton
Franka Cadée
Frances Day-Stirk
Jemima Dennis-Antwi
Elizabeth Duff
Barbara Kwast
Bridget Lynch
Nester Moyo
Sandra Oyarzo
Sally Pairman
Della Sherratt
Ingela Wiklund

[1] The titles and organisations represented by each individual are listed without dates for the time periods, reflecting why they were chosen and/or volunteered to be interviewed and contribute.
[2] The Authors take full responsibility for this list and any possible omissions.

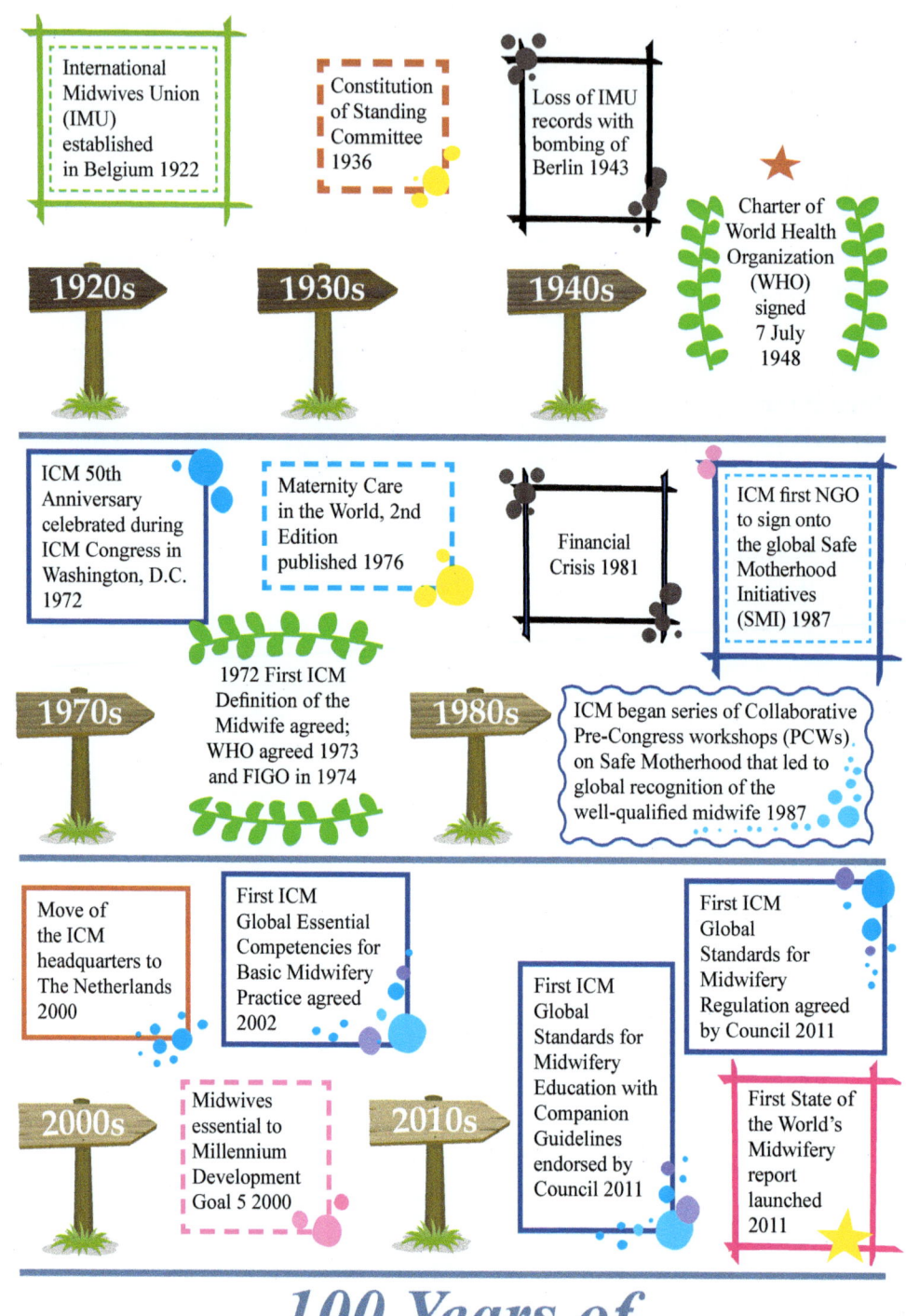

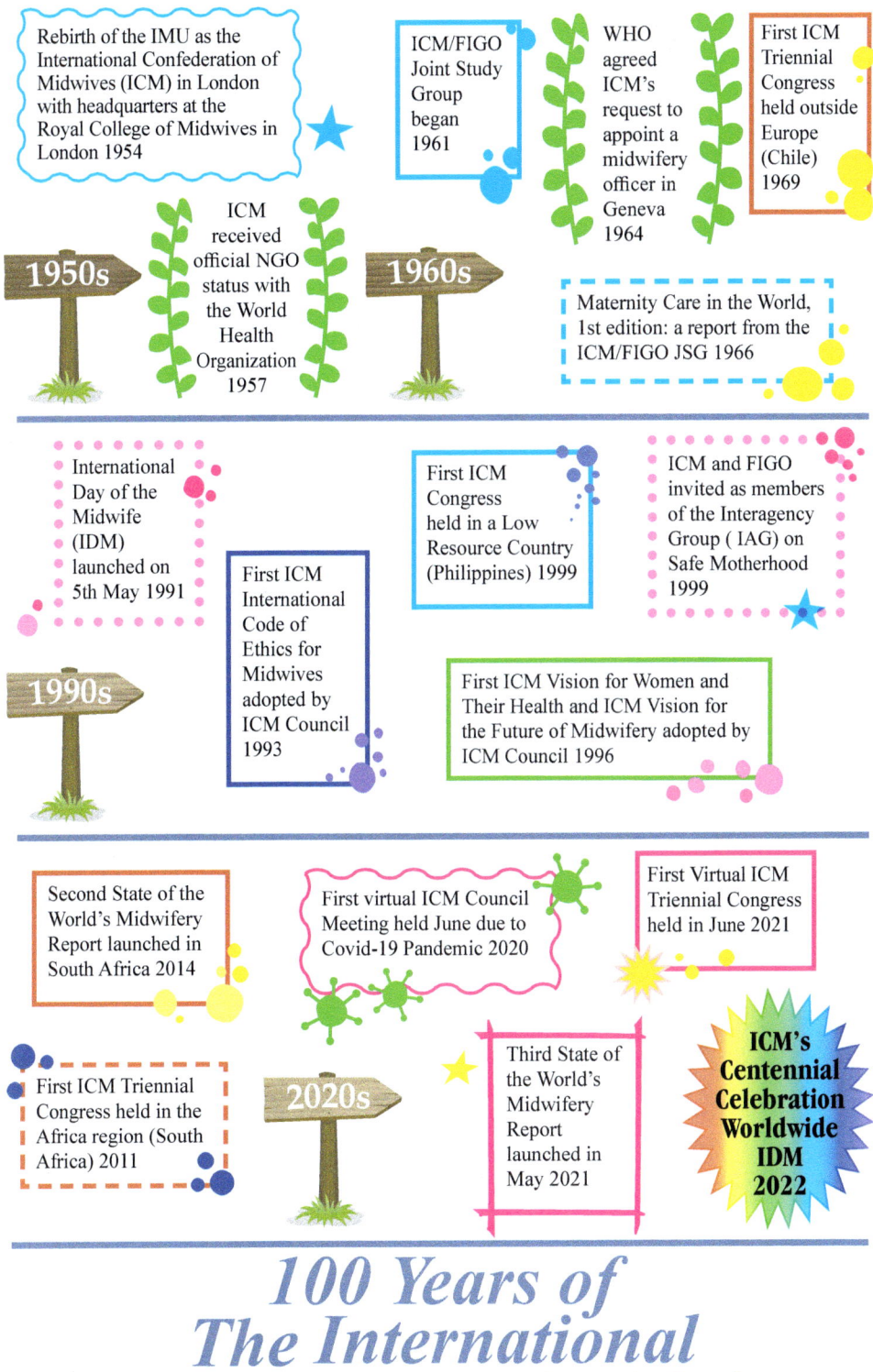

Table of Contents

List of Figures and Tables	24
Recurring Abbreviations	25
Preface by Her Royal Highness The Princess Royal	27
Foreword	29
Section I: Birth, Rebirth and Organisation of the ICM	33

Chapter 1: **Introduction** — 33
- a. Centuries of Midwifery Care — 33
- b. Approach to a Century of Collaboration and Empowerment Within the ICM — 35
- c. Key Themes During ICM's 100-Year Journey — 38
- d. The Legacy of the ICM — 38
- e. Summary — 39

Chapter 2: **Gender, Socio-Economic Status and Racial Influences on the ICM's Development** — 40
- a. Introduction — 40
- b. Suffrage, Women Workers and Their Rights — 40
- c. Feminism, Social Class and Midwifery — 42
- d. Post-World Wars Concerns for Mothers and Babies — 43
- e. Socio-economic Status of Women Affecting the ICM — 43
- f. Gender-Based Decision Making — 46
- g. Changing Global Trends — 47
- h. Summary — 47

Chapter 3: **Birth of a Global Midwifery Organisation: The International Midwives' Union** — 50
- a. Introduction — 50
- b. European Midwives' Efforts to Meet — 50
  - i. Development of Midwifery Associations prior to 1922 — 50
  - ii. Local, National and International Midwifery Meetings prior to 1922 — 51
- c. Overview of the International Midwives' Union — 52
- d. When Did the IMU Begin? — 52
- e. What Was the Name of the Organisation? — 53
  - i. What Did the Midwife Do? — 54
- f. What Was the Purpose of the Organisation? — 54
- g. How Did the IMU Function? — 55
  - i. Secretariat — 57
  - ii. Governance — 57

	iii. Subsequent Regulations	58
	iv. Officers of the International Midwives' Union	59
	v. IMU Affiliated Midwifery Associations/Members	60
	vi. Finances of the IMU	61
h.	Conferences/Congresses/Meetings	63
	i. Involvement of Obstetricians in the IMU	65
i.	Midwives for Peace and Healthy Mothers and Babies	66
j.	Summary	67

Chapter 4: Rebirth of IMU as the ICM — **70**

a.	Introduction	70
b.	Call for Rebirth of IMU	71
	i. 1949 IFMO Meeting	71
	ii. 1953 IFMO Meeting	72
c.	WHO Expert Committee on Midwifery Training, July 1954	73
d.	The ICM Congress in London: 4–11 September 1954	75
e.	ICM Council Decisions 1954	76
f.	1955–1956 ICM Activities	78
g.	The ICM Admitted into Official Relations with the World Health Organization – 1957	78
h.	Other Early Partnerships	79
i.	ICM World Congress in Stockholm – 1957	80
j.	Summary	80

Chapter 5: ICM's Constitutional Mandates and Structure — **84**

a.	Introduction	84
b.	Aims and Objects of the IMU/ICM Over Time (Purpose)	84
c.	Major Constitutional Mandate Changes	85
	i. The ICM Structure 1954–1981	86
	ii. The ICM Structure 1981–2008	87
d.	ICM Byelaws	88
e.	Constitutional Mandates/Powers Affecting the Structure of the ICM	89
	i. ICM Board: Qualifications and Responsibilities	89
	ii. Responsibilities of the Board of Management (BoM)	90
	iii. Executive Committee 1954–1981–2017; The Board 2017–present	90
	iv. Responsibilities of the Executive Committee	91
f.	Governance of the Confederation – the ICM Council	92
i.	The ICM Structure from 2023	93
g.	Actions and Responsibilities of the Council	93
	i. Criteria for ICM Membership	93
	ii. Setting Global Midwifery Policies and Standards	96
	iii. Selection of Host Associations for Congresses	96
	iv. The ICM Secretariat	97
	v. Responsibilities of the Secretariat	98
h.	Summary	98

100 Years of the International Confederation of Midwives

Chapter 6:	**The Search for Financial Stability/Viability**	**101**
a.	Overview	101
b.	Sources of ICM Income	102
i.	Membership/Capitation Fees	103
ii.	Congress Fees and Sharing of Proceeds/Profits from ICM Activities	104
iii.	Core Funding	105
iv.	Project Funding	106
v.	Special Funds	106
c.	Financial Support for Member Associations and Midwives	107
i.	Support for Council and Congress Participation	107
d.	Recurring Expenditures	109
e.	Financial Ups and Downs in the	
i.	1970s	110
ii.	1980s	110
iii.	1990s	111
iv.	2000s	111
v.	2010s	113
vi.	2020s	114
f.	Summary	114
Chapter 7:	**Support of ICM Business by the Secretariat**	**117**
a.	Introduction	117
b.	The ICM Secretariat (Headquarters/Head Office)	118
i.	Geographical Locations	118
ii.	Leadership of the Secretariat	119
iii.	Work of the Secretariat	120
iv.	Ongoing Work	122
v.	Staffing the Secretariat	124
c.	Communication with Member Associations	124
i.	Phone, Facsimile and Courier	125
ii.	Newsletters	128
d.	The *International Journal of Childbirth*	*130*
e.	The ICM Websites	131
f.	Representation of the ICM	132
g.	Summary	133
Section II: ICM: A CATALYST FOR GLOBAL RESPECT FOR MIDWIVES AND WOMEN		**137**
Chapter 8:	**ICM Vision, Mission and Strategic Directions**	137
a.	Introduction	137
b.	Vision Statements	138
c.	Mission Statements	142
d.	Strategy Documents	143
i.	Need for Outside Consultant – 1997	144
ii.	'Meeting of the Minds' – 2001	146
iii.	The Story Continues	147
iv.	Strategic Planning during 2008 Council Meeting	148
v.	New Approach in 2017	148
vi.	Strategic Directions Summarised	149
e.	Summary	151

100 Years of the International Confederation of Midwives

Chapter 9:	**Updating Midwives' Knowledge and Skills**	**154**
a.	Introduction	154
b.	Triennial Congresses: Scientific Meetings	155
	i. Locations of Congresses	155
	ii. Management of Triennial Congresses	156
	iii. Structure of Triennial Congresses	156
c.	Safe Motherhood Pre-Congress Workshops	158
	i. Purpose and Organisation of Pre-Congress Workshops	159
	ii. Pre-Congress Collaborative Safe Motherhood Workshops (Table)	162
d.	Mid-Triennium Executive Committee Meetings with Symposia	164
e.	ICM-Led Workshops During Congresses	166
f.	Regional Meetings/Conferences	167
g.	Country Workshops	169
	i. Burkina Faso	169
	ii. Ghana	169
	iii. Zimbabwe	170
	iv. Specific Country Efforts: 2005 and Beyond	171
h.	ICM Education for Midwifery Teachers	171
	i. Competency-Based Education Workshops	171
	ii. Strengthening Midwifery Education in French-speaking Africa	172
	iii. Global Standards for Basic Midwifery Education with Guidelines	172
	iv. Midwifery Education Accreditation Programme (MEAP)	172
	v. Additional education resources	173
i.	Summary of the ICM's educational efforts	174
Chapter 10:	**Strengthening Member Associations**	**177**
a.	Introduction	177
b.	The Work of the Confederation	177
c.	Member Association Issues Addressed	179
	i. Council Agreed ICM Policy, Position, Statement and Core Documents (Annex A)	179
	ii. Challenging Balance of Member Concerns	180
d.	Awards for Exemplary Midwives	181
	i. Marie Goubran Memorial Leadership Award – 1991 (Annex I)	181
	ii. Columbia University Award for Midwives and Their Associations – 2001	182
	iii. Saving Newborn Lives from Save the Children Award for Midwives – 2005	183
e.	Support for Country Activities	183
	i. Working Parties	183
	ii. Projects with Collaborative Partners/Donors	184
	1) Johnson and Johnson International	184
	2) Johns Hopkins Programme for International Education of Gynaecology and Obstetrics (Jhpiego)	184
	3) Sanofi Espoir Foundation [France]	185
	4) Laerdal Global Health	185
	5) Bill & Melinda Gates Foundation	185
	6) Direct Relief	185
	7) Strengthening Midwifery Services (SMS) with UNFPA	186
	8) Swedish International Development Agency (SIDA)	186

		9) White Ribbon Alliance	186
		10) MacArthur Foundation	186
		11) New Venture Fund	186
f.		Tools to strengthen Member Associations	186
	i.	Midwifery Association Strengthening	187
		1) Twinning Member Associations	187
		2) Young Midwifery Leaders Programme	187
		3) Member Association Capacity Assessment Tool (MACAT)	189
		4) Midwifery Services Framework (MSF)	190
		5) ICM RESPECT Toolkit	190
		6) ICM Advocacy Toolkits	191
		7) ICM's Inaugural Global Goodwill Ambassador	192
g.		ICM Standing Committees (SC)	192
	i.	Professional Practice Committee (PPC)	193
	ii.	ICM Research Standing Committee (RSC) – 1996	193
	iii.	ICM Education Standing Committee (ESC) – 2002	194
	iv.	ICM Regulation Standing Committee (RegSC) – 2008	196
	v.	Recent Standing Committees	197
h.		The International Day of The Midwife (5 May)	197
i.		Summary	200

Chapter 11:	**ICM's Core documents**	204
a.	Introduction	204
i.	What is a Profession?	204
ii.	Why Autonomy?	205
b.	*International Definition of the Midwife*	206
i.	Road to the First Joint ICM/FIGO/WHO *International Definition of the Midwife* – 1972	206
ii.	Updated *International Definition of the Midwife*	208
c.	*Scope of Midwifery Practice*	209
d.	*International Code of Ethics for Midwives* (1993)	210
e.	*Philosophy & Model of Midwifery Care* (2005)	213
f.	*Bill of Rights for Women and Midwives* (2011)	215
g.	*Definition of Midwifery* – 2017	216
h.	Summary	217

Chapter 12:	**ICM's Global Competencies and Standards**	220
a.	Introduction	220
b.	*Essential Competencies for Basic Midwifery Practice* (2002)	221
i.	Background	221
ii.	ICM Council Adopts *Provisional ICM Essential Competencies for Basic Midwifery Practice* – 1999	222
iii.	ICM Council Adopts ICM *Essential Competencies for Basic Midwifery Practice* – 2002	222
iv.	Updated ICM Essential Competencies – 2010/2011	223
v.	2017 Update of ICM Essential Competencies	224
c.	Midwifery Education Standards and Guidelines (2010)	225
i.	Background	225

		ii. Development of the Standards & Guidelines	226
		iii. ICM Adopts *Global Standards for Midwifery Education with Guidelines – 2011*	227
	d.	Midwifery Regulation Standards and Toolkit	230
		i. Background	231
		ii. Development of Regulation Standards	231
		iii. ICM *Global Standards for Midwifery Regulation (2011)*	232
	e.	Midwifery Regulation Toolkit (2016)	233
	f.	Summary	234

Chapter 13: **Regional Member Associations' Perspectives on the ICM** — 237

	a.	Introduction	237
		i. Number of Regions	237
		ii. Regional Survey Questions	238
	b.	Anglophone Africa	238
		i. Historical Background	238
		ii. Member Associations	239
		iii. Value/Impact of ICM Membership on Anglophone Africa MAs	240
		iv. Impact of Anglophone African MAs on the Growth and Development of ICM as an Organization	244
	c.	Americas Region: North America/Caribbean	245
		i. Historical Background	245
		ii. Member Associations	247
		iii. Value/Impact of ICM Membership on North American and Caribbean Midwifery Associations	248
		iv. Impact of the North America/Caribbean MAs on the Growth and Development of ICM as an Organisation	251
	d.	Americas Region: Latin America and Mexico	253
		i. Member Associations	253
		ii. Value/Impact of ICM Membership on Latin American and Mexican Midwifery Associations	254
		iii. Value/Impact of Latin American and Mexico MAs on the Growth and Development of ICM	256
		iv. Conclusion	256
	e.	Asia-Pacific/Western Pacific Region	257
		i. Introduction	257
		ii. Historical Background	257
		iii. Member Associations	258
		iv. Value/Impact of ICM Membership on Asia-Pacific/Western Pacific Midwifery Associations	260
		v. Value/Impact of Asia-Pacific/Western Pacific MAs on the Growth and Development of the ICM	261
	f.	Eastern Mediterranean Region	263
		i. Historical Background	263
		ii. Member Associations	263
		iii. Value/Impact of ICM Membership on Eastern Mediterranean Midwifery Associations	264
		iv. Impact of EMR MAs on the Growth and Development of ICM as an Organisation	267

100 Years of the International Confederation of Midwives

g.	Regional Expectations for the Future of the ICM	267
	i. Future Expectations of the ICM from Anglophone Africa MAs	268
	ii. Future Expectations of the ICM from North America and Caribbean MAs	268
	iii. Future Expectations of the ICM from Spanish-speaking Latin America and Mexico MAs	268
	iv. Future Expectations of the ICM from Western Pacific Region MAs	268
	v. Future Expectations of ICM from Eastern Mediterranean Region MAs	269
	vi. Common expectations from all Regions include	269
h.	Summary	270

Chapter 14: **Women, Midwives and the ICM** — **272**

a.	Introduction	272
b.	Women's Work	273
c.	Women as Members of ICM Member Associations	274
d.	The ICM's Vision for Women and for Midwive	276
	i. Listening to Women	276
	ii. ICM's Statement at the 4th World Conference on Women – 1995	277
	iii. ICM's Vision: Empowering Women, Empowering Midwives – 1993	277
e.	ICM's Commitment to Working with Women as Partners	278
	i. ICM's *Midwives, Women and Human Rights* – 2002	279
	ii. ICM's *Philosophy and Model of Midwifery Care* – 2005	280
	iii. ICM's *Bill of Rights for Women and Midwives* – 2011	280
	iv. The ICM's *International Definition of the Midwife* rev. 2011	281
f.	Organisations Sharing a Common Vision of Women and Midwives as Partners	281
	i. The White Ribbon Alliance	282
	ii. Other ICM Partnership Efforts	282
	iii. Partnerships with Global Health Groups/Agencies	283
g.	The ICM's Organisational Structure Supporting Women as Partners and Leaders	285
h.	Summary	286

Chapter 15: **United Nations (UN) Agencies and the ICM** — **289**

a.	Introduction	289
b.	The World Health Organization (WHO)	290
	i. The Who Expert Committee: *The Midwife in Maternity Care* – 1965	291
	ii. The ICM and the WHO: An Ongoing Relationship	293
	iii. Midwifery Technical Officers Within the WHO Assigned to the ICM	293
	iv. Meeting Challenges directly for *Health for All*	296
c.	The United Nations Children's Fund (UNICEF)	297
d.	The United Nation's Fund for Population Development (UNFPA)	298
	i. UNFPA-ICM Joint Initiative: Responding to a Decade of Action for Human Resources – 2008	298
	ii. Mutual Respect between ICM and UNFPA	299
	iii. Strengthening Midwifery Services	300
	iv. UNFPA/ICM Electronic Newsletter 2021: A Moment for Midwives	301
e.	The *State of the World's Midwifery* Reports (SoWMy)	302
	i. SoWMy 2011	302

		ii. SoWMy 2014	303
		iii. SoWMy 2021	303
		iv. Summary UNFPA/ICM Activities	305
	f.	Midwifery Expertise Shared with Partners	305
	g.	Summary	305

Chapter 16:		**Health Professional Groups and the ICM**	**309**
	a.	Introduction	309
	b.	International Federation of Gynecology and Obstetrics (FIGO)	309
		i. The FIGO/ICM Joint Study Group: 1961–1979	309
		1. Purpose of the FIGO/ICM Joint Study Group: 1961–1976	310
		2. *Maternity Care in the World*, 1st Edition: 1966	311
		3. Selected 1966 Outcomes Affecting ICM and Member Associations	312
		4. Continued Joint Study Group Efforts	313
		ii. European Working Party on Midwifery Training in European Countries – 1969	314
		iii. Second FIGO/ICM Project Aim and Objectives – 1972	314
		iv. *Maternity Care in The World*, 2nd Edition 1976	315
		v. Impact of the FIGO/ICM Joint Study Group on the ICM	316
		vi. The FIGO/ICM/WHO *Definition of the Midwife*	316
		vii. Ongoing ICM and FIGO collaboration	317
	c.	The International Pediatric Association (IPA)	317
	d.	The International Council of Nurses (ICN)	318
		i. Overview	318
		ii. Joint Efforts at the World Health Assembly (WHA)	319
		iii. Triad Meetings	320
		iv. Other ICM and ICN Collaboration	321
	e.	Partnerships for Maternal, Newborn and Child Health	322
		i. The Partnership for Safe Motherhood and Newborn Health (PSMNH) – 2004	323
		ii. The Partnership for Maternal, Newborn and Child Health (PMNCH) –2005	323
		iii. The Role of Health Professional Organisations in PMNCH	324
		iv. The PMNCH Work Plan and Board Members	325
	f.	ICM Joint Statements	326
		i. The Midwife as Prototype Skilled Attendant	327
		ii. Midwives and Nurses Call for Increased Skilled Attendance at Birth (2000)	330
		iii. Birth Registration (2003)	331
		iv. Prevention of Post-partum Haemorrhage (2004/2006/2008)	331
		v. Hammamet Call to Action: 'Scaling-up Midwifery in the Community' (2006)	331
		vi. A Global Call to Action (2010)	332
		vii. WHO/UNFPA/UNICEF/ICM/ICN/FIGO/IPA Definition of Skilled Health Personnel Providing Care during Childbirth (2018)	333
	g.	The *Lancet Series on Midwifery* – 2014	334
	h.	Summary	334

Chapter 17:	**ICM's Importance to Midwives, Women and World Health**	**339**
a.	Introduction	339
b.	ICM's Value/Importance to the Health of Women	340
i.	International Midwives' Perspectives	340
ii.	International Obstetricians' Perspectives	343
c.	Value of the ICM to Midwives and Midwifery Associations	344
i.	International Midwives' Perspectives	344
ii.	International Obstetricians' Perspectives	346
iii.	International Partners' Perspectives	346
d.	Importance/Value of the ICM to its Global Partners	348
e.	Lessons Learnt from History	351
f.	The ICM's Challenges Moving Forward	353
g.	Summary	355
Chapter 18:	**A Vision for the Future of the ICM and Midwifery**	**357**
a.	Introduction	357
b.	Strengthening Midwife Associations Is ICM's Core Business	358
c.	Autonomy of Women, Midwives and the ICM	359
i.	Women	359
ii.	Midwives	359
d.	ICM's Global Strategy 2020–2023: The Way Forward	361
e.	Summary	361
Annexes		364
A.	Member Association issues and resulting ICM Position Statements/Documents	364
B.	Countries Represented at each IMU Congress/Conference/Meeting 1922–1938	368
C.	Table of ICM Congresses and Themes 1954–2021	370
D.	Table of ICM Partners and Projects 1951–2022	374
E.	Wording of Objects/Aims in Constitutions of the IMU/ICM 1925–2022	379
F.	Table of ICM Appointed and Elected Officers 1954–2023	381
G.	Tables of ICM Member Associations by Regions 1934–2021	385
H.	Geographical Location of ICM Headquarters 1939–2022	398
I.	Winners of the Marie Goubran Memorial Leadership Award 1993–2020	399
Index		401

List of Figures and Tables

Table 3.1   IMU Congress Locations, Dates and Officers/Honorary Officers
Figure 5.1   The ICM Structure 1954–1981
Figure 5.2   The ICM Structure 1981- 2008
Figure 5.3   The ICM Structure from 2023
Table 7.1   ICM Secretary Generals & Chief Executive Officers 1922–2022
Table 8.1   ICM Strategic Directions 2008–2022
             ICM Strategic Directions with Objectives 2017–2023
Table 9.1   Pre-Congress Collaborative Safe Motherhood Workshops
Table 9.2   ICM Mid-Triennium Workshops/Symposia
Table 13.1   Anglophone Africa: Country, Name and Year Midwifery Associations Accepted for ICM Membership
Table 13.2   North America & Caribbean: Country, Name and Year Midwifery Associations Accepted for ICM Membership
Table 13.3   Latin America & Mexico: Country, Name and Year Midwifery Associations Accepted for ICM Membership
Table 13.4   Asia–Pacific: Country, Name and Year Midwifery Associations Accepted for ICM Membership
Table 13.5   Eastern Mediterranean: Country, Name and Year Midwifery Associations Accepted for ICM Membership
Table 15.1   WHO Midwife Technical Liaison Officers for the ICM

Recurring Abbreviations

ACMI = The Australian College of Midwives, Inc.
ACNM = The American College of Nurse-Midwives
BOM or Board = refers to a group of elected officers of the ICM
CBE = Competency-Based Education
CE = Chief Executive
Communications = *Communications of the International Midwives' Union* journal
Confederation = shortened for International Confederation of Midwives
Constitution = refers to the Constitution of the ICM
Council = Decision making body of the ICM consisting of two delegates from each Member Association plus elected Officers
DFID = UK government Department for International Development
EC = The ICM Executive Committee, i.e., Board of Management plus elected Regional Representatives from 1981 to 2005
ERA = ICM's three Pillars of Education, Regulation and Associations
FCI = Family Care International
FIGO = The International Federation of Gynecology and Obstetrics
GAGNM = Global Advisory Group of Nurses and Midwives to the WHO Director General
HQ = The ICM Headquarters, also referred to as Head Office
IAMANEH = International Association for Maternal and Neonatal Health
ICM = The International Confederation of Midwives
ICN = The International Council of Nurses
IDM = The International Day of the Midwife (5 May)
IMU = The International Midwives' Union
IPA = The International Pediatric Association
IPAS = International group that promotes safe abortion care and safe reproductive health
Jhpiego = originally known as the Johns Hopkins Program for International Education in Gynecology and Obstetrics; only the initials used now
JSG = The ICM/FIGO Joint Study Group
KSB = knowledge, skills, behaviour

MACAT = ICM's Member Association Capacity Assessment Tool
MA = An ICM Member Association as distinct from a country's midwifery association that is not an ICM member
MDGs = The United Nations' Millennium Development Goals (2000–2015)
MEAP = ICM's Midwifery Education Accreditation Programme
MEDPath = ICM's Midwifery education development pathway programme
MSF = ICM's Midwifery Services Framework
MMR = Maternal Mortality Rate
MNH = Maternal Neonatal Health
NGO = A Non-Governmental Organisation (more recently Civil Societies)
NZCOM = The New Zealand College of Midwives
PCWs = ICM's Collaborative Pre-Congress Workshops
PMNCH = The Partnership for Maternal, Newborn and Child Health
POPPHI = USAID's Prevention of Post-Partum Haemorrhage Initiative
PSMNH = The Partnership for Safe Motherhood and Newborn Health
PT = Part-time
Regions = the designated geographic regions of the ICM
RCM = The Royal College of Midwives
RMC = Respectful Maternity Care
SC = An ICM Standing Committee: e.g., R – being Research; E – being education; PP – being Professional Practice; Reg – being Regulation
SDGs = The United Nations' Sustainable Development Goals (2015–2030)
Secretariat = includes the ICM office location and staff
SG = Secretary General of the ICM
SIDA = The Swedish International Development (Cooperation) Agency
SM = Safe Motherhood
SMI = The WHO's Safe Motherhood Initiatives
SoWMy = The *State of the World's Midwifery* (reports)
UK = United Kingdom
UN = The United Nations
UNFPA = The United Nations Population Fund
UNICEF/Unicef = The United Nations Children's Fund USA = United States of America
USAID = The United States' Agency for International Development
WHO = The World Health Organisation
WWI = World War I
WWII = World War II
YML = Young Midwifery Leaders

BUCKINGHAM PALACE

I have had the honour of following in my Grandmother's footsteps as Patron of The Royal College of Midwives. In visits to countries across the world I have seen first-hand the esteem in which midwives are held and the care they are able to give to mothers and babies. This book sets out how, from small international beginnings, midwives across the world have worked together during the past 100 years to be better able to improve the health of women during their reproductive years and support them and their babies.

When three Midwives' Associations decided to work together in 1922, they could never have dreamed of how their collaboration has today helped midwives and childbearing women and their newborns in more than 120 countries. The Midwives Institute, forerunner of The Royal College of Midwives (UK), worked alongside midwives' associations in Belgium and the Netherlands in establishing the International Midwives' Union. Despite two world wars the midwives stayed strong and, in 1954, with The Royal College of Midwives playing a lead role, revitalised the international midwives' organisation as the International Confederation of Midwives (ICM).

I wish to applaud the International Confederation of Midwives and its leaders who accepted all the challenges that arose by being a female led organisation with a predominantly female workforce working for and with women in all corners of the world to become a valued health professional partner across the globe.

This book focuses on the value and impact of the International Confederation of Midwives, the only midwifery organisation representing midwives and the midwifery profession both individually and collectively, on the health of women and childbearing families. The Confederation has worked tirelessly with its member associations in countries, directly helping them with midwifery education, extending midwifery services to cover family planning, social and nutritional aspects as well as establishing legal frameworks. The help that associations give to each other has enabled a strong bond to develop, one of friendship as well as a professional one.

To understand this history is important to developing the future where midwives and midwifery can continue to progress and make a significant contribution to the health and wellbeing of nations.

Anne

Foreword

This book is a labour of love. It began in the 1990s shortly before the 75th anniversary with the bulk of archival searches beginning in earnest five years ago. Joan Walker is a UK midwife well-known to the Wellcome Collection Library staff[1] where she spent years searching through the archived International Confederation of Midwives' (ICM) papers and photos and putting those details in chronological order. Ann Thomson, also a UK midwife, was creative in her search of the archives at the Royal College of Midwives, The British Library, multiple nursing journals, many European country conference proceedings and conversations with individuals in order to reconstruct the history of the International Midwives' Union (IMU), the forerunner (grandmother) of the ICM. Her primary source documents were several issues of the Communications of the International Midwives' Union from 1925.[2] It was known that a significant number of documents pertaining to midwives and their associations were lost when libraries became collateral damage in the bombings throughout Europe during World War II (1939–1945).[3]

Margaret Peters, an Australian midwife, searched her own ICM files and directed the writers to key sources of information on the ICM, offering comments and insight on each chapter. Joyce Thompson, a USA midwife, searched her own files for ICM papers from 1990 to the present. Her writing was complemented by the archival material, personal papers and writings from Joan Walker.[4] In addition, interviews with key individuals and vignettes from former and current ICM leaders and partners provided much of the human-interest aspects. Additional primary source documents have been used when available, including Board and Council minutes, conference and workshop reports and correspondence. Three chapters are contributed by midwives recognised for their expertise in those topics.

100 Years of the International Confederation of Midwives

What this Book Is
This book is a brief narrative history of the International Confederation of Midwives (ICM) that, in 2022, completed 100 years of representing the world's midwives through strengthening and supporting its midwifery Member Associations (MAs) in order to protect and promote healthy newborns and empower women. The essence of this 'herstory' of the ICM revolves around a century of organisational development, growth and influence, especially related to women's reproductive health, rights and safe childbearing care.

Social Context
The 100-year history of the ICM would be incomplete without helping the reader understand the ICM's beginnings and ongoing development within the social context of what was happening, especially the challenges of gender, socio-economic status and race faced by its leaders and MAs. Though many of these challenges are woven throughout the book, Chapter 2 is included to offer insight into the social context of the International Midwives' Union (IMU) during 1922–1939, the forerunner of the ICM. Other discussion of social context is woven throughout later chapters.

Organisation of the Book
This content of the book is organised into two sections that address two major goals:
1) the description of the organisation beginning in 1922, and
2) the growth, accomplishments, and impact of the organisation globally.

The first section, titled Birth, Rebirth and Organisation of the ICM, is a chronological narrative beginning in 1922 of the ongoing development of the ICM as a female-led, female-oriented global health organisation. Content includes its efforts to address its dual aims to 1) promote and protect the health and well-being of women and childbearing families and 2) support its Member Associations to strengthen the education, regulation and practice of their midwives in order to attain the first Aim. A brief overview of the structure of the organisation and its financial ups and downs are included.

The second section of the book, titled ICM: A Catalyst for Global Respect for Midwives and Women, includes selected narrative details of the ICM's strategic activities and accomplishments that have strengthened its member associations and individual midwives. The ICM's reputation as a vital, collaborative partner in promoting reproductive health and rights, especially related to women and childbearing care, has been repeatedly supported by inclusion in several global reports contributing to Health for All.[5] The ICM has been a catalyst for change that has been and continues to influence major global organisations to take notice of the vital role that women and their health play in the health of all nations.

Language Used in Text

For the most part, the authors chose to use the generic 'midwife' throughout the text without attaching any gender. The word midwife in the original old English means with woman describing the work of midwifery and not the gender of the midwife. Therefore, midwife is a term that men in the midwifery profession can proudly use.

The newest challenge arose in the 21st century related to use of inclusive language.[6] As terminologies changed over the years the ICM has tried to be respectful of these. The ICM has always referred to adolescents or women when referring to those who give birth. The authors were advised recently that in some countries 'birthing people' is now a term used for those giving birth. In continuing to use the terms 'adolescents' and 'women' throughout this text when referring to childbearing, the authors accept that this now includes those who prefer to use 'birthing people'.

What this Book is Not

This book, however, is <u>not</u> the history of midwifery in the world, or in individual countries or regions, though some of that history is reflected in the narrative. It is also <u>not</u> an anthropological analysis or in-depth critique of the ICM as an organisation, though there will be some discussion of strengths, weaknesses and challenges faced. This book will <u>not</u> discuss all midwife leaders through the years, though a few who heavily influenced the development of the ICM and its global remit will be highlighted. Likewise, the book will <u>not</u> discuss every ICM position statement and core document, though a few will be highlighted. Annexes are provided that list these along with other ICM activities. Current documents can be found on the ICM website: www.internationalmidwives.org.

Authors' Biases

The authors acknowledge but do not apologise for our inherent biases as authors/editors of this history because of our personal involvement and leadership within the Confederation since the late 1960s. The writing style and content have been heavily influenced by the authors' interpretation of primary sources. The involvement of key players as authors brings many positives, including a passion and enthusiasm for the subject. The authors' personal involvement in many of the activities and issues/challenges discussed has resulted in more detail in some areas than others as is often the case in narrative writing. While the primary authorship is White/Caucasian, details and stories from the African, Asia-Pacific and Eastern Mediterranean regions are also included. However, the authors are not historians. We have done our best to tell the ICM 'story' as viewed through the lens of primary sources, interviews and our own personal experiences in an effort to highlight the significance, influence and global impact of the ICM on midwives and midwifery services that improve the sexual and reproductive health and rights of women, newborns and childbearing families in every corner of the world. Thus, the authors accept full responsibility for the content of this book based on available documents.

History is often written for learning so that mistakes are not repeated in the future to the detriment of the ICM, but positives are built upon. This book was also written to provide information for the current and future leaders of the ICM who will continue to demonstrate the ICM's strong and vibrant efforts to improve the health of young girls and women globally with well-qualified midwives supported by strong midwifery associations to benefit families and countries.

The Authors

1 The Wellcome Collection is the current name of the London-based organisation housing the ICM archives. During Joan Walker's ten years of gathering ICM history there, it was known as the Wellcome Institute Library.
2 Unfortunately, the 1925, 1926, 1927, 1928 and 1929 issues of the IMU-produced *Communications* have not been found, indicating how much midwives have lost of their early history as an international organisation.
3 Many details of the IMU history were lost when the organisation's papers were destroyed during bombing in Berlin in 1943 when the offices of the Deutscher Hebammen were hit.
4 Any personally-held papers relating to the ICM that are not already in the Wellcome Collection will be transferred to there after publication of this book.
5 A few examples of these reports include: World Health Organization. *World Health Report 2005*. Geneva: WHO, 2005. UNFPA. *Millennium Declaration and Goals, 2000–2015*. New York: UNFPA, 2000. UNFPA. *Sustainable Development Goals 2015–2030*. New York: UNFPA, 2015.
6 KD Gribble, S Bewley, NX Batick, R Mathisen, et al. Breastfeeding and Newborn Care: The Importance of Sexed Language. *Frontiers in Global Women's Health*. 8: Article 818858, February 2022. DOI: 10.3389/fgwh.2022.818856.

100 YEARS OF THE INTERNATIONAL CONFEDERATION OF MIDWIVES EMPOWERING MIDWIVES AND EMPOWERING WOMEN

Section I: Birth, Rebirth and Organisation of the ICM
Chapter 1: *Introduction*

'The global community owes a huge debt of gratitude to ICM for establishing midwifery as a respected profession, for standardization of [education], for being the voice of women for pregnancy and childbirth.'

Sabaratnam Arulkumaran (FIGO) – 18 March 2019

CENTURIES OF MIDWIFERY CARE

Midwives have been 'with women' for centuries, attending to their childbearing needs as well as providing birth-to-death care within the family and community, what today might be called primary health-care based on a public health model of health promotion and disease prevention.[1] Midwives were trusted members of their communities, held in high esteem by the people they served[2], yet sometimes feared and mistreated by those who did not understand the value of midwifery care and the 'mysteries' surrounding menstruation, birth and menopause. Midwifery work was frequently hard and challenging under difficult circumstances. It was also rewarding to the midwives who spent long hours, days and many years carrying out the mandate of their 'calling' / profession to promote the health and well-being of every woman and childbearing family they touched, and, whenever possible, to secure a safe outcome for every mother and newborn.[3] In other words, 'midwifery was a vital service for women at a critical moment in their lives, in the intimacy of their own homes'[4].

Midwives strived to do the best they could with the knowledge and skills available to them at the time, but never gave up on learning more. During different eras of feminism, the work of women, including midwifery, was highlighted along with the suffrage movements. Women's movements in many countries led to increasing demands for justice and basic human rights for adolescent girls and women. These movements affected midwives' roles and practise throughout the past 100 years, with a few instances addressed in this book. In addition, many women, particularly in resource rich countries, demanded their right to be more involved in decisions about their care. They identified actions needed to offset the lack of respectful care that modern technology and hospital births often brought about, and often sought the advice and support of midwives in their communities for a more humanised birthing experience.

Midwifery itself changed over the years with new demands for providing expanded services to save maternal and newborn lives (life-saving skills) beginning with family planning and other aspects of reproductive health care beyond childbearing. The search for new knowledge led to midwives' gathering in small and large groups to share stories, to learn from one another and to seek ways to improve the health of the women and families in their care.[5] However, until the end of the 19th and beginning of the 20th century, midwifery and midwives managed very well for thousands of years without the structures and complexity of a formal organisation.

What changed? European midwives' desire to formalise their efforts to share information as the demands for healthy childbearing increased following World War I (WWI) resulted in a decision to group together. The ICM's story organisationally began in 1922 in Belgium following WW1 when midwives when midwives from Belgium, England and the Netherlands met during a Flemish Scientific Conference and were encouraged by obstetrician Frans Daels to form an organisation (Chapter 2). World War II (WWII) 'silenced' organisational efforts from 1939 to 1948, with renewal of activities in the form of a Congress in 1954 in London. Initially, the organisation grew throughout Western Europe during the 1920s and 1930s. The ICM gradually expanded to include midwifery associations in high resource countries (United States, Australia) during the 1950s–1970s along with a few African groups. It was not until the 1980s that Midwifery Associations in Asia-Pacific and more recently in the Eastern Mediterranean region became members.

The ICM's dual aims throughout its history have been:
to promote and protect the health and well-being of women and childbearing families.
 to support its member associations to strengthen the education, regulation and practise of their midwives in order to attain the first Aim.
Though these aims have been addressed primarily through its member associations,

ICM leaders and members also agreed to support country midwives who did not yet have the benefits of an official midwifery association, often with the support of international health partners such as the World Health Organization (WHO), other United Nations' agencies, governmental aid organisations, global professional groups and private foundations.

Thus, the International Confederation of Midwives (ICM) was established (initially named the International Midwives' Union) in 1922 with the goal of midwifery associations working together to strengthen the profession of midwifery and protect and promote the reproductive health of childbearing women and their newborns. During the past 100 years, the ICM's efforts/activities have placed midwives and midwifery on the global reproductive health agenda throughout this narrative story as illustrated by the current ICM logo[6].

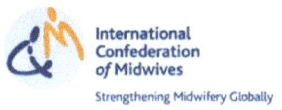 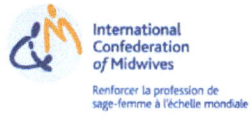 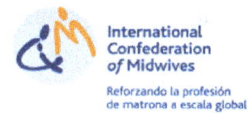

Current ICM logos – Used with permission of the ICM.

APPROACH TO A CENTURY OF COLLABORATION AND EMPOWERMENT WITHIN THE ICM

The content of this book focuses on key milestones (see Timeline) during the first 100 years of the ICM that have led to the modern-day organisation. Sentinel successes are part of the ICM story, including important global partnerships that share a common vision for healthy women and families. In many ways, the story of ICM reflects the story of women throughout the century who struggled for recognition, voting rights, respect and decision authority.[7]

The ICM's story reflects the influence of ICM leaders and its member associations over the past 100 years as they worked together to make sure women and childbearing families received evidence-based care from well-qualified, caring midwives in all corners of the world. ICM leaders also collaborated with international health partners in securing the ICM as a truly international, well-respected health professional organisation representing the profession of midwifery as distinct from other health professions.

Section One content begins with a brief overview of the social context into which the International Midwives' Union (IMU) was born in 1922. It includes the individuals who established the IMU and their struggles to maintain the organisation between two world wars. Content also briefly addresses the constitutional mandates of aims, vision and mission of the ICM that have remained relatively constant since 1954, along with its organisational framework, the struggle for financial viability and the vital role of the paid central office staff.

Section Two content addresses the ICM's educational and standard-setting role for midwives throughout the world leading to increased autonomy of the profession and its midwives and increased global respect for the role of the midwife in global health efforts. It includes educational workshops, Congress sessions and core documents that solidified the role of well-prepared midwives as primary care providers for women during their reproductive years. Of particular note for understanding ICM's development is that the period 1981-2000 was one of sustaining and stabilising the organisation financially, growing its membership into one that was more global, and gaining recognition from potential international agency partners that midwifery skills can and do provide the ways and means to improved outcomes for women in their reproductive years, especially in resource limited nations. This establishment of ICM's credibility provided the base from which in the next decades the ICM could move forward to develop standards and demonstrate its capacity to respond to needs of member associations with the 'tools' to more accurately measure the effectiveness of midwifery education and practice.

As the reader follows the ICM journey it is important to note that many of the successes of this global organisation were the result of thousands of volunteer hours and financial support from visionary midwife leaders at global and regional levels supported by a small paid staff of dedicated midwives/individuals. Financial support from governments and private foundations also contributed to the growth and development of the ICM as an organisation.

Midwives of the world understood that they alone could not meet the sexual and reproductive health needs of adolescents and women, nor could they save the lives of all mothers and newborns. Hence the emphasis during the ICM's journey on the importance of partnerships, beginning with the women themselves. Other key partners, such as the World Health Organization (WHO), the United Nations Children's Fund (UNICEF), the United Nations Fund for Population Assistance (UNFPA) and professional associations such as the International Federation of Gynecology and Obstetrics (FIGO), the International Pediatric Association and the International Council of Nurses, contributed both technical and/or financial support to the ICM's efforts in strengthening midwives and midwifery associations worldwide. This meant that the reproductive health of adolescents and women would be improved with well-qualified midwives and midwifery care. A few of these important partnerships are discussed briefly and illustrate the expanding remit of the organisation in sexual and reproductive health while maintaining a clear focus on strengthening midwifery associations and midwives providing evidence-based childbearing services where the need is greatest.

The closing chapter of the book reflects the 2022 ICM President Franka Cadée's view of the future of the ICM as an international health professional organisation committed to well-educated and appropriately regulated midwives who are empowered to lead global efforts in maternal, newborn, adolescent and Women's health and rights.

Key Definitions

In an effort to increase the reader's understanding of the ICM and its journey of empowering midwives and empowering women, three key questions are addressed.

WHO IS A MIDWIFE?
This book uses the title 'midwife' and 'midwifery practice' throughout representing a common understanding of both words and titles from the perspective of the midwives themselves. Though the first ICM agreed definition of a midwife was not endorsed globally until 1972[8], the intent throughout the book is to refer to those who were formally prepared for their role as a midwife in various countries and localities beginning in the 1700s. The ICM *Definition of the Midwife* became one of the most important documents for moving the ICM forward as an international organisation, with each iteration of the wording expanded to define 'formal' education and 'legal recognition' more clearly.[9] The ICM in the early years was not concerned with how or where midwives were educated, and thus accepted into membership groups of midwives based on the country's definition of who was a midwife and what that person provided in the way of midwifery services. This was a similar practice in many health professions in the 17th through to the 19th centuries[10], where the group itself defined the criteria and standards for practice of that profession.

WHAT DOES A MIDWIFE DO?
Key aspects of the midwifery scope of practice along with education and regulation standards followed from the *Definition*. Throughout its history the ICM has been

focused on the 'competencies' of the midwife and the 'way midwives provide care' (philosophy and model) so that health outcomes for women, mothers and babies worldwide are improved. The competencies were agreed by the ICM Council in 2002. This was an important milestone when one considers the goal of representing all the world's midwives who meet the international definition of a midwife.

HOW IS A MIDWIFE EDUCATED?
The ICM is less concerned about the pathway to education as a midwife (direct entry or post nursing programmes) or the type of recognition the graduate of the formal programme received (certificate, diploma, university degree). The ICM leaders focus on the content of that education, e.g. evidence-based competencies within a framework of competency-based education methodology. Agreement of the ICM *Global Standards for Basic Midwifery Education* in 2010 and ICM *Global Standards for Midwifery Regulation* in 2011 are discussed with some examples of their use in various areas of the world as governments and policymakers develop or update the midwife education programmes and legislative frameworks in their countries.

KEY THEMES DURING ICM'S 100-YEAR JOURNEY
Self-identity and the struggle for autonomy (self-governance) along with the ever-present discussion of whether midwifery is a profession distinct from medicine and nursing appear at various points in the story of the ICM. Other themes woven throughout include financial viability and disparate views of ICM Member Associations on whether the ICM was meeting the needs of midwives in low resource countries at the expense of the needs in high resource countries and vice versa. Stories that illustrate these struggles and themes are included throughout this book as one way to enhance understanding of the ICM today and its ongoing commitment to represent autonomous midwives within strong midwifery associations with women at the centre of all activities. This is how the ICM contributes to global health as defined within the United Nations' *2030 Agenda for Sustainable* Development[11] and the UNFPA *Global Midwifery Strategy 2018–2030*[12].

THE LEGACY OF THE ICM
The legacy of the ICM includes a foundation of strong midwifery associations and their midwives throughout the world who have the knowledge and tools needed (competencies, standards, etc.) and commitment to continue their partnership

with women and other organisations to advocate for the sexual and reproductive health and rights for all. The authors have highlighted the great strides that the ICM has made in strengthening midwifery associations and the status of midwives globally. Over the years, the ICM has also succeeded in expanding its influence beyond the Global North into the Global South and will continue so that every young girl and woman of reproductive age from the remotest corners of the world to the most modern urban centres has access to a midwife. In other words, the ICM has become the catalyst for improved health for women, newborns and families everywhere.

SUMMARY

The story of the ICM is a combination of the stories of its member associations, its leaders and its international partners working together to make childbearing safe, newborns healthy and women empowered with full human rights alongside the men of the world. As noted in the *Milestones* pamphlet produced in 1994, 'ICM's story is one of the emergence of a modern, public, health care profession from an ancient, private craft … closely linked to the educational, social and economic status of the women it serves'[13]. Welcome to the ICM story that follows. We hope you enjoy your journey through time.
The Authors

1 WHO, *A vision for primary health care in the 21st century: towards universal health coverage and the Sustainable Development Goals*. Geneva: World Health Organization and the United Nations Children's Fund, 2018.
2 The Swedish Association of Midwives. *300 Years in the Service of Life*. Sweden: Svenska Barnmorskeförbundet, 2011. Laurel Thatcher Ulrich. *A Midwife's Tale: The Life of Martha Ballard, Based on Her Diary, 1785–1812*. New York: Vintage Books, 1991.
3 Caterina Schraeder. *Memoirs*. In Hiliary Marland (Trans.) *'Mother and Child Were Saved': The Memoirs (1693–1740) of the Friesian Midwife Catharina Schraeder*. Amsterdam: Rodopi, 1987.
4 ICM. *Milestones in International Midwifery (pamphlet)*. ICM: London, 1994, p 2.
5 The first Section of this book discusses some of the known local and national meetings of midwives before the inception of the International Midwives' Union in 1922. These include 1900 in Berlin when the German midwives' association invited midwives from around Europe to attend their meeting.
6 The current ICM logo illustrates the ongoing efforts to strengthen midwifery globally. The use of the logos in this book was authorized by the ICM with the understanding that the content of the book is the sole responsibility of the authors and not the ICM.
7 Jean Donnison. *Midwives and Medical Men: A History of Inter-Professional Rivalries and Women's Rights*. New York: Schocken Books, 1977.
8 WHO, ICM, Unicef, *Midwifery Education Action for Safe Motherhood: Report of a Collaborative Pre-Congress Workshop, Kobe, Japan 5–6 October 1990*. Geneva: WHO Pub. #WHO/MCH/91.3, p 27 presents the Definition of a Midwife 'adopted by the International Confederation of Midwives (1972) and International Federation of Gynecology and Obstetrics (1973) following amendment of the Definition formulated by expert panels of the World Health Organization.' The WHO definition was initially agreed during the First *Report on Midwifery Training*, published by the WHO in July 1955, p 6.
9 ICM. *International Definition of Midwife*. Chiswick, London: International Confederation of Midwives, 1972.
10 John Wesley. *Primitive Physic: Or an Easy and Natural Method of Curing Most Diseases*. London: The Epworth Press, reprint 1970 of original 1791 document. Paul Starr. *The Social Transformation of American Medicine*. New York, NY: Basic Books, Inc. 1982.
11 https://sustainabledevelopment.un.org/sdgs
12 UNFPA Sexual & Reproductive Health Branch, Technical Division. *Global Midwifery Strategy 2018–2030* and *Implementation Guide Global Midwifery Programme Strategy 2018–2030*. New York: UNFPA, March 2018.
13 ICM. *Milestones in International Midwifery (pamphlet)*. ICM: London, 1994, p 4.

Chapter 2: *Gender, Socio-Economic Status and Racial Influences on the ICM's Development*[1]

'The voice on the other line asked if I could put her in touch with the midwife who supported her, as a poor single teen mother, and into whose hands her daughter was born. I was the midwife. She told her daughter the story of her birth and about 'her midwife' many times and she wanted the midwife to attend her daughter's surprise college graduation party. She shared that after the birth, she realized she had strength and completed high school and earned a college degree.'

Katherine Dawley, USA midwife.

INTRODUCTION

The post-World War I (WWI) founding of the International Midwives' Union (IMU)[2] in 1922 followed and occurred during decades of feminists organising in Europe, the United States, Australia and New Zealand.[3] In these countries and others, feminism focused on attaining the rights of women in marriage, in the arena of work and in eligibility to vote. Likewise, concern for mothers and babies following the world wars led to an increased interest in and a need for midwives, especially after WWII. Since nearly all midwives in the early 20th century were women, the social context of feminism, universal suffrage, women's rights and a reaction to the high numbers of maternal and newborn deaths led feminists and workers' rights activists into an important and natural coalition.

The content in this chapter includes a description of the social context during the early development of the global midwives' organisation, first named the IMU and after 1954 named the International Confederation of Midwives (ICM). Later chapters include ongoing discussion of the social context of that time. This social context is a complicated interface of feminism, race, gender and socio-economic status. In particular, the primary focus is on what was happening to women and midwives and how their lived experiences affected the ICM.

SUFFRAGE, WOMEN WORKERS AND THEIR RIGHTS

Progress toward achievement of universal suffrage/the right to vote in political elections bridged gender and class.⁴ In the late 19th and early 20th centuries men also struggled for the right of universal suffrage. Large numbers of working-class men and all women did not have the right to vote. In England the vote in Parliamentary elections at the turn of the 19th century was restricted to only 2/3 of all men. From the perspective of late 19th and early 20th century British and European social and political history, the linkage of suffrage and labour can be seen in the names and work of the suffrage organisations and in organisations for midwives and nurses.

In the 1860s the National Union of Women's Suffrage Societies became active in England. By 1903 they were joined by the Women's Suffrage and Political Union. After WWI in 1918 some British women attained the right to vote, but full suffrage was not achieved until 1928.⁵ In mid-19th and early 20th century Europe, as in England, feminism focused both on women's suffrage and work. Strong ties between Belgian feminists and socialists with neighbouring activists in France and the Netherlands shaped the struggle for women's suffrage in Belgium which began in the early 1890s. In France and in Belgium Catholic feminist organisations that focused on women's rights in work and education also developed. Within this context, the IMU was born (Chapter 3).

Universal suffrage was achieved at different times and for different social classes, first in New Zealand in 1893. The New Zealand campaign for women's suffrage was tied to the temperance movement. Campaigner Kate Sheppard argued moral reform would follow women's franchise.⁶ After the formation of the Australian Federal Parliament the right to vote in federal elections was granted to all white citizens in 1902.⁷ However, the 1902 Commonwealth Franchise Act excluded indigenous people who were not granted full suffrage until 1967.⁸ It is important to note that little was written/known of the situation of women on the continents of Africa and Asia regarding voting rights until the latter half of the 20th century.

National European feminist organisations for suffrage were linked through international congresses and organisations, the International Woman Suffrage Alliance, and the International Council of Women with 7 million members in 24 countries.⁹ WWI caused a hiatus in feminist activism. Like American feminists, such as Jane Adams, the war moved suffrage activism towards anti-war pacifism and work with the Women's International League for Peace and Freedom. This call for peace was prominent in the last IMU Congress in 1938 as noted in Chapter 3. Full Belgian women's feminist and suffrage activism returned after WWII though full women's suffrage there was not achieved until 1948.¹⁰

FEMINISM, SOCIAL CLASS AND MIDWIFERY

Feminist political activism extended beyond campaigning for the vote into improving conditions of women's work influenced by socio-economic conditions. In the 1880s feminists took up the cause of midwifery as a potential occupation for women.[11] In England Louisa Hubbard, a socialist and campaigner for suffrage, focused much of her work on improving education for teachers and organising national societies focused on women's employment in industry, teaching and midwifery. In 1882, nurse-midwives Zepherina Smith (nee Veitch)[12] and Rosalind Paget, with assistance from Paget's uncle William Rathbone, a member of Parliament, founded the Trained Midwives Registration Society which in 1885 became the Midwives Institute. In 1902 the Midwives Act was passed and the Central Midwives Board was established in 1903. The Act defined both education and practice standards and the Board set national certification examinations for midwives.[13]

In an era of feminist agitation for suffrage and improved working conditions, other countries in Europe saw the same movement related to midwifery. By 1803 French law established guidelines for midwifery education and a national examination. In Italy a national exam and diploma in midwifery was created in 1859.

Midwifery in New Zealand became a regulated profession with the Midwives Act of 1904 which established a system of registration and state control of midwifery.[14] In Australia, midwives were regulated by the individual state governments in different ways. The Midwives Registration Bill was passed in 1915 establishing the Midwives Board state by state or territory, regulating direct entry, or 'vocational' midwives, and those who entered midwifery through nursing. Over a period of several years, activity undertaken by nursing and medicine resulted in the elimination of the Midwives Board and in 1928 a new Nurses Act brought midwifery under the control of nursing. At this point nursing education was a prerequisite for midwifery education.[15] By this time colonialists had started introducing midwifery based on nursing elsewhere in the world reflecting what was happening in Western Europe. As Fahy[16] noted in her article, the power strategies used by medicine towards nursing and the 'state' in Australia needed to be understood so that midwives and the midwifery profession could avoid and/or overcome their subordination in the years that followed. Positive action resulted when the Australian Capital Territory was the first to recognise midwifery as a separate profession from nursing. In 2010, Australia established the Health Practitioner Regulation National Law[17] which provided national registration and a separate register for midwives and nurses. It was not until some eight years later that midwifery was recognised as a distinct profession in the National Law.[18]

POST-WORLD WARS CONCERNS FOR MOTHERS AND BABIES

As noted above, in the aftermath of WWI the IMU was formed to address a growing concern with the expansion of the midwives' role, place of birth, standards for education and working conditions, and high maternal and infant mortality, especially among the poor. Midwives were joined by public health reformers to address some of these concerns for improved maternal and child health for all childbearing families. On the eve of WWII, the last IMU midwives congress moved beyond professional concerns to issue a plea for peace. Globally, WWII raised many concerns about the eugenics movement as a driver of policy and law in Europe and the United States.[19] After the war eugenics policies declined. WWII interrupted activities of the IMU and national nurse-midwife organisations in the United States and in many other countries involved in the war.

Post WWII (1945 in Europe and the United States) there was renewed interest in national and international midwifery organisational development to share professional knowledge and improve the health of women, infants and childbearing families through standards for education and practice. The long-standing Royal College of Midwives (RCM) took on a vital role in the rebirth of the ICM in 1954[20] and in 1956 the American College of Nurse-Midwifery (ACNM) and Mary Breckinridge's American Association of Nurse-Midwives (AANM) were accepted as ICM Member Associations (MAs), with many similarities between the three organisations. For example, many of the ACNM members practised midwifery internationally and knew the importance of organisational membership for the strength of midwifery. This was the same with many members of the RCM working internationally in former British colonies in Africa and India, and many members of AANM were educated in and originally practiced in the British Commonwealth.

SOCIO-ECONOMIC STATUS OF WOMEN AFFECTING THE ICM

Prior to the 1970s midwives in many countries cared primarily for populations with the highest maternal and infant morbidity and mortality – the poor, those who were isolated in rural areas and minorities/immigrants. In 1987, the ICM joined global efforts to promote Safe Motherhood (Chapter 9) for all women at a time when needless maternal deaths were often characterised as the greatest 'social injustice' arising from a lifetime of abuse and neglect.[21] All women face a higher risk of abuse in pregnancy, and poverty increases this risk. Assessment for abuse is integrated into practice and for many midwives their work in this area expands to the policy level and to creating safe spaces for abused women.

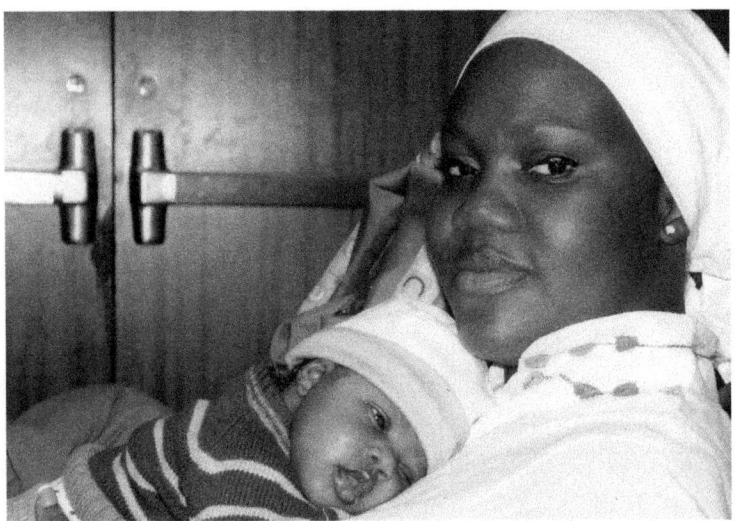

Healthy Mother and baby – Courtesy of Karen Guilliland

As noted by WHO leaders, the road to maternal death begins at birth for many of the world's women, especially those in low resource countries and those of limited income in high resource countries. This lack of basic human rights and gender-based violence supported the ICM's efforts to adopt position statements and core documents that set the standard for how women and midwives should be viewed in every society (Chapter 10).

The ICM's ongoing efforts to empower women and empower midwives since the 1990s have met with successes and many challenges (Chapter 14). The most difficult question that faced leaders over the years was how to set the standard for women's and midwives' ethical treatment following adoption of the ICM *International Code of Ethics* in 1993 (Chapter 11). At the time, there were such extremes of viewing women as persons with basic human rights among the MAs in High and Low Resource countries, and the way individual midwives were being treated in different societies. This struggle of women for basic human rights was also witnessed during the 1995 4th World Conference on Women and NGO Forum on Women in China:

100 Years of the International Confederation of Midwives

'The voices of women crying out for understanding, for justice, for peace, for basic health care were magnified a thousand times over as the days passed.'

Joyce E Thompson: Report on the 1995 NGO Forum on Women

As noted earlier, late-19th-century feminist activism for suffrage and improved conditions for working women including midwives continued well into the 20th century. But as much as conditions have changed, they remain the same. For example, in the mid-1990s a Minister of Health in a sub-Saharan African country met with a midwifery association leader and an international midwifery consultant. When presented with the poor working conditions of midwives including long hours, lack of needed supplies and meagre compensation – not enough to feed their family. He replied that since midwives were doing women's work, it was accepted in the health system that they did not need to be well compensated.

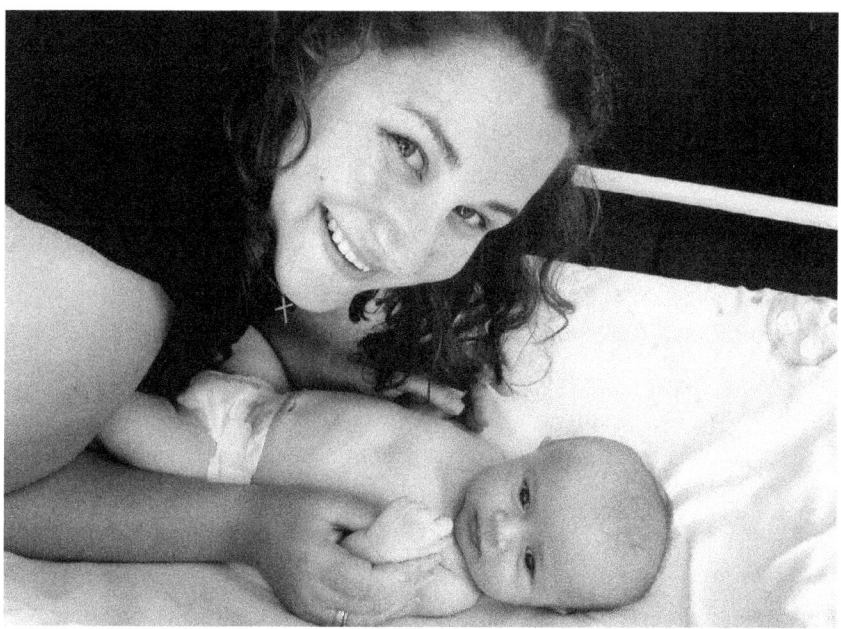

Healthy Mother and baby – Courtesy of Karen Guilliland

The evolving social status of women described earlier and its influence on the directions of the ICM were reflected during a 1997 ICM Strategy Planning Day facilitated by Mr Geoff Ribbens (Chapter 6). The outcomes of the Strengths, Weaknesses, Opportunities and Threats (SWOT) analysis revealed ongoing factors of gender that were influencing the organisation, both positively and negatively. For example, the ICM's professional demarcation of midwifery as 'women's work' along with a predominantly female profession and the 'volunteer structure' of the ICM with strong commitment from elected leaders, who often paid their own expenses and offered expertise without compensation, was noted as both a strength and a weakness. This was similar to the downside of women's work not being recognised because it was not paid.[22] As of 2022, none of the ICM Board members are paid a salary for their time and effort, though the President, Vice-President and Treasurer receive a 'stipend'[23] and all members of the Board continue to be reimbursed for travel and accommodation for meetings.

GENDER-BASED DECISION MAKING

The appointed and/or elected midwife Presidents/Directors of ICM for the past 90+ years have been female midwives, primarily English-speaking (though not always their first language) and Caucasian (Global North). Though there are men in the midwifery profession in many countries today, other countries do not allow them or struggled to have male midwives educated and accepted. One historical example was the 1975 Act that banned sex discrimination in employment, allowing men to become midwives in the UK. Bowing to pressure from this Act, the UK government permitted men to train as midwives in two experimental training programmes – one in Islington School of Midwifery, north London, from 1977, and another at Forth Valley Midwifery School in Stirling, Scotland, the following year.[24] However, there are few male midwives who have become leaders of the profession or within the ICM. One exception is Vitor Varela (Portugal) who was an ICM regional representative and then elected as the ICM Treasurer in 2020.

Though race, culture and language are important considerations in any global organisation, the ICM was at a disadvantage until the 1970s when an increasing number of MAs from Africa and SE Asia became active in the organisation. The ICM attempted to represent all races, cultures, genders and language groups in its many deliberations and with the development and agreement of key position statements and core documents (Annex A). These were discussed and agreed within ICM Council meetings where all MA delegates had a voice (when time for translation was allowed) and vote (Chapter 5). Partnerships with the WHO, FIGO and other groups over the years have increased the ICM's understanding of the world from a variety of perspectives, including those of men and individuals from low resource countries.

One organisational weakness identified in 1997 (Chapter 8) was the limited voice of midwives in general and the tendency of Council delegates to make decisions with their 'heart' rather than sound business principles (e.g. sites of Congresses or mid-triennium meetings were chosen to support a nation or association experiencing challenges, but, in reality, there would be fewer participants). In addition, the unequal leadership and managerial expertise in elected Directors along with financial/resource instability led to less-than-optimal decisions at times. These weaknesses were also reflected within the ICM as an employer of women. In addition, some of the weaknesses reflected the status of women at the time as well as the lack of understanding of what is required for a predominantly women's organisation led by women to function well. Each of the ICM's strengths and weaknesses could be viewed as inherent in the way women thought and worked at various times during the past 100 years, sometimes allowing the ICM to be successful and at other times limiting its ability to meet its aims, vision and mission.

CHANGING GLOBAL TRENDS

The 21st century could be described as 'Age of Upheaval', similar to that described by David Brooks in his description of Edwardian Politics 1899–1914.[25] It is a world in need of new leadership approaches and styles; a world that seeks stability, peace and health for all; a world that has and will continue to heavily impact the ICM and its Member Associations. Some of the major trends include digital distribution (information communication technology such as online distance learning MHealth); shifting demographics; increase in non-communicable diseases; the quest for the next generation of knowledge workers (e.g. migration, attracting potential midwives to the profession along with non-practising midwives); quality of (respectful) care; equity and sustainability. In 2020 the world was hit with the COVID-19 pandemic, calling on the ICM and its MAs' midwives around the world, nimble female (and some male) professionals skilled in responding to emergencies, into action. The ICM and its members responded quickly in their efforts to lead and support safe midwifery services for both women in their care and the midwives themselves through the accelerated use of virtual communication methods (Chapter 18).

SUMMARY

Some ICM leaders may not have had the expertise needed to manage an international organisation with its wide remit and very few staff, yet the ICM survived many challenges and became a strong international health professional organisation throughout the past 40–50 years. Feminist activity, human rights and the pledge to avoid inherent biases within the organisation have contributed to the development and growth of the ICM and its Member Associations. Progress on gender, socio-economic disparities, race and language use reflected where the world stood on these issues throughout the ICM's history. During the raising its status in the eyes of regulatory bodies and the world. This progress was incremental and made under the influence of strong, vision-oriented, pioneer women.

With the renewal of feminism in the mid-1990s midwives brought this perspective to the development of core documents, standards and position statements along with a concerted push toward autonomy of the profession. Likewise, during a period of revitalised global interest in gender equality, women's basic human rights and health issues in the early 2000s, the ICM embraced working more closely with and including women and childbearing families in the promotion of midwifery. All women involved in establishing and maintaining the ICM did so in the environment of their day. Some goals were therefore harder to reach than others but all those working to keep the ICM relevant and progressive remained true to the belief that good midwifery care made a positive difference in the well-being of adolescents, women, newborns, families and nations. It is important to keep these perspectives in mind as you read this 100-year story of the ICM. You are also encouraged to draw your own conclusions about the influence of the societal context of gender, socio-economic status, race, language and human rights on the ICM over the years.

100 Years of the International Confederation of Midwives

1. This chapter was written by Katherine Dawley, a nurse-midwife with doctoral preparation in the history of midwifery in the United States. It was edited to fit the format and context of the book.
2. The International Midwives' Union established in 1922 in Belgium was the predecessor of the International Confederation of Midwives with the latter name of the organisations adopted post-WWII in 1954.
3. Contributors of this book also noted similar feminist activities in Australia and New Zealand, though no specific references were found at this time.
4. Diane Atkinson. *The Suffragettes in Pictures.* London: Museum of London, 1996.
5. Diane Atkinson. *The Suffragettes in Pictures.* London: Museum of London, 1996, pp xiii–xiv.
6. Brief History. https://www.nzhistory.govt.nz/politics/womens-suffrage/brief-history (Ministry for Culture and Heritage), updated 5 July 2018. Accessed 3/6/21.
7. Michelle Arrow. 1902: Commonwealth Franchise Act gives women the vote in federal elections. David Hunt. *Defining Moments: Women's Suffrage.* State Library of Australia, 1894: Women's Suffrage South Australia. https://www.nma.gov.au/defining-moments/resources/franchise-act Accessed 3/6/21.
8. Kathleen Fahy. An Australian history of the subordination of midwifery. *Women and Birth* 20:1 (Mar 2006), pp 25–29. https://www.Doi:10.1016/j.wombi.2006.08.003 *Suffrage in Australia.* Accessed from Wikipedia on 8 March 2021.
9. Anne-Laure Briatte. 'Feminism and Feminist Movements in Europe XIX–XXI.' *Enclyopedie pour une histoire numerique de l'Europe'* [online], ISSN 2677-6588, published on 22/06/20, consulted on 09/02/2021. Permalink: https://ehne.fr/en/node/12314. p 5).
10. Julie Carlier. 'Entangled Feminisms. «Rethinking the History of the Belgian Movement for Women's Rights Through Transnational Intersections.' *Revue belge de Philologie et d'Histoire* tome 90, fasc. 4, 2012: 1339–1351.
11. Jean Donnison. *Midwives and Medical Men: A History of Inter-Professional Rivalries and Women's Rights.* New York: Schocken Books, 1977.
12. Wikipedia accessed online 2/15/21.
13. Jean Donnison. *Midwives and Medical Men: A History of Inter-Professional Rivalries and Women's Rights.* New York: Schocken Books, 1977. B Cowell and D Wainwright, *Behind the Blue Door: The History of the Royal College of Midwifery 1881–1981.* London: Bailliere Tindall, 1981, pp 33–34.
14. Jane Stojanovic. Midwifery in New Zealand 1904-1971. *Contemporary Nurses* 30:2 (October) 2008, pp 156–167. Doi: 10.5172/conu.673.30.2.156 Karen Guilliland. Midwifery in New Zealand. *Birth International.* Accessed website 4/4/21. https://birthinternational.com/midwifery-in-new-zealand/
15. Kathleen Fahy. 'An Australian history of the subordination of midwifery,' *Women and Birth*, 20:1, 2007, pp 25–29.
16. Kathleen Fahy. 'An Australian history of the subordination of midwifery,' *Women and Birth*, 20:1, 2007, pp 25–29.
17. The Health Practitioner Regulation National Law (the National Law) was enacted in each state and territory of Australia in 2009 and 2010. The goal of the National Law was to create a national registration and accreditation scheme for registered health practitioners (the National Scheme). Downloaded 21 May 2022 from: https://www.nhpo.gov.au/legislation#:~:text=The%20Health%20Practitioner%20Regulation%20National,practitioners%20(the%20 National%20Scheme%20).
18. Email from Margaret Peters, 20 May 2022.
19. Allan Chase. *The Legacy of Malthus: The Social Costs of the New Scientific Racism.* New York: Knopf Publishing Company, 1977.
20. After several years of searching archival records and requesting information from current European Member Associations who did not respond, the authors accept that the 1954–1956 ICM membership list is very incomplete. It is thought that many of the Western European midwifery associations rejoined the ICM as of 1954, especially midwives from France and Sweden who initiated discussions of the rebirth with Miss Edith Pye and Marjorie Bayes.
21. Rebecca J Cook. *Women's Health and Human Rights.* Geneva: World Health Organization, 1994.
22. Joan Walker, former ICM Secretary General, remembered Sonja Sjøli, the ICM honorary president hosting the 1996 ICM Council Meeting and Congress in Oslo, Norway, had a lot of difficulty getting Norwegian midwives to volunteer as Tellers and other helpers during Council and for other jobs needed during Congress as their culture expected payment for such activities.
23. *Ingela Wiklund note to Joyce Thompson*: As of the early 2010s, the ICM president, vice president and treasurer have a small allowance. April 2021.
24. BBC News, 1978.
25. David Brooks. *Age of Upheaval: Edwardian politics 1899–1914.* Manchester, England: Manchester University Press, 1995. There was great political unrest at the time within the context of social and economic change, stimulated in part by the fervent feminist movement in the early 20th century in England.

Chapter 3: *Birth of a Global Midwifery Organisation: The International Midwives' Union*

'Only by indefatigable stamina the profession of the midwife will achieve the height which according to our society regulations seems to be the ideal aim to us — only with united power will we be able to improve the midwife's social position.'

Frau Olga Gebour, President Berlin Congress, 1900

INTRODUCTION

As described in the Bible and by midwives and their teachers in Ancient Egypt[1], women have received assistance during birth, usually from other women. As noted in the Introduction, many of these birth assistants became known as midwives. It is not the intention to write a history of midwifery in this chapter but to demonstrate how midwives met internationally and worked together, forming a strong international midwives' organisation.

Today midwives meet at the International Confederation of Midwives' (ICM) Congresses, conferences and workshops, but where did it start, when did it start, who started it and how has it got to where it is today? The first part of this chapter is a brief overview of European meetings of midwives that led to the founding of the International Midwives' Union (IMU), the forerunner of the ICM. The second part a somewhat detailed description of the IMU is presented, beginning with its founding in 1922 and its contribution to the story of the current ICM.

EUROPEAN MIDWIVES' EFFORTS TO MEET
Development of Midwifery Associations prior to 1922

European midwives in various countries had been organising into associations since the latter quarter of the 19th century and early 20th century. Examples include the Royal College of Midwives (initially entitled Midwives' Institute) that was formed in 1881, the Swedish Association of Midwives founded in 1886[2], the Belgian midwifery association beginning in the late 1910s and the Luxembourg midwifery association starting in 1919. In addition, it appears obvious from a series of articles in Nursing Notes (forerunner of the Midwives' Chronicle and Nursing Notes) and the official journal of the Midwives' Institute in England, that knowledge about midwifery in European countries and some other parts of the world was available at this time. The organisations began after groups of midwives had met for conferences, congresses etc.

Local, National and International Midwifery Meetings prior to 1922
In Germany there were meetings in Berlin (1890) and Leipzig (1895) for German and Austrian midwives[3]. In a personal communication the Deutscher Hebammen Verband reported that among the topics discussed were midwives' pay, midwifery education and selection of students. On 25 August 1898, Mme Bocquillet, founder and secretary of the Syndicat General des Sages-femmes de France, was elected an honorary member of the 'Manchester & District Midwives Association' when she attended their meeting. Unfortunately, it is not reported why she was given this honour.

In 1900 Frau Olga Gebour organised a meeting of the Berlin Midwives' Association in Berlin. To this meeting she invited midwives from around Germany and midwives from Denmark, Holland, Hungary, Russia, Sweden, Romania and Switzerland.[4] Apparently the invitation to midwives in England arrived too late for travel arrangements to be made. There has been confusion about the number of midwives who attended with reports of 1,000 midwives being present. However, the German Midwifery Journal stated that there were 993 attendees (not known if all were midwives) present over the three days (30 August–1 September) of the meeting, with just over 500 on each day, not a total of 1,000 midwives.[5] Representatives from countries outside Germany all gave papers on the second day. To have organised a meeting of this size without the benefit of the electronic communications that are available in 2022 was a truly amazing feat. Topics discussed were pension schemes for midwives, the new disinfection policy, differentiation between midwife and post-partum carer.[6]

The Italian Midwives' Association held a conference in Bologna in 1909 but no report of the Proceedings was found. The German Midwives' Association held a conference in Dresden in 1911 and reported the results of a survey sent to 600 Midwifery Training Institutions on workforce issues.[7] The Austrian Midwives' Association intended to hold a conference in Vienna in 1914 but the outbreak of World War I stopped it.

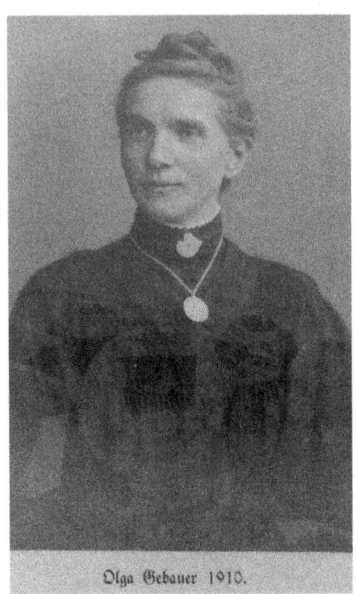

Olga Gebour (1910) – Organiser of midwives' meeting in 1900.
ICM Archives at Wellcome Collection

The annual Flemish Scientific Organisation and its Congresses were attended by teachers, social workers, nurses and midwives. It appears that midwives were present in Bruges in 1919. At the 1921 meeting midwives from Belgium, Holland and England were present. Miss Perneel from Ghent led the midwifery discussions and a base was laid for an international midwives' organisation.

OVERVIEW OF THE INTERNATIONAL MIDWIVES' UNION

The International Midwives' Union (IMU) was born during the Flemish Scientific Conference in Bruges in 1922.[8] It was the forerunner of the International Confederation of Midwives (ICM) and functioned until 1939 as reconstructed from the IMU-produced *Communications of the International Midwives' Union (Communications)* from 1925.[9] In the 1932 issue (Vol 6) Professor Frans Daels, a Belgian obstetrician who was one of the movers for the organisation, reported the early IMU history.[10] These *Communications* were published in English, French and German, and sometimes in Flemish. It was intended that they were to be published in Italian after the 1942 Congress in Rome.[11] There are occasions when the volumes do not appear to be internally consistent. For example, in 1932 Daels reported that the organisation commenced in Bruges in 1922[12] but in his report as General Secretary at the Berlin Congress in 1936 he stated that the IMU commenced in 1919.[13]

WHEN DID THE IMU BEGIN?

As noted above, there has been confusion over when the IMU began. It was reported in *Communications* that the first International Midwives' Congress, not an organisation, occurred in 1919.[14] However, there is no evidence of any Constitution at that time nor any subsequent meetings. It is reported to have been founded as a result of midwives from Belgium, the Netherlands and England meeting at the Flemish Scientific Congress in Bruges.[15] A News item in the Nursing Notes reported that the International Midwives' Union (IMU) began in Bruges, Belgium, in 1922.[16] It started in Europe and was an organisation for Midwifery Associations, not for individual midwives.

There are other reports confirming the 1922 start date – in the introduction to the conference programme for the ICM Congress in America in 1972, celebrating the 50th anniversary of ICM,[17] and again in the ICM Pamphlet of 1981.[18] After presenting evidence of the start date from these sources, the 2014 ICM Board accepted the birth date of 1922.[19] Whilst it is accepted that the organisation was set up in 1922, Daels reported that the initial suggestion for the formation of a midwifery organisation came from Frau De Graaf Van den Elst at the 1921 International Scientific Meeting in Bruges.[20]

Whilst the IMU was started in Europe, mostly Western Europe, by European midwives, from the beginning it was entitled 'International' implying that it was for midwives and their associations all over the world, not just the countries in Europe. However, a communication from the Ghana midwives' association (GCMA) puts into question the perceived remit of the IMU being beyond Europe in its early years. In 1933, a Ghanaian midwife, Madam Fredrica Kwarley Aba Addo, visited the United Kingdom (UK), contacted the Midwives' Institute, briefed them about the Gold Coast[21] Midwives' Association (GCMA), and sought information about how to join the IMU. She was informed that despite the organisation's title it was only for European-based associations.[22] This appears confusing because America and India were in postal communication with the IMU in the early days, though possibly they did not ask to join the union. The first person from outside Europe to attend an IMU Congress was a midwife from India (Mrs Mitra) who not only attended the Congress in London in 1934 but also gave a paper on the organisation of obstetric services in British India.[23]

WHAT WAS THE NAME OF THE ORGANISATION?

The first proposed title of the organisation in 1922 was the International Association of Midwives. Daels' proposed title during the meeting was the International Union of Midwives. The name finally agreed by those midwifery associations present was the International Midwives' Union (IMU). One example of the lack of internal consistency from reports in the Communications was illustrated in reported different names for the organisation[24] that ranged from

IMU to use of terms such as 'League', 'Federation' or 'Associations'. No evidence has been found in any Communications of a formally approved name change so it can only be presumed that these differing names were due to translational difficulties. In the material searched there was no inconsistency in the reporting of materials or individuals working within the organisation, suggesting that despite the differing names it was the same organisation.

What Did the Midwife Do?

In order to understand the IMU organisation it is important to understand the profession of those meeting together. Though a formal contemporary definition of 'midwife' was not found in existing documents, it appears that member associations 'knew' what a midwife did or did not do.

The role/scope of practise appeared to vary somewhat in the different countries, including whether the midwife worked in the community, cared for women in their homes or worked in hospital. It appears that in the organisation's initial history the midwife was always a woman. There were no references to men practising midwifery in available records. 'Professors of Midwifery' are referred to, but they were most likely obstetricians, as was Frans Daels. Some are referred to as being in charge of Schools of Midwifery. All doctors who have appeared in the literature related to the IMU were men, which is surprising when, for example, women doctors were practising at this time in the UK and, in particular, in maternal and child health.[25]

At the beginning of the organisation it was accepted that midwives looked after women during labour and at birth.[26] Subsequent arguments chronicled in the *Communications* suggested that midwives cared for women in the postnatal period, and there were separate proposals for midwives to look after 'nurslings'. Later there were suggestions that midwives should look after women during pregnancy. In addition, there was an argument for midwifery to be separated from nursing,[27] an argument that continues in the 21st century. The overriding issue that appeared throughout the early history is that midwives should be concerned with the social aspects of maternity, not just the clinical aspects.

WHAT WAS THE PURPOSE OF THE ORGANISATION?

Following the presentation of the paper (The Conditions of Midwifery in Holland) in 1922 in Bruges by Frau De Graf Van Den Elst reporting the poor situation of

Dutch midwifery at the time, Professor Frans Daels proposed the following motion:

> 'This convention of Nursing and Social Medicine, having 800 members (nurses and midwives), of whom 400 are present at the general meeting on August 7th, 1922, taking in consideration that the standard of the profession of midwives ought to be put on a high level by raising that of midwifery as a whole, set forward a demand to have secretaries organised in Holland and in Flanders by their respective associations; that they would bring a report about the social-medical activities of both countries. It is also calling immediately for the assistance of the present representatives (English, Dutch and Flemish) to institute an *International Association of Midwives*.'[28]

The motion was passed and Professor Daels was elected President of this possible 'International Union of Midwives'. The intention was to invite international delegates to a meeting later in 1922 to 'point out the line of study and activities'.

In the report of the Congress in Prague in 1925[29] the following was given, stating that this was in the account of the first Midwives' Conference in 1922:

> 'Experiments are being made in different countries as to the best organisation of a Midwifery consideration, been neglected partly because of the attraction of the new office of Visiting Nurse. It is considered that no uplifting of the Nurse's status in general is possible without a joint uplifting of the Midwives' status and that the well-regulated Activity of any institution of social medicine demands that the Midwives' task should be recognised with its full extension. The International Midwives' Union wants to carry out studies on (the) above questions with a complete devotion of heart and spirit to the cause of the protection of motherhood.'

It is not known where this quotation originated but it is possible it was in one of the earlier Communications that have not been found. The quotation suggests that these midwives were concerned about the status of midwives and midwifery; that it was not just newly qualified doctors encroaching on midwives' territory but nursing as well. However, their overriding concern was to protect motherhood, what would today be referred to as preventing maternal mortality.

HOW DID THE IMU FUNCTION?

From the beginning the IMU functioned by conferences/congresses every two years, except for 1930 when there were no funds to support one. It was recognised from the beginning that sending information to member associations was also vital. This was performed by circulating *Communications of the International Midwives' Union [Communications for short]*. However, throughout the five editions available there are constant apologies for late publication. This was mostly due to the difficulties in producing the documents in at least three languages. There is no information on how the international meetings were funded. Today midwives expect to pay a conference fee to the organising committee to cover the costs of the venue, hire of meeting rooms, use of visual aids etc. None of this is reported in any of the Communications. In one instance there was a report of a modest lunch being provided, on another occasion participants were asked to pay and book in advance for refreshments. At the 1938 Congress in Paris the Nestle Foundation supported a conference reception.[30] In some of the invitations to the Congresses potential participants were asked to let the secretariat know as soon as possible of their intention to attend so that inexpensive accommodation could be secured.[31]

Following identification of the venue of the next Congress, the affiliated (member) association elected a President, secretary and local organising committee. The organising committee would be responsible for arranging meeting halls etc. That committee would function during the build-up to Congress and during Congress, until the next Congress venue was selected and a new

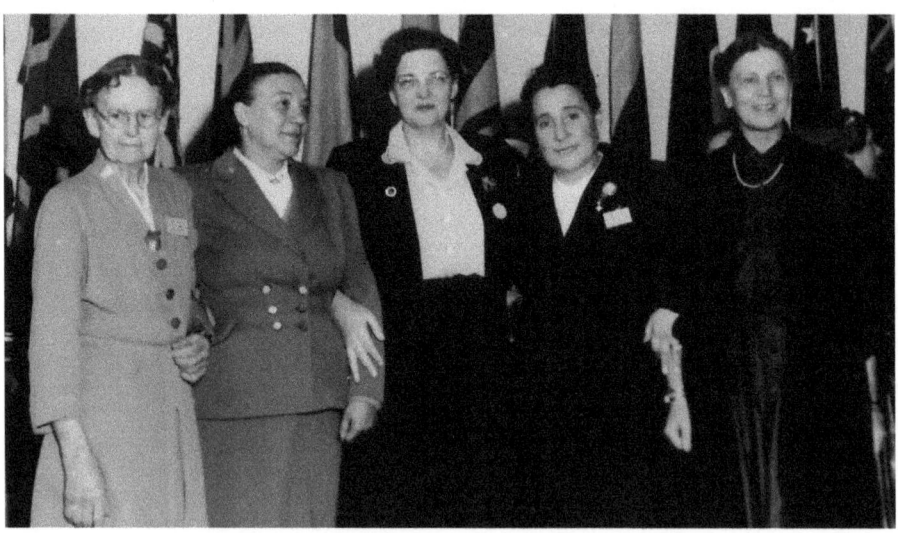

Five early International Midwives Union Presidents (1934) – Left to right Miss E. M. Pye (Great Britain); Madame M. Jay (France); Miss N. B. Deane (Great Britain); Signora V Luzzi (Italy); Miss E Erup (Sweden).
ICM Archives at Wellcome Collection

organising committee would take over. The committees were also responsible for identifying the topics, such as newborn care, place of birth, education or regulation of midwives, that were to be discussed at the Congress. These topics were circulated to each member association and they would be asked to return a report giving information on the topics of the situation in their country. The reports had to be returned at least two months before the Congress, so that a document containing the information could be sent to the participants before arriving at the Congress. However, that did not always happen.[32] These reports were then summarised by a member of the organising committee before presentation to the Congress. Following this the conference took decisions on the matters discussed and the results were sent in the following Communications to each Midwifery Association to be circulated as appropriate in their own country.

There has been some confusion as to whether the President and the rest of the Committee were in post for just the congress or for the whole period until the next Congress.[33] However, following the redaction and revision of the regulations that took place in Vienna at the 1928 Congress it was stated that the President was chosen for two years.[34]

Secretariat

From the beginning of the organisation the secretariat was set up by the midwifery association where the next congress was to be held. This was not efficient, in particular because of the lack of continuity. Therefore, at the 1932 Congress a decision was taken that there would be a permanent secretary's office in Ghent and it would not move with each Congress.[35] The Secretariat would be under the direction of Professor Daels with a Flemish midwife working with him.[36] It was hoped that, with a permanent and better organised secretary's office, increased contact between the various midwives' organisations would ensue. However, no evidence has been found that a permanent secretary's office was actually established at this time.

Governance

In the early years of the organisation governance can only be described as 'developing'. This was because the function of the organisation changed according to the host country of each Congress. As noted above, the host country midwifery association elected/appointed a President and Secretary. A meeting was held in Antwerp in 1923 (it is presumed that this was the meeting that should have been held in 1922) at which it appears the original regulations were drawn up. No regulations of the IMU have been found in the very early literature; however, at the meeting in Prague in 1925 the following regulations were agreed. It is believed that this is how the IMU was governed from the beginning:

1) A union of all midwives' associations of the whole world is instituted under the name: International Midwives' Union.
2) The aim of the union is: 1) protection of maternity and nursing of the baby; 2) the scientifical (sic), maternal, social, and ethical elevation of the midwife standing.
3) The seat of the international union is the dwelling-place of the international secretary.
4) The union is obliged to organize at least once every other year an international congress. The order paper of each congress is defined by the president, after having consulted the different national associations. Social questions on protection of maternity and nursing of the babies will be discussed. The necessary financial help must be rendered by the affiliated associations. The chairman of the international midwives' union convenes the meeting in understanding with the affiliated unions.
5) The direction of the international union is composed by the president, chosen by the international congress, the international secretary, and two deputies in each affiliated union, if there is only one association in the country; when there are two associations each of them sends one deputy if the association has at least 200 members. The office has a right to take still other councillors.
6) Each affiliated union is obliged to pay yearly at least 5 dollars as a contribution to the international union.
7) These regulations are to be examined again at the next congress.
8) The delegates at the international congress of Prague constitute the office of this one and have been authorized to do so by their unions.[37]

Subsequent Regulations

No changes in the regulations of IMU were reported as a result of the 1932 Congress. At the 1934 Congress it was noted that if items in the regulations were not reported to have changed then the latest regulations would remain in practice.

However, notwithstanding the name change reported in the 1934 Congress notes, the changes in the regulations were mostly to do with wording. The frequency of Congresses was to be reduced to every three years but this did not occur while the IMU existed. The languages remained at English, French and German. An organising committee appeared at this Congress with the task of organising the future Congress. The annual subscriptions were to be reviewed at each Congress but the amount of the subscription was not changed in 1934.[38] The protection of the mother and child remained its primary objective and therefore the efforts and activities of the IMU were to be directed towards the scientific, moral, social and economic improvement of the profession of midwife. The IMU was to again stand firmly apart from all questions concerning politics, race or religion. It aimed at maintaining unity among all the Associations and all countries while avoiding all discussions on these subjects.

For the first time, Decisions Concerning Internal Administration of the IMU resulted from the 1934 Congress.[39] These decisions referred to 1) the presentation of the accounts, 2) membership fees that should be paid on a fixed date each year, 3) the Secretary General (Professor Daels) should be in charge of the material reported in the international journal (*Communications*), 4) the frequency of publication of *Communications*, 5) the number of copies of *Communications* that each Association should receive and 6) that each association was to urge the relevant administrative authorities to give effect to the resolutions passed at each Congress.

During the 1936 Congress it was decided that, because of the increasing importance of the IMU on the international stage with regard to the health of mother and baby, a permanent Standing Committee should be instituted. It would consist of the Presidents of previous congresses, the President of the last Congress, the General Secretary of the Federation and certain persons who have taken part in Congresses and therefore knew the different subjects discussed and the decisions made.[40]

Officers of the International Midwives' Union

There was no consistency in Communications in the reporting of personnel and job titles, and who fulfilled those jobs or titles. Table 3.1 has been compiled to the best of the author's ability from what is reported in the Communications.

Table 3.1

IMU Congress Locations, Dates and Officers/Honorary Officers 1922–1938

No	PLACE	YEAR		Other Officers of IMU Country
	IMU Congress Locations and Year		Individuals Appointed/Elected President of IMU	Other Known Officers
3	Antwerp, Belgium	1922/3	Mme De Graef van den Elst Mlle Perneel[41]	Dr Putto (secretary)
4	Prague, Czech Republic	1925	Mme Liscova	Mrs Cuhelova (secretary)
5	Vienna, Austria	1928	Mme Berthe Hubel	Paulina Kraegel (secretary)
6	Ghent, Belgium	1932	Mme Block	
7	London, UK[42]	1934	Miss Edith M Pye	
8	Berlin, Germany	1936	Frau Nanna Conti	
9	Paris, France	1938[43]	Mlle Mossé: Organisation Nationale des Syndicats de Sages-Femmes	Secretary: Mme Godillon, Niort (Deux-Sevres)[44]

IMU Affiliated Midwifery Associations/Members

To be affiliated with or be a member of IMU, the Midwifery Association had to pay an annual fee. In the early days these fees sometimes did not arrive, or if they did, they arrived at varying times. According to *Communications*, in 1932 the following countries had midwifery organisations which joined the International Midwives' Union: England, Germany, Holland, 'Flemish', Poland, Hungary, Denmark, Yugoslavia, Latvia, Austria and Tcecho-Slovakia.[45] The report also noted that the Prussian Midwives' Union, the Moravian Midwives' Union and the Silesian and Slovakian National Midwives' Union asked to become members but these requests were referred to the Congress for a decision because it appeared that the activities of existing member associations in their countries were the same. No information has been found as to whether decisions were taken on these Associations. The IMU encouraged the Swiss League of Midwives to join.[46]

In addition to the listed associations above who had paid their membership fees, there were several other countries' midwifery associations reported to be in communication with the IMU Secretariat. They were Argentina, Chile, China, Estland, Finland, Greece, Italy, Portugal, Turkey and a few separate German midwifery groups as well as a group from Bucharest, Romania, showing IMU's reach outside Europe.

Mme Mosse (1938) – Sage-Femme en Chef honoraire de la Maternité de Paris. Présidente d'honeur de la Confédération Nationale des Syndicates de Sages-femmes Françaises, Présidente du 8me Congrès international des accoucheuses. (Paris 1938). ICM Archives at Wellcome Collection

Finances of the IMU

From the beginning of the organisation to the end of the 1939 period the IMU finances were unstable. As already noted, there were reports of private donations coming to the rescue of the organisation.[47] Based on the Regulations redacted in 1925 all affiliated associations with 200 members paid $5 (USA) annually.[48] At the 1928 Congress the subscriptions were increased for those with more than 200 members. They were required to pay $1 more for each extra 500 members.[49] Whilst it is noted at this time that subscriptions were in American dollars, the payments are recorded in Belgian francs except for the English where it was usually reported in pounds sterling![50]

Whilst fees were supposed to be paid annually, the finances reported in *Communications* were only reported for the years of Congresses and the statements do not include fees for the years between Congresses. In the seventh issue of *Communications* there is a request for all subscriptions to be sent as a postal cheque to the organisation's Central Office, care of Professor Daels at a Belgian Post Box. This request was made because apparently there had been 'numerous enquiries' as to where subscriptions should be sent. If affiliated associations had been unsure where to send subscriptions perhaps that was the reason for the poor finances. At the 1934 Congress the decision was made that subscriptions were to be paid on the first of April[51] each year so that the organisation had some stability in the amount of money in the bank. There is no evidence of a treasurer during this 1922–39 period and oral accounts may have been presented at the Congresses. It was reported that a decision had been taken that, as in previous years, the accounts were to be presented to the Committee annually.[52] However, the accounts only appeared in the *Communications* in the reports of the last two congresses (Berlin 1936[53], Paris 1938).

The report of the 1928 Congress noted, 'When the direction of the International Congress of midwives was taken over the finances were very low'.[54] The major financial problem was translation of the *Communications* into the three languages. After the London Congress in 1934 cash in hand amounted to 378 francs. The sum of 2,449 francs had been received. The expenses for publication was 4,616 francs. The large deficit had been made good by private donations. In 1937 it was reported that the IMU funds were exhausted. Countries with a low rate of exchange wished to fix the subscription accordingly. It would, however, have been technically difficult to abandon the dollar as a basis and subscriptions continued to be calculated on the gold dollar. The reports of the number of countries paying fees in 1936 and 1937[55] did not tally with the number of countries being affiliated that year. The information about the financial situation of the organisation came from the last meeting of the Standing Committee in 1939. 'Since the publication of the last number of the International Journal, the National Unions of Austria, Estonia and Denmark had also paid their subscriptions so that the receipts of International Headquarters amounted to 7,134 Belgian Francs since the previous Congress. The publication of the last number of the International Journal cost 6,354 Belgian Francs. Postage expenses amounted to 275 francs, making a total of 6,629 francs. The present balance is 505 francs'.[56]

There is no evidence of any fees being paid for the secretarial assistance used by Professor Daels in Ghent. Neither is there any evidence of funding of the secretarial assistance for each of the Congresses. In Conti's description of the activities of the Berlin Office[57] funding must have been obtained from somewhere. Because of Conti's close working relationship with the German Ministry of Health[58] it is presumed that this came from the German government.

CONFERENCES / CONGRESSES / MEETINGS

As already reported, IMU held conferences/congresses in Antwerp (1923), Prague (1925), Vienna (1928), Ghent (1932), London (1934), Berlin (1936) and Paris (1938). There was a meeting of the International Standing Committee in Ghent in June 1939.[59] Following this all activities of the organisation were stopped by WWII.[60] The organisation mostly functioned through the conferences/congresses held in Europe. The number of countries' midwifery associations represented at each meeting grew from three in 1922 to 23 in Berlin in 1936, though only 16 in Paris in 1938 (Figure 3.1 in Annex B).

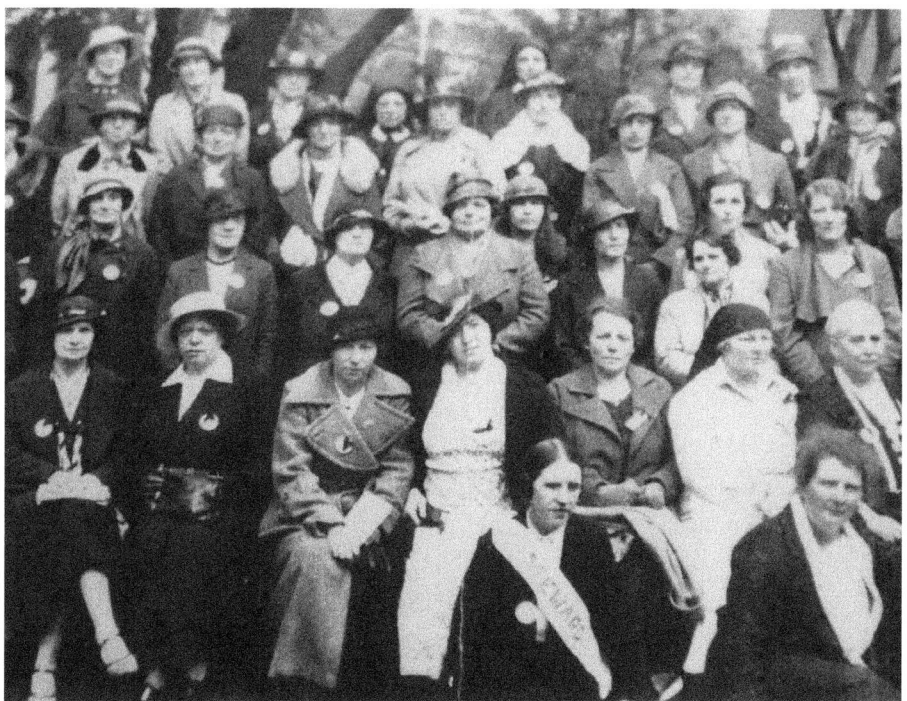

Group 1 Delegates at the 1934 International Midwives' Union Congress – ICM Archives at Wellcome Collection

From reports in the *Communications* only 15 countries were represented at the last congress before WWII, but Edith Pye reported that there were 20 country representatives in 1938 in Paris.[61] Russia is not in the list of represented countries at the 1932 Congress in Ghent, and yet in the Congress report their representatives are noted to have asked a representative of the Soviet Institute for the Protection of Mothers and Children in Moscow to communicate with the IMU.[62]

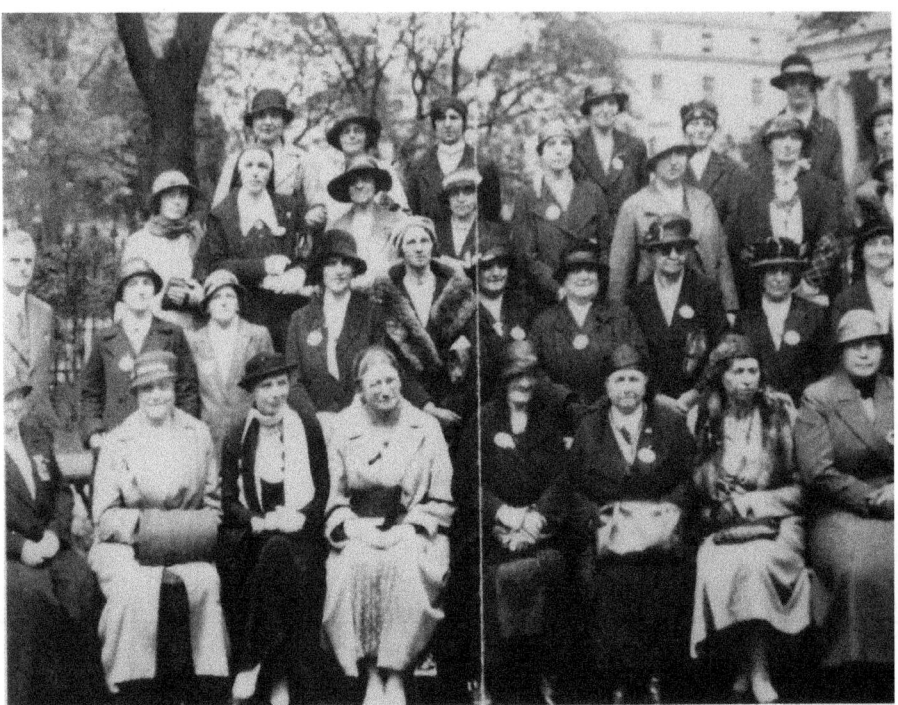

Group 1 Delegates at the 1934 International Midwives' Union Congress – ICM Archives at Wellcome Collection

Whilst fewer countries (15) were represented in 1938 in comparison to the previous year (23), more individual delegates from outside the country attended Paris (355) in comparison to Berlin. The greatest number of attendees during an IMU Congress appears to have been in Berlin in 1936 when there were 200+ participants from outside Germany and 1,000 German midwives.

In summary, the number of country midwifery associations participating in the meetings increased over the 17-year period of the IMU (Annex B). At the first meeting in 1922 a reporter said that the meeting gave workers of all nationalities the opportunity to exchange knowledge and ideas. Over the years the IMU addressed many topics. Amongst those addressed regularly were regulation of midwifery, midwifery practice, midwifery education, salary for midwives, pensions for midwives, place of birth and care of the unmarried mother. Most of these topics have persisted through the next six decades of the ICM.

The final activity of the IMU took place on 13–14 June 1939 in Ghent.[63] It was not a conference or congress, but a meeting of the Standing Committee. Decisions were taken on the place of the next Congress, Rome, the publication of *Communications*, the format of the Congress and the congress programme. The plans were to meet again in Rome in 1942. It was again stated firmly that no question of politics or religion should in any way be considered by the Federation of Midwives' Unions.[64] However, with the beginning of WWII in Europe, the IMU fell silent until the late 1940s when a few midwives in Europe questioned when the group could reconvene (See Chapter 4).

Involvement of Obstetricians in the IMU

From the beginning of the organisation obstetricians from all countries where midwifery associations were in membership with IMU worked with midwives to assist in the setting up of the organisation and then to help it grow. Whilst it is not stated, the reports of private donations to the organisation leads the reader to presume that these were given, or obtained, by doctors. In the *Communications* reporting all the conferences/congresses there are reports of Obstetricians being present, giving papers and contributing to discussions. Whilst there were many it is necessary to report on one in particular.

Professor Frans Daels was a Belgian obstetrician. He was instrumental in assisting the development of the Belgian Midwifery Association.[65] He was present at the Scientific meeting in Bruges in 1922 and he proposed the motion which brought the International Midwives' Union into being. He was the first President, but later was also the Executive Secretary. He was very supportive of this organisation and in the early days provided accommodation in his home for early meetings of the organising committee.[66] In the early years the organisation was short of money and it is presumed it was he who was instrumental in obtaining the private funds that made up the shortfall. He attended all the conferences and congresses, giving papers at most of them.

In her history of the IMU, Miss Pye[67] reports that Daels disappeared during WWII as did 'his' papers. At the 1932 Congress it had been agreed that there would be a permanent Secretariat in Ghent, where Professor Daels lived. Ghent was subjected to a lot of Allied bombing at the beginning of the war so it is possible that he thought the IMU papers would be safer elsewhere. According to Peters[68] he asked Frau Conti to take over the position of Secretary in 1942. This was unconstitutional as Daels did not have the right to do this and Madame Mossé, who was still the President of IMU at this time, was not consulted, let alone informed. All the IMU papers were transferred to Berlin at the same time. Frau Conti kept the papers in the office of the Deutsche Hebamme, which was bombed in 1943.

Miss Pye did not know what had happened to Professor Daels because he had escaped to Switzerland in 1945. This was to avoid impending legal action due to his work with the Nazi regime.[69] There is no evidence of his involvement with the rebirth of the midwifery organisation after his return to Belgium in 1951.

MIDWIVES FOR PEACE AND HEALTHY MOTHERS AND BABIES

The IMU started shortly after the end of WWI and was stopped at the beginning of WWII. Therefore, it is not surprising that the effects of the previous fighting and the potential for more fighting would have been on the minds of members of the midwifery associations. Some of the comments reported in Communications follow.

In 1932 Mlle Merle from France stated, 'Too often the nations incite themselves to discover perfected means for killing men. I salute this Congress wich (sic) has assembled us in order to look for better means of giving birth and of assuring a better life to **the children of all countries**' (bold as in original). Miss Pye followed by stating, 'We believe that international gatherings are valuable because they increase friendship and understanding between our different nations, and by making the experience and knowledge of each available for all, they promote the welfare of the Mothers and infants of our respective countries whose interests are our first consideration'[70].

In Paris (the final IMU Congress in 1938), M Justin Goddard, a former Minister, addressed the meeting and said:

> 'This is an international gathering. By your singleness of purpose and by the eagerness which you have all shown to come together, you evince a deep feeling of unity, which brings you together, but a feeling of unity amongst women, passing beyond and above all frontiers. Looking upon you now, I cannot but be moved by the thought that I am in fact in the presence of those who are the good harvesters of humanity, those who reap the harvest of life, directing it from the first moment towards Health and happiness. I cannot refrain from thinking of others who destroy life. I am reminded that horrible wars are actually in progress in the world at this moment and this humanity is ever haunted by the grim spectre of war. Ladies, in the name of that life which you serve, in the name of that life which means to us public men the future of our countries, remain united in defence of life and of humanity'.[71]

At this final Congress, Miss Pye proposed the following Motion:

> 'The VIIIth International Midwives Congress declares that if the catastrophe of war overwhelms the world again, it will be against the wishes and desires of the mass of the people in every country and above all against those of the Mothers.
>
> Midwives, whose work is the preservation of life deplore the wilful destruction of it through the use of scientific knowledge for destructive instead of constructive ends. The Congress asks Midwives everywhere, whatever the future may bring forth, to remember the bond which unites them to one another in working in the same spirit for Humanity.'[72]

This motion was passed unanimously.

SUMMARY

In the first 17 years of existence, the IMU grew from three midwifery associations in membership in 1922 to 36 who were present at the 1936 Congress. Whilst the IMU started in Western Europe, midwifery associations in Eastern Europe and North Africa attended the Congresses by 1939. However, IMU leaders were also in communication with midwifery associations in South and North Europe, South America, India, the USA and China. The organisation kept in contact with midwifery associations by producing The Communications of the International Midwives' Union. The midwifery associations used the content of these Communications to provide information to their governments as appropriate. In response to requests for information on midwives from international organisations, such as The United Nations, a Standing Committee was formed to attend to these requests. The IMU's existence from 1922 to 1939 was a considerable achievement for a women's organisation that began with no funds in 1922 and little in the way of organisational support.

100 Years of the International Confederation of Midwives

1. Genesis 35:17. The Bible. Rosalie David's paper on College of Midwifery in Ancient Egypt presented at ICM Congress in Toronto, 2017.
2. Personal email from Ingela Wiklund, historian and member of Swedish Association of Midwives, April 2021.
3. Examples include: June 1886, p 83, reports of receipt of Journal des Sages Femme and Hebammen Zeitung; Aug 1896, p 109 report on Midwives in Chicago; Aug 1897, p 110 report of Item from Hebammen Zeitung; Nov 1898, p 157 Report on Dispensary Midwives in Paris; 1 Jan, 1901, pp 9–10 – The Position of Midwives in Germany; 1 June 1901, pp 84–85 Midwives Defence Union & German midwifery; 1 June, 1903, pp 78–79 ; 1 Nov, 1903, p 154 Foreign Midwives & their work – France, Spain, Germany, Bavaria, Saxe-Coburg and Gotha, Hesse, Baden, Saxony, Austria, Hungary, Italy, Russia.
4. Nursing Notes, Dec 1900, p 176. Austria is also listed in the 1954 ICM Programme as having attended.
5. Vereinigung Deutsche Hebammen-Zeitung 15:18, pp 287–288.
6. Personal communication from Deutchher Hebammen Verband.
7. Personal Communication from Deutscher Hebammen Verband. ICM. Programme of 1954 Congress in London. History of ICM section.
8. Scientific Flemish Conference. Nursing Notes October 1922, p.127.
9. In the 1932 issue (Vol 6) Professor Frans Daels, a Belgian obstetrician who was one of the movers for the organisation, reported the early IMU history.
10. Communications 6, 1932, pp 14–21. Other sources of IMU history were gathered from reports from English, German and Polish journals.
11. Communications 10, 1939, p 121.
12. Communications 6, 1932, p 14.
13. Communications 9, 1937, p 18.
14. Communications 6, 1932, p 6.
15. Nursing Notes, 1922, p 127; Communications 6, 1932, p 14; Private papers of Edith Pye in Royal College of Midwives' archives.
16. Nursing Notes, 1922, p 127.
17. ICM. New Horizons in Midwifery: XVIth Congress, Washington DC, USA. Printed in USA: ACNM, p 7. ICM President's Greeting, 'Fifty years ago, in 1922, we were struggling to bring together and formally organize little groups of midwives who had labored since the late 1800s to establish their organization and develop their objectives of better care for mothers and babies.'
18. The International Confederation of Midwives pamphlet, 1981, p 7: History of the International Confederation of Midwives.
19. ICM. 50th Anniversary Celebration of the ICM Banquet Programme. ICM Congress, Washington, DC, USA. May 1972, on loan from Carmela Cavero, ACNM President and host of the 1972 ICM Congress. ICM. (SA/ICM/R/4). Wellcome Collection. Marjorie Bayes' History of the ICM. First 50 years. Miss Bayes, ICM Secretary General in 1972, confirmed the 1922 start of IMU in her history document. The confusion appeared when ICM celebrated its 75th anniversary in 1996 using the 1919 start date of IMU, most likely confusing the 1919 Congress of midwives as the beginning of the IMU, though no organisational details were found.
20. Communications 6, 1932, p 14. Whilst Daels reports Miss Perneel as the founding midwife of the IMU, in the report of the 1932 conference in Ghent it is stated that Miss De Graaf Van Elst of Haarlem was the Founder in 1922.
21. The Gold Coast was the name of the country that took on the name 'Ghana' at the time of independence in 1957.
22. Personal communication Jemima Araba Dennis-Antwi, ICM Regional Representative for English-speaking Africa. 2020
23. Communications 10, 1939, p 72.
24. This is one example of the difficulty in tracking the early history from Communications as a primary source due to lack of meeting papers destroyed during WWII.
25. However, as late as the early 1980s in the UK some University Chairs of Obstetrics were entitled 'Chair of Midwifery' e.g. Glasgow.
26. Communications 7, 1934, pp. 32, 37, 39.
27. Frau De Graf Van Den Elst. Communications 7, 1937, p 36.
28. 1922 Scientific Flemish Congress October, Nursing Notes, p 127.
29. Conference at Prague September. Nursing Notes, 1925, p 141.
30. Communications 10, 1939, p 72
31. Communications 10, 1939, p 72
32. Frans Daels. Communications 7, 1934, p 37.
33. Anja Peters. Nanna Conti (1881–1915). Unpublished dissertation: Eine Biographie der Reichshebammn fuhrerin. Unpublished thesis, der Ernst-Meritz-Arndt – Universitat Greifswald, 2014. Anja Peters' personal communication to AT, 2020.
34. Communications 6, 1932, p 18.
35. Communications 6, 1932, p 3.
36. Communications 7, 1934, p 27.
37. As there is no evidence of any meeting in 1924 it is presumed that these regulations resulted from the 1923 meeting in Antwerp.
38. This is one example of the inconsistency of naming the organisation within the published Communications.
39. Communications 8, 1936, p 62.
40. Communications 8, 1936, p 61.

41 ICM. (SA/ICM/R/4). Wellcome Collection. This document lists Mlle Perneel as the President of the IMU in 1922/1923.
42 Betty Cowell & David Wainwright, Eds. Behind the Blue Door: The History of the Royal College of Midwives 1881–1981. London: A Baillieree Tindall book published by Cassell Ltd, 1981, pp 55, notes that 'the International Midwives Union held its sixth Annual Congress in London.' Miss Edith Pye was President of the host association, the Royal College of Midwives. This numbering of the IMU Congresses was in conflict with other sources that stated the London Congress was the seventh.
43 ICM (SA/ICM/R.4). Wellcome Collection. This document lists a meeting in Rome in 1950 presided over by Signora Schimmenti, and a 1953 meeting in Paris presided over by Mme Jay. Unable to know whether these were official meetings of IMU or its successors or a scientific conference for those in Europe able to attend. There is some evidence that the 1953 meeting was the organising one for the official ICM meeting in 1954 in London.
44 Communications 10, 1939, p 5.
45 Communications 6, 1932, p 30.
46 Communications 6, 1932, p 30.
47 Communications 9, 1937, p 20, when Daels gives this information in his report to Congress.
48 Communications 6, 1932, p 17.
49 Communications 6, 1932, p 19.
50 Communications 9, 1937, p 90.
51 Communications 8, 1936, p 62 ; Communications 10, 1939, p 50.
52 Communications 8, 1936, pp 61, 62.
53 Communications 9, 1937.
54 Communications 6, 1932, p 30.
55 Communications 9, 1937, p 90.
56 Communications 10, 1939, p 51.
57 Communications 9, 1937, pp 78–80.
58 Anja Peters, 2014.
59 Communications 10, 1939, p 121.
60 Communications 10, 1939, p 121. Private papers of Miss Edith Pye in the archives of the RCM.
61 Edith M Pye. Personal papers held in the RCM archives, undated but text suggests 1949.
62 Communications 7, 1934, p 34.
63 Edith M Pye. Personal paper 1949 held in RCM archives.
64 Communications 10, 1939, p 121.
65 ICM archival letters in Wellcome Institute Library.
66 Communications 6, 1932, pp 14–21.
67 Edith M Pye. Private papers, 1949, held in the RCM Archives. Miss Pye was a member of the Royal College of Midwives and President and Host of the 1934 IMU Congress in London, England.
68 Anja Peters. Nanna Conti (1881–1915). Unpublished dissertation: Eine Biographie der Reichshebammnfuhrerin. Unpublished thesis, der Ernst-Meritz-Arndt – Universitat Greifswald, 2014.
69 https://nl.m.wikipedia.org/wiki/Frans_Daels accessed 3 April 2021.
70 Communications 7, 1934, p 30.
71 Communications 10, 1939, p 52.
72 Communications 10, 1939, p 72 & 75.

Chapter 4: *Rebirth of the IMU as the ICM*

Miss EM Pye, President of the IMU London Congress in 1934, in handwritten notes in 1949, wrote that with the disappearance of Dr Daels and all his papers from the international scene during WWII, it was 'necessary for us [Midwives] to decide upon our future for ourselves with regard to an international body, and it is for this purpose that we have called together a few of those midwives in other countries with whom we have been in contact, in order that we may decide whether there is an advantage in an International Midwives Union, and if so whether we should try to organize such a Union.

INTRODUCTION

Acknowledging the vision and energy of obstetrician Frans Daels in bringing the IMU into being with Frau De Graf Van den Elst, Edith Pye stated that Daels' disappearance during WWII made it necessary for midwives to decide upon their own future, hence the meeting in 1949.[1] And that is just what midwives have been doing since the rebirth of the IMU as the International Confederation of Midwives (ICM) in 1954.

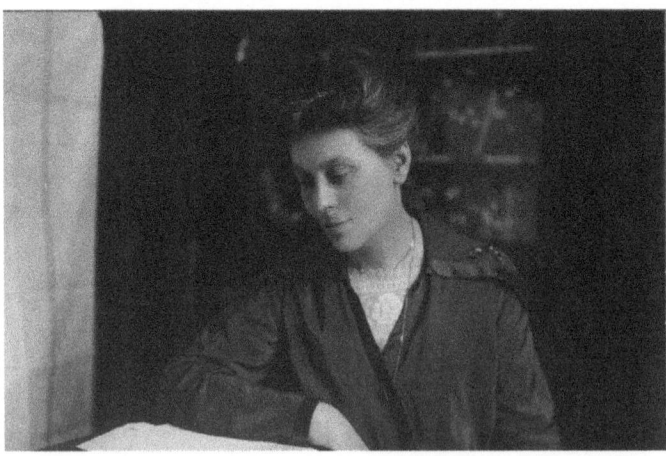

Edith Pye, as a younger woman at her desk (date unknown) – President 1934,
Reproduced with permission from: Royal College of Midwives. RCM/PH2/2/P/6/1 Trimmed black and white photograph of RCM President.

In this chapter the who, why and where the rebirth of the IMU happened and the importance of collaboration with the WHO and renewed Triennial Congresses beginning in 1954 are discussed.

CALL FOR REBIRTH OF IMU

At the end of World War II, the Swedish Association of Midwives[2] wrote to the Royal College of Midwives (RCM) asking whether the pre-war international conferences of midwives could be revived.[3] Miss Pye at the RCM was most interested in joining with other midwifery associations to resume meetings to share stories, learn new approaches to childbearing care, and discuss efforts to improve the status and work environments for midwives.

1949 IFMO Meeting

This request resulted in the RCM hosting an international meeting of midwives representing eight countries that coincided with the 1949 Maternity and Child Welfare Conference in London. Edith Pye appeared to summarise the reason for the 1949 meeting of midwives when she wrote:

> 'In 1939 there was a meeting in Belgium of a committee to prepare for the Congress planned for 1941 – that was the last meeting of our international organisation. But we did not forget that promise [midwives working in the same spirit for Humanity deplored the wilful destruction of life]. The purpose of our gathering today is to try to find out how to join up again the bonds severed by war that unite us as a profession, so that together we may share our knowledge and experience for the benefit of the mothers and infants in all our countries to whom our service is devoted.'[4]

The first post-war European-based meeting of midwives, now called the International Federation of Midwives Organization (IFMO), was reconstituted by Miss Edith Pye in 1949 with Headquarters based in France,[5] though there is some debate as to whether this meeting included European midwives who were previously involved in the IMU or midwifery associations interested in meeting together. The RCM was asked to appoint an acting secretary of the IFMO[6] in 1949 and Congress secretary in 1953. That midwife was Marjorie Bayes[7], who was the assistant to the General Secretary of the RCM at the time.[8]

One of the midwives attending the 1949 meeting was Frieda Riede from West Germany. She reported that:

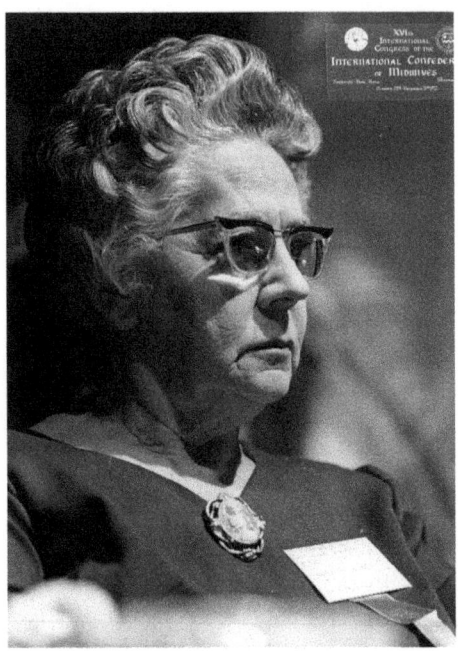

Marjorie Bayes, Executive Secretary, at 16th International Congress, Washington, DC, 1972. – ICM Archives at Wellcome Collection

'It has been recommended that the former International Federation of Midwives Union, founded in the year 1922 as the International Midwives Union, should be revived and from now on called by the title, 'International Federation of Midwives Organization (sic).'[9]

No evidence of this meeting was located in existing archives in Europe. Five years of planning followed with much of the groundwork carried out by Miss Bayes in preparation for the International Congress in 1954.

1953 IFMO Meeting

In 1953 the delegates from Germany, Sweden, Finland, the Netherlands, Denmark and the UK met in London. Riede and Schwietzke[10] noted that an international union of midwives had existed since 1900[11] and 'was revived by the Belgian midwives in 1922'. This group felt that a lot of valuable, good work had been accomplished in the meetings over the past two decades and that 'by no means the connection to this shall be ended'. They also reported that they 'agreed that the official name of this union shall be: International Council of Midwives. By this there shall be in no way a new founding of the international midwives' association.'

Miss Bayes' noted that this change in name was a response to debates as to whether the IFMO should join with the International Council of Nursing (ICN), an early, yet ongoing, debate on whether midwives and nurses should join together. Midwives present agreed that midwives and midwifery practice were different from nurses and nursing practice, thus agreeing the name as the International Council of Midwives (ICM).[12] Though the initials ICM were the same as the present-day organisation, the International Confederation of Midwives became the official name of the organisation in 1954[13], remaining the same for the past 68 years.

WHO EXPERT COMMITTEE ON MIDWIFERY TRAINING, JULY 1954

At the same time as the events leading to the rebirth of the ICM, the World Health Organization (WHO), established in 1948 as part of the United Nations, was continuing its interest in the work of midwives as it addressed maternal and neonatal mortality and morbidity in the world.[14] The collaboration between the ICM and the WHO began formally with the establishment of the WHO *Expert Committee on Midwifery Training* in August 1954 following a recommendation made by the WHO Expert Committee on Maternity Care to consider the training of midwifery personnel at all levels. The agreement to include midwives on the Expert Committee was pivotal in the ICM's story.

This Committee was to focus primarily on areas of the world where maternity services were less developed, with a paucity of midwife professionals so that auxiliary personnel were required. This was a joint committee drawing members from the WHO Expert Advisory Panels on Nursing and on Maternal and Child Health. Dr NJ Eastman, a US obstetrician, was elected Chairman and Miss N Goffard, a Belgian midwife, Vice-Chair.[15] The first meeting was held in The Hague, the Netherlands 2–7 August 1954. The depth of review of this history-making expert committee helps the reader to understand the WHO's long-held views and support for midwives and midwifery practice along with ICM's early efforts to collaborate with and help the WHO understand the difference between a fully qualified midwife and others providing maternity care services.[16]

The beginning of the Expert Committee meeting included adopting the WHO 1952 definition of maternity care[17] and reminding each other that the acceptance of maternity services and health personnel depended not only upon technical knowledge but also on knowledge, understanding and respect of culture, traditional beliefs and customs. The group also understood that maternity care included a wide range of personnel providing needed services, including physicians, midwives, nurses and auxiliary personnel – a position that some ICM leaders and member associations in the 21st century tended to discourage, including a statement adopted by the ICM in 2017 that stated only midwives practised midwifery.[18] The 2017 position statement was adopted, in part, to advocate for midwives as the primary caregiver for childbearing women.

The Expert Committee defined the types and functions of midwifery personnel (except physicians) including the traditional birth attendant (TBA)[19], auxiliary midwife and the fully trained midwife. The fully trained midwife included the 'trained midwife, nurse/midwife, and public health-nurse/midwife'[20], noting that in some countries nursing was required prior to midwifery education and that the public health nurse/midwife often had supervisory responsibility for auxiliary midwifery personnel. Nearly 70 years later, this situation of midwifery personnel remains in many countries.

The remainder of the report described in detail the general principles of preparation for the fully trained midwife and auxiliary midwife, following prior reports from the Expert Committee on Nursing noting that the principles were essentially the same for both nurses and midwives.[21] The midwifery training committee also agreed the attitudes, knowledge and skills desired of midwifery personnel [essential competencies][22]; criteria for the selection of students; classroom and clinical facilities needed; residential accommodation; transport to community sites; methods of teaching that focused on active learning and preparation of the midwife teacher for the clinical as well as classroom settings.[23] The group reinforced the importance of accepting the Traditional Birth Attendant (TBA) as a member of the maternity care team and her role as a respected member of the village with the responsibility to transfer women to the fully trained midwife when needed.

One of the final recommendations of the Committee was related to the need for legislation that supported the practice of midwifery in each country, requiring flexibility as changes indicated. Another recommendation of note to the ICM in future years was:

> 'That at appropriate times the WHO should promote the holding of regional conferences which will evaluate the expanded training and use of midwives in relation to the maternity care programmes. These conferences should be based on exchange of information on the experience that is now being gained throughout the world.'[24]

The Committee's final recommendation was that the WHO arrange research and studies to promote better understanding of the problems and help make training [sic: education] programmes more realistic. This Committee's recommendations were carried out in large measure in collaboration with the ICM following its official UN recognition as a Nongovernmental Organisation (NGO) by the WHO in 1957.[25] This initial collaboration between the ICM and the WHO became an important building block for future collaboration between the two organisations in order to face the challenges of post-war concerns for healthy mothers and babies that continues to the present day.

THE ICM CONGRESS IN LONDON: 4–11 SEPTEMBER 1954

After tentative discussions and meetings in Rome, Paris and London, a decision was made to relaunch the midwives' organisation as the International Council of Midwives (ICM) with a secretariat based in London and a new constitution. This partially fulfilled the long-held dream of Madame Mossé, the pre-war IMU President, of the organisation reforming in France, for which she had made provision in her will for premises as a home for the ICM. Her death in 1949 left the project for France without a champion and the Royal College of Midwives in the United Kingdom stepped in to set about organising the first full-scale congress after the war. Records do not reveal whether Madame Mossé's provision for the premises ever came to fruition, possibly due to the delay between her death and the agreement to restart based in London, or the money could have been used in France in maintaining some communication in order to hold the meetings enabling the restart. We are left to form our own opinions on this, though the idea of having paid housing for the Secretariat over the past 70 years could possibly have alleviated some of the financial woes of the organisation.

The RCM, with its headquarters based in London, hosted the 1954 ICM Congress from 4 to 11 September at the Tuke Hall, Bedford College London[26], with 800 midwives from 46 countries in attendance. The Congress theme was 'The Midwife – Her Training and Professional Responsibilities' under the Congress-adopted motif of 'The Family'.[27] There was great enthusiasm among midwives with lots of sharing of midwifery stories and practices along with social interactions for the long-awaited goal to gather together again to discuss midwifery in the world.

Edith Pye, immediate past-President of the RCM, presided over the Congress and Council meetings as the ICM President. The Royal Patron of the RCM was Her Royal Highness the Duchess of York.[28] Her daughter, who became Queen Elizabeth II, was the Patron of the 1954 ICM Congress.[29] The opening ceremony featured Nora B Deane, described as Congress President.[30] British midwifery was highlighted by the Minister of Health, the Rt Hon Ian McLeod, who said, 'If there is one feature of our British Health Services in which we feel unrestrained pride it is our midwifery services.'[31] Indeed, in many ways, British midwifery was a standard bearer for quality midwifery education and practice globally, and the RCM was and continues to be a strong supporter of the ICM to the present time.

The 1954 ICM Congress drew not only midwives but in attendance were obstetricians, international health organisations and governmental officials. A WHO representative attended for the first time, although European midwives had been working with the WHO for many years prior to 1954 on various topics related to maternal and child health.[32] This meeting helped to formalise the relationship of the ICM with the WHO. During the 1954 Congress, Professor Nicholson J Eastman paid tribute to midwives as not only present at the time of childbirth, but as potential apostles of hygiene for the populace at large. He added that if midwives are to serve their highest function in relation to world health, then their main task is teaching.[33] Other international speakers from outside Europe, including Sitt Howa Ali El Bassir from Sudan and Rachel Blecher Zvi-Tov from Israel, positively reinforced the wider inclusiveness of the ICM at that time. In addition, the recognition by the WHO and a renowned obstetrician/gynaecologist put the ICM in the position of leading the midwives of the world in efforts to promote health for all.

With midwives from beyond Europe attending this conference, a significant increase in membership began, though the archival resources could not determine the actual numbers. Such was the enthusiasm that with the appointment of a voluntary, part-time ICM Secretary, events were able to be organised between congresses and the organisation was becoming established on the political scene. It will become clear to all who read this book that the hosting of Triennial Congresses around the world raised enthusiasm among midwives to know more about each other and to share experiences, and, in some cases, reinforced the value of midwives to governments such as in Vancouver and Durban. The various themes of each congress (Annex C) reflected what was of particular interest to midwives and/or to the country hosting at that particular time. As a consequence, the ICM responded by developing resources to aid its member associations in working with governments in their development of education, ethical and competent midwifery practise, and legal frameworks that facilitated this practise. The meetings between congresses sought to take forward the outcomes of each congress, providing a voice for midwives at country and regional levels.

ICM COUNCIL DECISIONS 1954

During this Congress, a formal Council meeting was held. Miss Pye chaired the meeting for the delegates from 22 countries who met as the Executive Council. The four General Officers (President Deane, two Vice Presidents and an Honorary President) and an executive committee of 12 were among the 39 official member association delegates representing 22 countries making up the Council. One of the first decisions of the Executive Council was to rename the International Council of Midwives to the International Confederation of Midwives (ICM) with its headquarters placed in London at the RCM. Miss Marjorie Bayes had been selected by the RCM to be the ICM Secretary in response to the group who met in 1953.[34] There is a suggestion that the Secretary position was a voluntary one initially and Miss Bayes was an employee of the Royal College of Midwives. The ICM office was a desk in a basement room at the RCM.

Another important outcome of this 1954 ICM Executive Council meeting was the adoption of a new British-based Constitution[35] that defined the General Officers, the International Council, the Executive Committee, Triennial Congresses and the three official languages of English, French and Spanish.[36] General Officers at this time included Miss Deane (UK) as President; Miss Ellen Erup (Sweden), Vice President; Madame Luzzi (Italy), Vice President; Mme Jay (France) as Honorary President (immediate Past President) and an Executive Committee of 12.[37] The newly agreed Constitution defined the policymaking body as the ICM Executive Council that included the General Officers, Executive Committee members and two delegates each from the rest of the member associations.

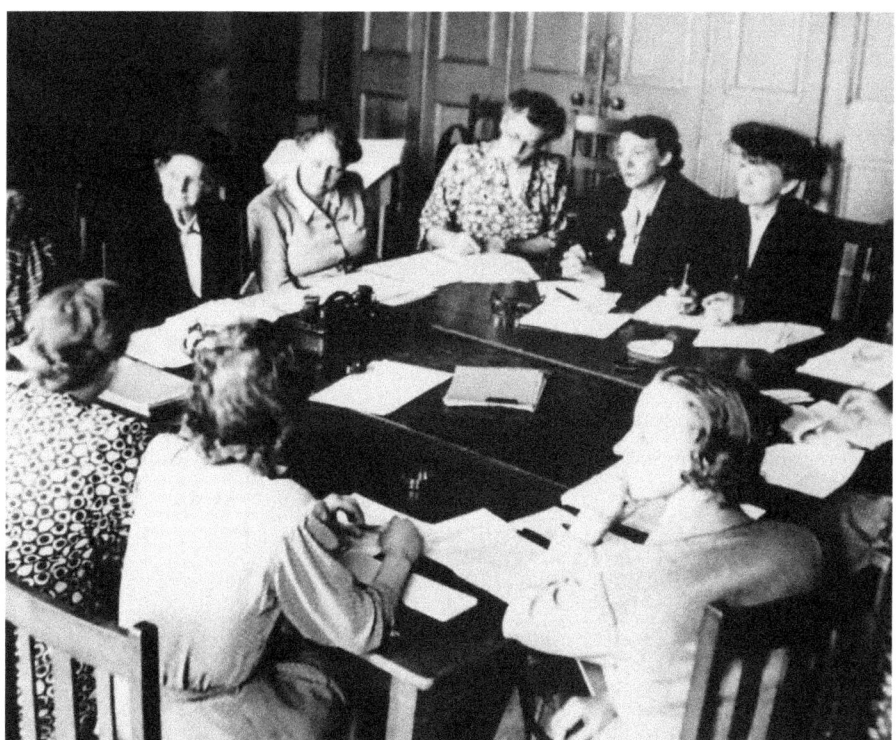

Meeting of Executive Committee of 12 (1950s) – ICM Archives at Wellcome Collection

1955–1956 ICM ACTIVITIES

The Executive Committee of the ICM met in 1955 and approved more than one association per country to join as long as each association:
1. Met the terms of reference in the 1954 Constitution:
    a. The Organisation should be non-political
    b. Midwives recognised by their governments as competent to practise midwifery
    c. Association's Constitution and Byelaws in harmony with those of Confederation
    d. Proposed and seconded by two member groups and accepted by majority vote of Council[38]
2. Represented a reasonable proportion of midwives in their country, and
3. The total number of representatives on the Council did not exceed that of another country, in keeping with the intent of the 1954 Constitution.[39]

This decision led to many debates during the next 50 years as countries with more than one midwifery association in membership with two votes each at Council meetings could overwhelm needs and interests of another country's single member association. This Committee also added the word 'Executive' to the title of 'Secretary' in line with other international organisations at the time.[40] The report[41] also mentions a General Officers' meeting at the same time who agreed the promotion of exchange visits and the collection of data in regard to midwifery training and practice, although no archival evidence of this over the following five years was found.

In 1956 the General Officers met again and reported a total membership of 24 associations from 21 countries representing over 101,000 midwives and continuing to increase.[42] This increase in membership was reflected at the Congress held in Stockholm in 1957 when midwives from low resource countries (LRC) were present for the first time since the rebirth in 1954, demonstrating the ICM's determination to make the Congresses and organisation for more than European midwives.

THE ICM ADMITTED INTO OFFICIAL RELATIONS WITH WORLD HEALTH ORGANIZATION – 1957

During early autumn 1956, the ICM prepared and sent materials on the organisation, including its officers and membership list, to the WHO headquarters in

Geneva to request official status within the WHO. On 30 January 1957, MG Candau, Director-General of the WHO, sent the following response to Marjorie Bayes, ICM Executive Secretary:

> 'I have the honour to refer to my letter of 19 September 1956 and to inform you that after considering the report of its Standing Committee on Non-Governmental Organizations [NGOs], the WHO Executive Board at its nineteenth session decided to admit the International Confederation of Midwives into official relations with the World Health Organization. I feel sure that this relationship will lead to closer collaboration and fruitful work between the two organizations.'[43]

This official relationship was reviewed along with all NGOs every two years, though apparently the ICM was admitted in an 'off' year for these reviews as they were asked for updated activities in August 1957, barely a year into the official relation.[44] However, on 10 February 1958, Dr Candau sent a letter to the Executive Secretary of ICM stating:

> 'I now have the pleasure of informing you that the Board, on the recommendation of its Standing Committee on Non-Governmental Organizations, has approved the maintenance of official relations with your organization on the basis of the criteria established by the World Health Assembly. I should like to express my very real satisfaction at this decision, which confirms the usefulness of our relations in the past and ensures their further development in the future.'[45]

Miss Bayes' response on 14 February 1958, noted, 'It will be my great pleasure to report this to my General Officers when they meet in March, and I can assure you that it is our earnest wish to work as closely as possible with the WHO whom we admire for the wonderful work you are doing.'[46] Later in ICM's story some of the challenges of working with the WHO are highlighted.

OTHER EARLY PARTNERSHIPS

With ICM becoming an officially recognised NGO with the World Health Organization in 1957[47] consultative status with the United Nations Children's Fund (UNICEF) was applied for and received in the early 1960s. With the record stating that the ICM finances were very weak at this time, the decisions the General Officers made in 1958 suggested they were looking ahead to international collaboration as one way to seek financial support (a strategy that continues to the present time). The

General Officers agreed a decision to work with the International Federation of Gynecology and Obstetrics (FIGO) in 1959. At the same time, the WHO had requested the ICM's assistance in a worldwide collection of data on midwifery training and practice. It took ICM leaders a year to decide to work with the WHO on this task that resulted in agreeing to an FIGO/ICM Joint Study group (see Chapter 16 for details). The ICM took the initial lead by circulating questionnaires prepared by the WHO to 61 countries.[48] The outcomes of these and other joint efforts and funding support for the ICM are described throughout this book (Annex D has complete list of Partners).

ICM WORLD CONGRESS IN STOCKHOLM – 1957

> 'Another impression concerns the quality of the [ICM] educational programs. Whatever limitations and frustrations exist, whatever changes may seem desirable, there is no question that there have been wise leadership and excellent opportunities for continuous exchange of worthwhile ideas and ideals.'
>
> Coates and Strachan, *Impressions of 1957 Congress in Stockholm.*

The ICM Congress in Stockholm, Sweden, included small groups of midwives from less developed countries for the first time.[49] Ellen Erup was the ICM President at the time and helped the group understand that dual training in nursing and midwifery was necessary as hospital births increased rapidly and district nurses became competitors for midwifery services in child welfare.[50] Marjorie Bayes noted that membership in the ICM had almost doubled since 1954, with 31 Member Associations from 21 countries, representing over 107,000 midwives (Brazil, Greece, Iceland and Turkey associations were accepted into membership in 1957).[51]

SUMMARY

The decade of the 1950s was pivotal in the history of the ICM for many reasons. First and foremost was the rebirth of the organisation in 1954 with a stable headquarters for the Executive Secretary within the Royal College of Midwives. Second was the name change to the International Confederation of Midwives that has remained the same to this day. In addition, the ICM now had a formal Constitution describing aims and other details of the organisation and its decision-making bodies, including agreement for triennial congresses. Finally, the decade began official relationships with UN agencies and FIGO that contributed to the development and strengthening of the ICM and its voice as a legitimate global health professional organisation. All these important milestones for the ICM were firmly built upon the foundation of the IMU and its fearless leaders following two world wars – leaders who continued to work towards healthy women and childbearing families with well-prepared midwives providing needed services.

1 Edith M Pye. Private papers, 1949, held in the RCM Archives.
2 The Swedish Association of Midwives. *300 Years in the Service of Life*. Stockholm, Sweden: Svenska Barnmorskeförbundet, 2013, pp 33–35. The Swedish Association of Midwives was founded during a meeting of 191 midwives on 10 July 1886 (p 23). Swedish midwives had a long tradition of becoming involved in low-income countries in order to reduce maternal and newborn mortality while promoting sexual and reproductive rights for all, especially in Africa and India (p 127). Thus, it was important for these midwives to push to open the ICM to midwives and their associations beyond Europe, especially in resource-limited nations.
3 In B Cowell & D Wainwright, *Behind the Blue Door: The History of the Royal College of Midwives 1881–1981* London: Bailliere Tindall, 1981, it was noted that Swedish midwives asked that the pre-war midwifery conferences be revived in 1949 'that resulted in the 1954 Congress in London when 800 midwives from 46 countries gathered. In 1955, the International Confederation of Midwives was formed, and its headquarters placed in London, at RCM, with Miss Bayes as its executive Secretary.' (pp. 69–70).
4 Edith Pye handwritten letter without date or location. Given reference to the disappearance of Dr Daels during WWI and all his papers along with mention of the death of Mme Mossé that occurred in 1949, it is thought this letter was written in 1949 in English. [Ann Thomson personal files]
5 ICM (SA/ICM/R/4). Wellcome Collection. *Marjorie Bayes' Draft History of ICM, 1st 50 years,* p. 2.
6 It was difficult to know exactly what name the formal organisation of midwifery associations carried throughout its early history. Depending on the primary source material used, including Dr Daels' IMU *Communications* journal, the name varied from International Midwives' Union, International Midwives Organization Union, International Federation of Midwives Union, etc. It is possible that some of the variations in the name of the organisation was due to translation errors into English. Authors of this book attempted to use the name as reflected in the source being used, wherever possible.
7 ICM (SA/ICM/R/4). Wellcome Collection. *Marjorie Bayes' Draft History of ICM, 1st 50 years,* p. 2.
8 Title confirmed by former General Secretary, Miss Ruth Ashton on 7 February 2022. Miss Ashton also noted that Miss Bayes' title changed to Deputy Secretary sometime between 1954 and 1969.
9 Frieda Riede. 'Bericht uber die Stzung der Internationalen Delegierten zur Wiederbelebung der Internationalen Hebammnvereinigung' In *Deutsche Hemabben-Zeitung*, 1, Jg, 1949: 151 (Translated from German by Anja Peters).
10 Frieda Riede and Magdalene Schwietzke. 'Internationale Tagung der Hebammen am 24 Marz 1953 London.' In *Deutsche Hebammen-Zeitung*, 1953, p 129. (Translated from German by Anja Peters)
11 There was no archival evidence found that substantiated the German reflection that the 1900 meeting was a 'union' of midwifery associations.
12 ICM (SA/ICM/R/4). Wellcome Collection. *Marjorie Bayes' Draft History of ICM, 1st 50 years.*
13 ICM (SA/ICM/R/4). Wellcome Collection. *Marjorie Bayes' Draft History of ICM, 1st 50 years.*
14 The World Health Organization was founded as one arm of the United Nations. Together WHO and UNICEF were leaders in addressing the high maternal, neonatal and child deaths in the world that had been overlooked during the wars. Hence the development of several Expert Committees to address these deaths, with midwives as one of the primary providers of maternal and newborn services.
15 WHO. 'Expert Committee on Midwifery Training: First Report' *WHO Technical Report Series No 93* (Geneva: WHO, 1955), p 3. There were representatives from Belgium, England, Japan, India, Indonesia, Netherlands, Senegal, Sudan, Sweden and the USA.
16 ICM applied for official relations as a Non-Governmental Organisation shortly after reorganising in 1954. That official UN status was granted in 1957, another recognition by WHO of the important role that ICM and the midwives played in international maternal and child health.
17 WHO. 'Definition of Maternity Care', *WHO Technical Report Series No 51* (Geneva: WHO, 1952), p 3.
18 ICM. *Definition of Midwifery*. The Hague: ICM, 2017.
19 The TBA generally learned her knowledge of birth and skills from her mother/grandmother, passed from generation to generation.
20 WHO. 'Expert Committee on Midwifery Training: First Report' *WHO Technical Report Series No 93* (Geneva: WHO, 1955), p 6.
21 WHO. 'Expert Committee on Nursing', *WHO Technical Report Series 24 (1950) and 49 (1952)*. (Geneva: Who), pp 24, 9. Historically this is another example of the apparent confusion within WHO circles of the difference between the profession and practice of midwifery and the profession and practice of nursing – a theme that permeates until the present time.

22 The definition of knowledge, skills and behaviours from the 1954 Expert Committee preceded the ICM *Essential Competencies for Basic Midwifery Practice* adopted in 2002, 47 years later.
23 WHO. 'Expert Committee on Midwifery Training: First Report' *WHO Technical Report Series No 93* (Geneva: WHO, 1955), pp 7–18. This discussion reflects similar themes expressed in the ICM *Global Standards for Midwifery Education* that were first adopted by ICM in 2010, 55 years later.
24 WHO. 'Expert Committee on Midwifery Training: First Report' *WHO Technical Report Series No. 93* (Geneva: WHO, 1955), p 21.
25 *Candau letter to ICM Executive Secretary (Miss Bayes), 30 January 1957*. WHO archives with copy sent to Joyce Thompson.
26 Betty Cowell and David Wainwright. *Behind the Blue Door: The History of the Royal College of Midwives 1881–1981*. London: Bailliere Tindall, 1981, pp 69–70.
27 Wellcome Institute Library SA/ICM uncatalogued Box 6 reports of Congresses.
28 The Duchess of York was the mother of Queen Elizabeth II, thus the Queen Mother in 1954. She was patron of the RCM for over 50 years.
Betty Cowell and David Wainwright. *Behind the Blue Door: The History of the Royal College of Midwives 1881–1981*. London: Bailliere Tindall, 1981, p 55. 1954 Congress bulletin includes of photo of Queen Elizabeth II with a note that she was the Patron on the ICM Congress in 1954.
30 *Programme of the 1954 ICM Congress*. Personal papers E Duff.
31 Betty Cowell and David Wainwright. *Behind the Blue Door: The History of the Royal College of Midwives 1881–1981*. London: Bailliere Tindall, 1981, p 69.
32 Lyle Creelman, Chief, Nursing Section, WHO, letter to Marjorie Bayes, Executive Secretary, ICM, dated, 8 February 1957, stated, 'I am sure you will have had an official letter informing you that the International Confederation has been granted official relationships with WHO. I am very glad of this and look forward to a continuance of the close co-operation we have had in the past … I know we shall be calling on you for information and assistance in obtaining suitably qualified personnel for posts in our programmes.'
33 Lucille Woodville. Historical Background on the International Confederation of Midwives. *Bulletin Nurse-Midwives* XVI:2 (May 1971), p 38. Marjorie Bayes. *Draft History of ICM, first fifty years*. Wellcome Institute Library document SA/ICM/R/4, p 2.
34 Betty Cowell and David Wainwright. *Behind the Blue Door: The History of the Royal College of Midwives 1881–1981*. London: Bailliere Tindall, 1981, pp 69–70.
35 ICM. *The International Confederation of Midwives Constitution Agreed by Council on September 10th, 1954*. London: ICM, 1954, pp 1–2. [Personal papers of Joyce Thompson]
36 ICM. *The International Confederation of Midwives Constitution Agreed by Council on September 10th, 1954*. Regulation 5. Official Languages, p 3. [Personal papers of Joyce Thompson]
37 There is a discrepancy in Marjorie Bayes' History notes as to when the official name was adopted so the authors went with the earlier date of 1954 confirmed by the Congress programme and other articles.
38 ICM. *The International Confederation of Midwives Constitution Agreed by Council on September 10th, 1954*. London: ICM, 1954, pp 1–2. [Personal papers of Joyce Thompson]
39 ICM (SA/ICM/R/4). Wellcome Collection. *Marjorie Bayes' Draft History of ICM, 1st 50 years*, p. 2. ICM. *The International Confederation of Midwives Constitution Agreed by Council on September 10th, 1954*. London: ICM, 1954, pp 1–2. [Personal papers of Joyce Thompson].
40 ICM (SA/ICM/R/4). Wellcome Collection. *Marjorie Bayes' Draft History of ICM, 1st 50 years*, p. 2.
41 The terminology of General Officers at this time of ICM history appears to refer to the immediate past president, current president, and two vice-presidents according to Miss Bayes' history notes. A constitutional change at the 1978 Council meeting in Israel changed from Honorary Officers to General Officers.
42 ICM (SA/ICM/R/4). Wellcome Collection. *Marjorie Bayes' Draft History of ICM, 1st 50 years*, p. 2.
43 *WHO Director General Candau letter to ICM Executive Secretary (Miss Bayes), 30 January 1957*. Letter in WHO archives sent to JET by Jill Caughley, researching history ICN in 2007.
44 *Letter of Marjorie Bayes, ICM Executive Secretary, to MG Candau, Director-General, WHO, dated 13 November 1957*, apologising for the delay in responding to his letter of 30 August 1957 requesting information on ICM. In that letter, Miss Bayes explains that since all the ICM details had been presented for the WHO Executive Committee vote in January 1957 to admit ICM into official relationship with WHO and the Congress held in Stockholm, her response was delayed. The membership list was attached to her letter. WHO Archives.
45 *WHO Director General Candau letter to ICM Executive Secretary (Miss Bayes) 10 February 1958*. WHO Archives.
46 *Bayes letter to MS Candau, Director General, WHO, 14 February 1958*. WHO Archives.
47 Lyle Creelman, Chief, Nursing Section, WHO, letter to Marjorie Bayes, Executive Secretary, ICM, dated 8 February 1957, stated, 'I am sure you will have had an official letter informing you that the International Confederation has been granted official relationships with WHO. I am very glad of this and look forward to a continuance of the close co-operation we have had in the past.' 'I know we shall be calling on you for information and assistance in obtaining suitably qualified personnel for posts in our programmes.'
48 ICM (SA/ICM/R/4). Wellcome Collection. *Marjorie Bayes' Draft History of ICM, 1st 50 years*.
49 ICM (SA/ICM/R/4). Wellcome Collection. *Marjorie Bayes' Draft History of ICM, 1st 50 years*.
50 The Swedish Association of Midwives. *300 Years in the Service of Life*. Stockholm, Sweden: Svenska Barnmorskeförbundet, 2011, pp 86–89.

51 Again, the discrepancy of numbers in Miss Bayes' history, since she recorded 39 delegates from 22 countries in 1954 Congress, but then reported a doubling of membership in 1957 though the numbers were less. Without primary source documents available, it was impossible to determine who was a member and who was not.

Chapter 5: *ICM's Constitutional Mandates and Structure*

The selection of new member Israel to host the 1978 Congress caused an uproar among the eight African countries with ICM membership, as noted by Mrs RO Sosanya. 'African countries are quite ready to concede [Congress Host] to elder member countries in ICM, but we find ourselves unable to accept the nomination of a junior member particularly in the manner that Israel, a most junior member of ICM, was voted in for the next Congress. We consider this an affront and an injury to us and a damage to the faith and respect we have for the ICM and we therefore ask the Congress to reconsider this decision in favour of Nigeria, particularly since an ICM Congress had never been held in the African continent.'

INTRODUCTION

Most groups who choose to formally organise, whatever the reason, will develop and agree a structure, that allows them to function. In this chapter a brief overview of the organisational structure of the ICM, functioning as an international health organisation through the years in keeping with its dual aims and objectives is provided Without a structure and supportive foundation, the ICM would have never survived its first 100 years. The value of a formal Constitution and Byelaws to a non-profit organisation sets the purpose and rules of operation.[1] In other words, such documents provide order in the midst of potential chaos among good-hearted individuals wishing to make the world a better place. For the ICM, its Constitutions and Byelaws over time provided clearly stated aims/objects with generic activities to meet those aims; criteria for membership; description of its officers and how elected and the governing body with the rules for conducting meetings.

AIMS AND OBJECTS OF THE IMU/ICM OVER TIME (PURPOSE)

As noted in Chapters 3 and 4, the International Confederation of Midwives (ICM) began as a union of midwifery associations in 1922 following great efforts to restart international scientific meetings among European midwives that had ceased during WWI. The International Midwives' Union (IMU)[2] drafted, revised and adopted in 1925[3] the early byelaws which included:

> 'The aim of the union is:
>
> protection of maternity and nursing of the baby;
>
> the scientifical (sic), maternal, social and ethical elevation of the midwife standing.'[4] In addition, the regulations stated that IMU was 'a union of all midwives' associations of the whole world.'[5]

The ICM operated using these Byelaws until 1954 when a new Constitution was developed as described later in this chapter. Annex E illustrates the changes in wording of the Aims/Objects from 1925–2022, noting how the various Council decisions over the years viewed the importance of women's health either in general or just those women who were bearing children. The emphasis during the 1970s when Family Planning was high on the agenda can be compared with the mid 1990s when the focus on sexual and reproductive health was limited in the stated aims and mission statements, again reflecting the views of various Council delegates at a given point in history.

Given that well-qualified midwives were needed to improve the quality of care for women and childbearing families, the ICM Council adopted a revised Constitution in 1981 that, since that time, viewed the work of the ICM as twofold:
1) Strengthening midwives and midwifery associations.
2) Improving the standard of care for women and childbearing families.

MAJOR CONSTITUTIONAL MANDATE CHANGES

In this section three major Constitutional changes are highlighted, all affected by a concern for financial viability, that changed how the organisation functioned. The first was the adoption of the 1954 Constitution with the rebirth of the IMU as the ICM.[6] The 1954 Constitution[7] mandated:
a) Triennial Congresses (Chapter 9) that provided the updated scientific knowledge and sharing of global midwifery practices sought after by midwives.
b) An Executive Committee that consisted of eight General Officers and 12 national members elected by Council. In addition there were up to four additional vice- Presidents co-opted from continents not currently represented among the elected Executive Committee. This meant that the

Executive Committee had 24 members with each one having a vote. This was a large group to organise for meetings, leaving the General Officers and/or President of the day to make needed decisions in between Council and Executive Committee meetings. It was important to note that from 1954, each elected officer had the responsibility to represent the international community of midwives, not their own midwifery association/country[8], remaining the same in 2022 (See Figure 5.1).

The ICM Structure 1954–1981: Figure 5.1

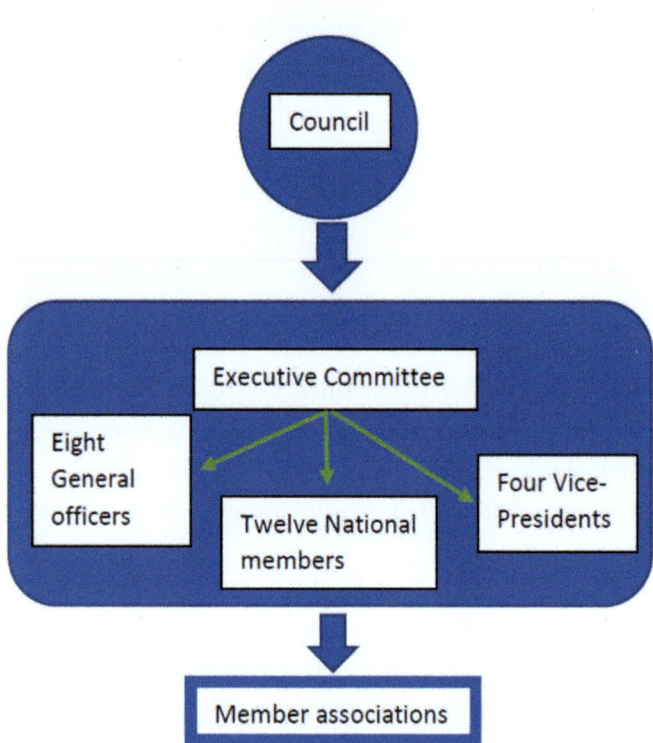

The second major Constitutional change occurred in 1981[9] when the governance structure of the organisation was changed.[10] Margaret Peters, the ICM Appointed President 1981–1984, noted that the 1981 Constitution was redrafted as a key action taken to address the financial crisis at that time, when the United States' Agency for International Development (USAID) grant funds ended in December 1979. The financial crisis was caused by unrealistic expectations of the 1981

Congress revenue, poor advance planning in view of the end of USAID project funding, and a serious misuse of the ICM funds by its Financial Advisor.[11]

The 1981 Constitution more clearly identified the lines of authority and responsibilities of a smaller decision-body in between Triennial Council meetings, notably a three-member Board of Management (BoM) and 11 Regional Representatives in comparison with the 24-member Executive Committee of 1954.[12] See Figure 5.2.

The ICM Structure 1981–2008 Figure 5.2

However, the Constitution did not specify any qualifications for the elected officers beyond holding membership in an ICM Member Association (MA) in good standing. This lack of qualifications led to a variety of leadership strengths and gaps, depending on who was elected and what experience they had in organisational management. Margaret Peters also noted that the financial crisis of the early 1980s required action to not only reduce the size of the Executive Committee but also the need to relocate the ICM Headquarters from the palatially sized one on Victoria Street, London, to an attic on Lower Belgrave Street [London]. She went on to say that the part-time employee (Executive Secretary) was retained to keep the ICM functioning during the financial crisis. Both actions averted bankruptcy and the newly acquired UK charity status was retained.[13] This was an early recognition that finances dictated, in part, not only the activities that the ICM could carry out, primarily with external financial aid, but also its headquarters' location and staffing levels.

The third major Constitutional change began in 1999 when the ICM Council agreed the move of the ICM Headquarters (HQ) from the UK to the Netherlands, again prompted, in part, by a financial concern as it was becoming increasingly expensive to maintain the ICM HQ in the London area. An additional incentive was that the Village Council of The Hague offered financial assistance for the move and the government of the Netherlands promised core funds for ongoing support of the ICM if sited there. This move required a change in governance documents to meet Dutch legal requirements.[14] A Foundation (Stitching) was formed and carried out the governance of the ICM until 2005 when a decision was made to meet the legal requirements for an Association.[15] The UK Charity Commissioners agreed that as long as the ICM would use any funds in UK accounts for charitable activities and that the Dutch Foundation was established with identical objects and aims, they would release such funds as a grant from the UK Charity to the Dutch Foundation. In addition, the UK Charity Commission agreed to be the outpost legal entity with the UK ICM Constitution in force until a new Dutch ICM Constitution could be adopted.[16]

The agreed 2005 Constitution[17] mandated the ICM governance and activities (essentially the same since the 1950s) through 2022 with two important changes. These included:

a) The mandate for yearly Council meetings to approve financial matters and the change of titles of elected officers as of 2008.

b) The ICM Council elected a President (formerly Director) and Vice President (formerly Deputy Director) along with a Financial officer (Treasurer) with responsibilities essentially the same as the former Board of Management. Bridget Lynch was the first elected President of the ICM and Frances Day-Stirk was the first elected Vice President under the Dutch Constitution (Annex F: ICM Officers).

ICM BYELAWS

The Byelaws are important tools for explaining and expanding on how the work of the Confederation is accomplished, providing needed details to carry out Constitutional mandates. In addition, Byelaws are easier to change than the Constitution of an organisation, so they provide an avenue for Member Associations (MAs) to change them as needed to reflect the times. The ICM Byelaws address such things as financial management of profit and losses of the ICM sponsored activities, definition of the ICM Regions and representation (beginning in 1981), details of rights of membership, voting delegates and timing of Council meetings, how election of officers are conducted and host associations selected for Congresses, the role and responsibilities of elected officers and the calculation of membership dues. Each Byelaw is referenced back to the Constitution so it is in line with the intentions of the Constitution.

CONSTITUTIONAL MANDATES/POWERS AFFECTING THE STRUCTURE OF THE ICM
ICM Board: Qualifications and Responsibilities

From 1954 until 1981 the eight General Officers were responsible for the day-to-day management, changing in 1981 to the three midwife Board of Management (BoM) members elected by Council as noted above. The qualifications to be an elected officer were very general in both the Constitution and Byelaws, noting only that they needed to be 'a member of an association enjoying full rights.' This lack of specific qualifications meant that many elected leaders lacked the essential expertise for managing the wide-ranging affairs and activities of the Confederation. A prime example being that the Constitution noted that the Treasurer was expected to reside in the country of the ICM secretariat, though there was no mention of financial expertise needed. This resulted in a decision by the BoM beginning in the 1990s with Sr Anne Thompson, Treasurer, to have a volunteer group of financial experts, as advisors, whom she lovingly called the 'wise men'. The BoM drafted detailed Position Descriptions for elected leaders beginning in 1999, though these were not always used during most elections.

An integral part of the growth and development of the ICM as a female-led organisation was reflected in the leadership of its elected officers. European midwifery leaders from strong midwifery associations with a Western European understanding of midwifery were the elected officers of the ICM until 1984 when Margaret Peters from Australia was elected Deputy Director of the BoM.[18] As membership grew from other continents, elected officers came not only from Australia (Peters, Brown), but the USA (Thompson), Africa (Malata), Canada (Lynch), the Caribbean (Lewis), Portugal (Varela) and Chile (Oyarzo). Refer to Annex F: Table of ICM Appointed and Elected Officers since 1954.

With Headquarters based in the Hague, the Netherlands, the final adoption of the Dutch-based Constitution for the ICM in 2008, the process having begun in 2005, resulted in the election of a President, Vice-President and Treasurer, who took on the prior roles of the elected Director, Deputy Director and Treasurer (BoM).

Responsibilities of the Board of Management (BoM)

The responsibilities of each BoM member were detailed in the Constitution and Byelaws, including Powers, Duties, Meetings, Notice and Quorum for meetings. The BoM was charged with managing and controlling the revenue, expenditures, credits, investments and property of the Confederation; authorising Confederation publications; creating and overseeing the terms and conditions of service of the Secretariat, including appointments and terminations; delegating necessary authority to act on its behalf; and 'all other acts which may be necessary to give effect to the aims of the Confederation'. The first Executive Committee Manual of 1998 was updated in 2003 with core ICM documents included as part of the orientation for new members. The BoM manual had job descriptions and HQ staff policies included for their work with the Secretary General/Chief Executive.

A Triennial report of activities of the BoM was required at each ICM Council meeting, facilitated by a 6-year Plan of Work constructed/adjusted after each Triennial Council meeting. The Plan of Work addressed the geographical area, title of project(s), description of activities and resources, linkages, expected outcomes, funding required and sponsors, beginning in 1987.

Executive Committee 1954–1981–2017; The Board 2017–present

In 1981 the Executive Committee was reduced in size from the 24 members of 1954 in total to three Council elected BoM members plus 11 elected Regional Representatives. From 1981 to 2017, each Regional Representative was the MA voted to take on the role by MAs within each region. The MA would then name an individual midwife to carry out this role.

The ICM Byelaws often made mention of the need for a division of the world into geographical regions. The number of Regions within the ICM beginning in 1981 remained steady for many years at four (Africa, Americas, Asia-Pacific[19] and Europe), with all but Europe having two Regional Representatives. Europe had five representatives initially, and then in 2005 the number was reduced to three.[20]

In 2014 a third Regional Representative was added in the Asia-Pacific Region[21], and in 2017, some of the European MAs transferred from the European Region to create the Eastern Mediterranean Region (Refer to Membership Charts in Annex G). During the 2020 virtual Council meeting, delegates agreed that the number of Regions would be the same six as those of the WHO with realigned numbers so that the final Board would include the Eastern Mediterranean region and the divided Asia-Pacific region that was among the largest by geographic area.[22] This decision moving forward meant that Regional Representatives would be reduced to one per region as of 2023 making a total of nine Board members (three Officers plus six Regional Reps) with all being involved in every meeting throughout the triennium moving forward.[23] It will be important to evaluate this change going forward given the multiple language groups in many regions, including the Confederation's official languages which are under discussion as of 2022.[24]

Responsibilities of the Executive Committee
The ICM Regional Representatives take responsibility for maintaining contact with each MA in their region, keeping the Board and Secretariat updated on MA issues and successes, and participating in Executive Committee meetings, usually held mid-triennium and at each Triennial Council (now Annual Council) where Council mandates were considered and acted upon. Reports from Regional Representatives to the Secretariat were shared with the BoM and often appeared in the newsletters informing all MAs. Each Regional Representative also provided a summary of MAs' issues during the Triennial Council Meetings, often leading to the introduction of new position statements and/or comments on core documents. They were expected to cast votes during Council meetings that reflected their region, not their own MA.

The Asia-Pacific region and its representatives led the way in demonstrating the value of and opportunities for advancing midwives and midwifery in the region with meetings and conferences, many of which were sponsored in part by the governments of Australia and Japan, along with their MAs and New Zealand NGOs. In the early years, other regions with the exception of Europe did not have the resources to host regional meetings.

Over the years the Executive Committee (Board of Management and Regional Representatives – now the Board) have been responsible for advising Council delegates on professional policies and philosophical foundations of Confederation activities. They also had the power to create terms of reference for individuals and standing committees, name subcommittees for specific activities, appoint representatives to other organisations, and suggest agenda items for the Triennial Council meetings. The designation of the ICM regions fell to the Council and changed over the years, being static at four for many years, Africa, Americas, Europe and Asia, then expanding to six, then 11 and back to six, Africa, (Anglophone and Francophone), Americas (North America and Caribbean and Latin America), Western Pacific, Eastern Mediterranean, South-East Asia, Europe (Northern, Central and Southern), as of 2020.

GOVERNANCE OF THE CONFEDERATION – THE ICM COUNCIL

So, how is the ICM managed? Simply stated, the ICM Council, made up of two delegates from each MA in full membership at the time of the meeting, determines the ICM's strategic directions and policies, elects the officers and endorses the regional representatives chosen by each region of the Confederation. In other words, the ICM Member Associations decide and direct the policies for the organisation and establish midwifery standards. The ICM Board (Officers and Regional Representatives) is mandated to act on behalf of the Council's interests, and to implement its decisions in keeping with the Vision, Mission and Global Strategy (Strategic Directions) of the Confederation.[25]

From 2023 it is anticipated that with a smaller group of elected Regional Representatives (six) down from 11, and the three elected Officers, the ICM Board (formerly BoM and Executive Committee) will function as a whole at all times, making for increased input from all members as well as more transparency. These changes did not alter the governance responsibility of the ICM Council to set the aims, objectives, vision and strategic goals for each triennium as these remained constant throughout all the changes within the BoM and Executive Committees over the years (See Figure 5.3).

The ICM Structure from 2023 Figure 5.3

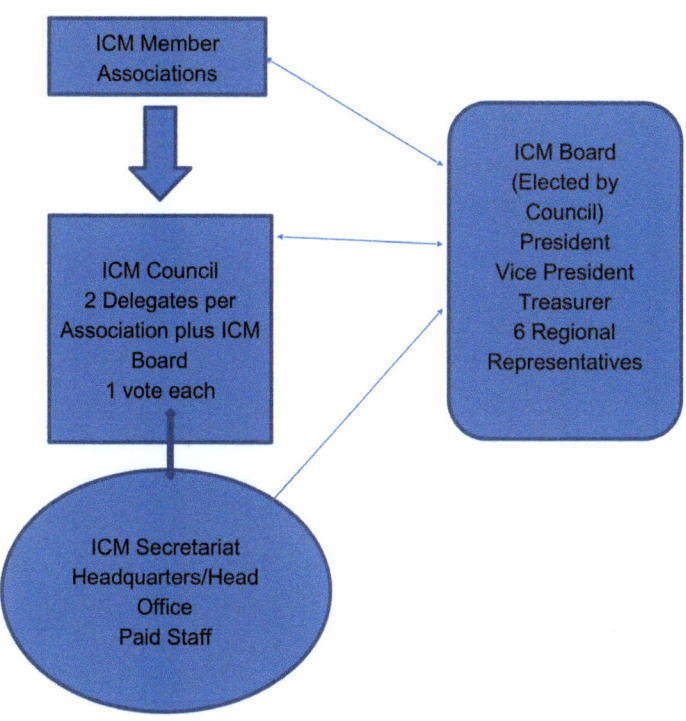

ACTIONS AND RESPONSIBILITIES OF THE COUNCIL
Criteria for ICM Membership

One of the most contentious and long-standing debates within the ICM Council, reflected in both the Constitution and Byelaws over the years, recognised members as midwifery associations in a given geographic area and the number of MAs from each country that could be accepted by the ICM.[26] Throughout all of the Council discussions of constitutional matters since 1954, the qualification for full membership remained. Those qualifications included midwifery associations whose:

1. midwives who meet the international definition of the midwife as of 1972;
2. midwives are legally recognised to practise in their country; and
3. who agree to pay financial dues in such form and within such time limits as may be decided by the Council.

Examples of additions/changes in membership criteria began in the 1981 Constitution, Article 5.

'Members of the Confederation shall be:
(i) associations of midwives, herein after called 'associations';
(ii) In countries where midwives and nurses belong to the same association, that association, or that section which represents the interest of midwives, may become a member provided
   (a) *a midwifery section exists with its own chairman and*
   (b) *meetings for the conduct of midwifery affairs are held separated from those of nurses.*'[27]

The membership eligibility clause in Article 5, (ii) in the 1993 Constitution remained unchanged[28] in spite of efforts during the 1990 Kobe Council meeting 2 October 1990 to adopt a proposed amendment to the Constitution suggesting that EACH country should have the same number of votes irrespective of number of midwives or number of associations.[29] These debates continued through 2020, though no new decision has been taken.[30] At the same Kobe Council meeting, the New Zealand College of Midwives (NZCOM) proposed allowing associations with women/consumers as part of their association members to be recognised. This was defeated (Chapter 14). With the Asia-Pacific region's persistence, the ICM Council in 1996 adopted the addition of a single word that allowed consumer members in midwifery associations. It read, in part, that a member 'shall consist primarily of midwives' and also acknowledged student midwives who were part of a MA.[31]

In 2014, three additional categories for membership without voting rights were added.

1. Collective: Associations that have formed a collective group to apply for full ICM membership (e.g. a small island in the Pacific with three midwives has no capacity to form an association but may form a collective association with the other islands).
2. Associate: Associations applying for full ICM membership that have not yet met the criteria required for becoming a full member. For example, some associations lack a regulatory framework in their country. These associations would be allowed six years to meet the ICM criteria. During this time, they would not have any voting rights, but would be allowed to participate in Council as observers.
3. Affiliate: This category is specifically for regional associations (e.g. Confederation of African Midwives Association or Confederation of

European Midwives Associations). These associations pay a symbolic fee and have no voting rights during Council.[32]

How the Council agenda needed to be organised, the processes of debate and voting were clarified in 1995 when the *Procedures for International Council Meeting* were adopted.[33] One of the most challenging aspects of Triennial Council Meetings for decades was how to deal with the variety of groups whose first language was not English and/or who were not used to following parliamentary procedures[34] for attending to the business of the meeting. Though Spanish and French translation was provided with the Japanese providing their own translator during the Council meetings, it took time for that simultaneous translation to be completed, causing problems when native English speakers called for a decision to be made ('called the question') before the proposal was fully translated, as illustrated in the text box below.

The 2005 ICM Council meeting was my first experience of working with midwives from over 70 countries speaking a variety of languages other than English. I understood the Rules of Order being used but was surprised and angered when those rules were used to deny full discussion of one issue, that of supporting the ICM/FIGO joint statement on prevention of Postpartum Hemorrhage. The New Zealand delegation put forth an agenda item related to withdrawal of ICM's participation in such joint statements, and without time for discussion, the Radical Midwives delegation 'called the question' effectively ending any discussion. I felt this action was a travesty of justice and totally disrespectful of our midwife colleagues who did not speak English and who were waiting for translation of the original agenda item. Many delegations were confused about what just happened, so I asked for a point of order to explain the process. I reminded the Council members that in 2002 actions they had asked the ICM Board to proceed with this joint statement, which they did. The Council was asked if they wished to revisit this agenda item for discussion. Council members agreed the need for further discussion, and the agenda item was defeated. I learned a lot during this meeting, including how difficult it is to include all Council delegates in discussion of items and how I, as a native English speaker, needed to be respectful of the time needed for this to happen.

Kim Campbell, Canadian Association of Midwives

The July 2005 the Executive Committee at the end of Council addressed five actions to improve Council meetings:
1. Listen before commenting
2. Support each Member Association wishing to speak (wait for language translation)
3. Work as a unified whole
4. Improve the communication link with MAs and regional representatives
5. Complete a feedback loop.[35]

These steps were essential to completing the business of Council with a balance of decisions that affected all members. In addition, a Council Handbook was created early on to facilitate participation during Council meetings and to understand the order of business to be conducted.

Setting Global Midwifery Policies and Standards

Among the most important decisions made by Council delegates related directly to what should be the priorities for action to carry out the agreed dual Aims. The result of Council decisions since 1954 are discussed in several chapters in this book, framed within the Council's agreement on three essential strategic directions:
1. Address women's health globally
2. Strengthen the midwifery profession
3. Promote the organisation internationally

The ICM's Vision and Mission statements are discussed (Chapter 8) as they relate to these three strategic directions. A variety of ICM Policy and Position Statements are listed in Annex A, Core ICM Documents beginning with the Code of Ethics are found in Chapter 11 and the ICM global standards for the education and regulation of midwives are discussed in Chapter 12 all relating to or implementing the strategic directions.

Selection of Host Associations for Congresses

The selection of the Triennial Congress site and Host Association from 1954 onward was generally agreed by Council members three to six years in advance to provide time for planning. Refer to Annex C: Table of ICM Congresses and Themes. The

Council delegates' selection of the Congress site had definite financial implications (registration fees were a main source of ICM income needing lots of attendees and the cost of contracts with hotels, etc. to meet expenses). For example, one of the hotly debated topics in 1975 occurred when the ICM Council selected the National Association of Midwives of Israel to host the 1978 Congress, an association accepted into membership at the same meeting (refer to text opening this chapter). Miss Bayes, Secretary General at the time, noted that since the ICM Council voted by ballot, no change could be made. It would appear that this decision by Council was based on the potential for financial success. At times, the ICM Council members made their decision based on their collective 'hearts' rather than just on financial viability, such as happened in the selection of Manila, the Philippines, in 1999, that resulted in a financial loss.

A Host Association contract was agreed beginning in the mid-1990s, including the per registrant fee percentage returned to the ICM and the equitable division of proceeds/profits and more clearly defining responsibilities of the ICM and the Host Association. However, as the cost of registration for participants and estimated costs of running the Congresses continued to rise, the ICM Council agreed that from 2020 forward, the ICM Board will select the Congress sites based on a detailed cost analysis, estimated attendance, and ease of international attendance (visas, etc.).[36] This decision was meant to move the ICM forward into the next decade, facilitated by global internet capabilities and other communication technologies not available in earlier years.

It was not until 2011 that an ICM Congress was held on the African continent (Durban, South Africa). Though overt discussion of racial discrimination evident in decisions on hosting Congresses, the conduct of Council meetings and the ongoing rich versus poor nations varying priorities within the ICM rarely occurred, there is evidence of such realities over the years.

The ICM Secretariat

The ICM Constitution defined the Secretariat as consisting of an Executive Secretary until 1990, with a name change to Secretary General (SG) until 2014, then Chief Executive (CE) appointed by the Board of Management/Board. From 1954, the Secretariat had an official 'office' in the London area until the end of 1999, then in The Hague, the Netherlands, beginning in January 2000 (See Annex H for location of ICM Headquarters).

Responsibilities of the Secretariat

At the direction of the ICM Council or Executive Committee/Board, the SG/CE managed the Confederation's day-to-day affairs.[37] In addition, the SG/CE was/is responsible for hiring and supervising staff needed to carry out the activities of the Secretariat in keeping with financial resources available for core activities in collaboration with the BoM. The Secretariat also prepared all papers for BoM, Executive and Council meetings. Throughout the 1990s and beyond, the three languages of the Confederation were supported by staff employed at headquarters with those language skills as well as the expanding language groups represented among Board members. Chapter 7 gives further details.

SUMMARY

What has remained consistent over the past 50 years is, 'The final authority for the policy and management of the affairs of the Confederation shall be the International Council …'[38]. That is, the top-level of decision authority remains in the hands of the Member Associations who make up the ICM Council. An overview of the aims/objects of the Confederation and a brief overview of by whom and how those aims and objects are carried out has been provided here. Additional chapters in this book provide evidence of the work of the ICM Council, the Board and the Secretariat to carry out its dual mandate of empowering women and empowering midwives

100 Years of the International Confederation of Midwives

1. The constitution of an organisation contains the fundamental principles which govern its operation. The byelaws establish the specific rules of guidance by which the group is to function. All but the most informal groups should have their basic structure and methods of operation in writing.
2. Refer to Chapter 3 for details on the beginning of the IMU.
3. News. *Nursing Notes*, 1922, p 127.
4. *Communications of the International Midwives' Union*, 1932.
5. *Communications of the International Midwives' Union*, 1932, p 1.
6. ICM. *The International Confederation of Midwives Constitution Agreed by Council on September 10th, 1954*. Regulations: Official Languages p 3. ICM (SA/ICM/R/4). Wellcome Collection. *Marjorie Bayes' Draft History of ICM, 1st 50 years*. ICM. *Constitution of the International Confederation of Midwives*. Chiswick, London: 1996, p 13 records amendments agreed during Council in 1987, 1990, 1993, 1996 following the major changes in 1981.
7. ICM. *The International Confederation of Midwives Constitution Agreed by Council on September 10th, 1954*. Personal papers of Helen Varney Burst sent to Joyce Thompson 4/2021 and will be sent to the Wellcome Library ICM archives. Article III referred to membership, Article IV ultimate decision authority of ICM Council that would meet triennially (p 2); Article V General Officers that included a President, Honorary President, two Vice-Presidents, three honorary recording secretaries and an honorary Treasurer (p 2). Article VI Executive Committee was elected by International Council to carry out directives between Council meetings (pp 2–3) and consisted of General Officers and 12 national representatives elected by Council who could then in secret ballot co-opt up to four additional members as vice-Presidents from any continent who did not have other members on the Executive Committee. Official languages of the Confederation shall be English, French and Spanish: #5. Under Regulations, p 3.
8. ICM. *The International Confederation of Midwives Constitution Agreed by Council on September 10th, 1954*. Article V: General Officers 1: p 2. 'These General Officers shall not consider themselves as representing their own country. Their duties are not national but international.'
9. ICM. *The Constitution of the International Confederation of Midwives, September 1982*. London: ICM, 1982. Note that the date on the Constitution was September 1982, though the decision was made by the ICM Council in 1981 to adopt the changes and there were no Council meetings in 1982. Most likely, it took some time for ICM Executive to finalise wording and the Secretariat to finish the council minutes and then type the new Constitution for Member Associations (email from Margaret Peters to JET, 16 May 2021). Miss Peters was at the 1981 meeting as Appointed President of the ICM in preparation for the 1984 Congress held in Sydney, Australia.
10. ICM. (SA/ICM/C/1/18/2). Wellcome Collection. *Executive Committee meeting minutes and paper 12–18 September 1981, Brighton 1 of 2*. Members were concerned with the new constitution including fears of losing Charitable status (worth £700–800 per year). Note: the ICM was not given official charitable status until 10 February 1983 as the first application sent in 1981 had been rejected.
11. ICM. (SA/ICM/H 7-10). Wellcome Collection. *Correspondence Margaret Peters Nov 1981–September 1988 (1 of 3) 25 March 1982*. ERROR – Mr Smith had used ICM cheque book to pay his own staff £7118.00), money retrieved with difficulty and cheque book returned to HQ and an unpleasant letter from Mr Smith, no apology.
12. Margaret Peters. *Written note to Joyce Thompson*, 4 April 2020.
13. Margaret Peters. *Written note to Joyce Thompson*, 4 April 2020. Charity status was obtained on 10 February 1983. Source: Charity Commissioners website downloaded 10 March 2021.
14. ICM. *ICM Minutes Council Meeting Manila, May 1999*. Agenda 99.19.7/8: Amendments to Constitution and Bye Laws, p 17.
15. ICM. *Letter to all Member Associations from Joyce Thompson, Director of the Board of Management*. November 1999, p 1. [Personal papers of Joyce Thompson].
16. Petra ten Hoope-Bender. *Email to Maria Spernbauer, Joyce Thompson and Judith Brown*. 23 November 1999. [Personal files of Joyce Thompson].
17. ICM. *ICM Council Meeting Minutes, Brisbane, Australia*, 18–21 July 2005. MIN. 05.23.1 Title: Authorisation of execution of deed of recording articles in the Netherlands, pp 20c21.
18. Margaret Peters' personal notes to Joyce Thompson. Margaret was present during the 1975, 1978, 1981 ICM Congresses and noted that the same people from Europe were ICM officers during those years. They appeared to be very friend-oriented rather than management oriented. They enjoyed social gatherings but did not appear interested in the mission, aim and objects of the Confederation. ICM also did not seem to mean a lot to many individual organisations at the time.
19. ICM. *ICM Council Meeting Minutes, Kobe, Japan, 1990*. Amendment to Bye-Laws 5ii, p 11, changed Western Pacific Region to Asia Pacific Region in 1990, and then in 2017 ICM Council split the Asia-Pacific into South-East Asia and Western Pacific regions. ICM. *Minutes of ICM Council Meeting, June 14, 2017, Toronto, Canada*. The Hague: ICM, Item 7.5 ICM Regions, pp 38 c40.
20. ICM. *Council Meeting Minutes, Brisbane, July 2005*. Proposal from European Region to realign five representatives to three: North, Central and southern Europe.

21 ICM. *ICM Council Meeting Minutes 27–30 May 2014 Prague, Czech Republic*. The Hague: ICM, 2014. Item 8.1., p 15, agreed third Asia-Pacific representative.
22 ICM. *Council Meeting Minutes, June 14, 2017, Toronto, Canada*. The Hague: ICM, Item 7.5 ICM Regions pp 38–40.
23 ICM. *ICM Council Meeting Minutes June 2020*. Agenda 4.2: Approval of change in regional board members from 10 to 6, p 4.
24 Franka Cadée, ICM President, noted that the ICM Board is discussing the official language(s) at the present time.
25 ICM. Refer to the ICM Constitutions and Byelaws, 1981, 1982, 1993, 1999, etc., Section of *Management of the Confederation*.
26 These two questions were addressed during the early years of the IMU as noted in Chapter 3. As of 2021, the ICM Constitution remains 'silent' on the number of Member Associations per country, in part, because member fees provide the core of ICM finances – more members equal more money.
27 ICM. *Constitution of the International Confederation of Midwives*, September 1982. Article 5, p 3.
28 ICM. *Constitution of the International Confederation of Midwives*, 1993. Article 5 (ii), p 2.
29 ICM. *ICM Council Meeting Minutes Kobe, Japan, October 9, 1990*. Minute 90/6.1, p 3. Also, 24 July 1990 letter from Marie Goubran. [Personal papers of Joyce Thompson]
30 ICM. *ICM Council Meeting Minutes, 2020*. Discussion item: Member Associations per Country, pp 30–31.
31 ICM. *ICM Constitution of the International Confederation of Midwives, 1996*. Para 5ii. ICM. *ICM Council Meeting Minutes Oslo, Norway, 1996*. Record 96.54, Agenda 44.3, p 22.
32 ICM. *ICM Council Meeting Minutes 27–30 May 2014 Prague, Czech Republic*. The Hague: ICM, 2014, pp 17–18, 19 for vote.
33 ICM. *Procedures for International Council Meeting*. Chiswick, London: ICM. 1995.
34 *Roberts Rules of Order* were based on UK Parliamentary law, and hence familiar to the founders of the ICM. In the Council Handbook they were called Rules of Order.
35 ICM. *Executive Committee Minutes*. 24 July 2005.
36 ICM. *ICM Council Meeting Minutes, June 2020*. Agenda 4: Changes for a more sustainable and equitable ICM, p 4.
37 ICM. *Constitution*. The Hague: ICM, 1999. This example was cited as it is the most recent Constitution under Dutch law.
38 ICM. 'Article 13'. *Constitution of the International Confederation of Midwives*, September 1982, p 5.

Chapter 6: *The Search for Financial Stability / Viability*

During a 1983 Executive Committee meeting in West Germany, ICM President Margaret Peters urged members to address financial issues facing the ICM 'coolly and logically to come to a considered solution to problems, and to consider the task ahead as a stage in ICM's maturity and to see the meeting as a coming of age leading to vigorous adulthood.'[1]

OVERVIEW

The ICM accomplishes most of its work through its Member Associations (MAs) and in close collaboration with global partner organisations, in keeping with ICM Council agreed policies.[2] ICM partners and donors are discussed throughout chapters that follow. The emphasis in this chapter is how the ICM's work has been affected by the ups and downs of income and expenditures and their relationship to international markets over the years. Financial viability and stability has been one of the greatest challenges for the ICM throughout its 100-year history.

Financial viability is a key aspect of organisational development and sustainability and, when joined with strategic planning and action, leads to a strong organisation with a future. The last 50 years of the ICM's development has been both strengthened and weakened due to its financial dependence on irregular income and generous donors/partners. The Royal College of Midwives (RCM) deserves a special note of thanks for its instrumental role in the revival of the ICM, supporting the early ICM Secretary Generals (Bayes, Hardy) and providing headquarters' space within the RCM for many years (1954–1972).

During times of positive reserves, the organisation planned for a bright though not always realistic future. Sometimes this meant that the addition of HQ staff or Board members' travel and ICM representation expenses exceeded income, resulting in use of reserve funds to keep the organisation afloat or the need for downsizing HQ staff[3] and limiting travel to meet available income. At other times, Congresses failed to meet expenses, such as in 1981 when the Host Association (RCM) had to dip into their own reserves to cover the shortfall.[4] Having more staff than the current funds allowed, required representation at global meetings that were not always sponsored by the outside organisation and global economic downturns were all challenges faced by the ICM Board members of the time, many of whom had little financial management experience and/or were not prepared to handle large budgets. Thus, several Boards beginning in the mid-1990s established Finance Advisory Committees[5]/Groups with financial experts who volunteered their services to the ICM over the years and helped in periods of financial recovery, as well as encouraging better planning for potential shortfalls or good management of funds during highly profitable years. The financial group became a standing committee in 2020.[6]

For many ICM leaders, the core business of the ICM focused on strengthening MAs so they could upgrade their midwifery workforce to provide quality care to improve the health of women and newborns and save lives! This focus on supporting members was very challenging as leaders sought innovative ways that were relevant to more than a single MA considering the great diversity of culture, languages and needs. At times desperate searches for external sources of income threatened to overshadow MAs' needs when project monies were sought that did not always support or strengthen the ICM's core business. These and other challenges to financial viability throughout the history of the Confederation to develop and maintain a strong international health professional association are highlighted in this chapter, beginning with sources of income and common expenditures.

SOURCES OF ICM INCOME
The ICM consists of national MAs and is dependent on membership fees, Congress income both from Registration fees and trade exhibitors, and fundraising undertaken by its Officers, Secretary General/Chief Executive and HQ staff. Income was augmented at various times by donations from individuals, midwives and selected MAs. Donors became an important contributor to ICM's income beginning in the 1970s and the number of donors expanded greatly in the last 20 years (See Annex D – Partners/Donors). During the 2017 ICM Council Meeting in Toronto, Canada, the ICM interim Treasurer, Ingela Wiklund, 'explained the importance of the stakeholders, donations and grants, which are essential to the future of the ICM because the membership fees only account for a small portion of the total income'[7]. She went on to note that a Stakeholder Engagement meeting in 2015 had attracted new funds and in-kind donations, and the ICM needed

to continue this approach so that it could be a flexible organisation matching activities to income at any given time.

Membership/Capitation Fees

The most stable source of unrestricted income for the Confederation since its beginning in 1922 through the present time has been the yearly Union Dues (IMU)[8] through the 1930s and Capitation Fees (ICM) since 1954 assessed on MAs.[9] For example, during the 1920s–1930s, the fee was a flat $5 per association with 200 members or less, and a modest increase of $1 for memberships over 500.[10] This concept of banding was continued in the ICM years with modest increases for every 200 members through 1993.[11] The pattern of assessing member fees based on the number of midwives in membership of the association that began in 1922 continued, though the formula became more complex once leaders realised that very large associations could/should pay higher fees than very small associations.[12] The idea of allowing only one national association per country was raised in 1995 with risks and benefits assessed by the Board of Management. It was defeated in Council primarily based on the ICM's goal to represent as many of the world's midwives as possible. A secondary fact was the greater financial value of adding more members from high resource countries (HRC) such as Japan, UK and the USA.[13]

Dependence on annual membership fees, even though less than half of an annual budget most of the time since the 1960s, was problematic throughout ICM's history. Many of the lesser developed members waited until the final year of each triennium to physically bring their outstanding fees (sometimes attempting to pay with beautiful cloths or nuts) so that they could attend the Congress or hoping only to pay that year's fees and fulfil the prerequisite for voting during the Council meeting.[14] In 1999, The Executive Committee agreed a membership fee category for 'least developed countries' (LDC) based on the poverty level of that country.[15]

This move allowed for the addition of many new ICM MAs from LDCs but did not necessarily add to the financial stability of the organisation due to the minimum amount paid by these LDC MAs. In addition, the requirement that fees be paid by the beginning of each year was not always met, so the ICM HQ and Board never knew exactly what capital they would have to work with from month to month.

Membership Trends Since 1954: Though MA Capitation Fees provided smaller and smaller percentages of the ICM budget over the last 50 years, it is important to understand the value of such membership to the organisation. Marjorie Bayes noted that despite the fact the ICM was making a name for itself during the 1970s with activities supported by FIGO, the WHO and USAID, its membership numbers hardly changed.[16] In fact, using the 1957 number of MAs (31)[17], there was very slow growth during the next 39 years to only 68 MAs in 1996[18] with a few modest increases in 1987 and 1993. In 1999 there were 80[19] ICM MAs, by 2008 the number of MAs reached 94[20], and in 2011 there were 109[21] ICM MAs with most of the increases from low resource countries (LRCs) in Africa and South-East Asia, who paid the least amount in member fees. The biggest jump in numbers was between 2014 (115)[22] and 2020 (143)[23], most likely due to increased electronic communication, an increased range of member services including access to global standards and competencies, and in-country projects highlighting the value of the ICM to its members.

Congress Fees and Sharing of Proceeds/Profits from ICM Activities

Another important source of ICM's income since the 1980s came in years when the triennial Congresses were well attended and resulted not only in a per-registrant Capitation fee paid to the ICM but also a sharing of proceeds with the ICM and the MA hosting the Congress once bills were paid. The ICM monies from these Congresses were to be spread equally during the next triennium, though not always recorded that way in the accounts, and used to fund core expenses unless otherwise designated. Several examples of profitable Congresses included the 1972 Congress in Washington DC ($70,000); the 1984 Congress in Australia (large donation beyond that agreed[24]); the 1987 Congress in The Hague (£18,121[25]); the 1990 Congress in Kobe ($150,000) and the 1993 Congress in Vancouver (£77,940[26]).

Following the success of the 1990 Kobe Congress, a generous donation of $24,000 from the Midwives Division of the Japanese Nursing Association went to the Midwives Association of British Columbia, Canada (MABC) for start-up costs (small loan as seed money) of the 23rd Congress, and MABC continued this spirit of generosity by sending $30,000 via the ICM Headquarters to the 24th Congress Organising Committee in Oslo, Norway.[27] The intent was that this small loan would be returned to the ICM at the end of each Congress separate from any registration fees or profits, and would continue as a start-up loan for future Congresses.

Core Funding

Core funding came from several external sources. The ICM attained charity status in the United Kingdom in 1983 which allowed for some support for activities of the office and meagre staff, though any activities had to fit the charitable category.[28] The move to the Netherlands at the end of December 1999 resulted in a small grant from the Village Council of The Hague for moving expenses, and significant core funding from the Dutch government from 2000 to 2007[29] for Secretariat activities in carrying out ICM Council mandates. A new wave of Core Funding came through the Swedish Government in 2010 with strict rules for use of the funds.[30] One question for the next approach to the ICM's core funding beyond 2022 is whether a virtual office might be a better choice. To a certain extent this has been experienced during 2020–2021 with the global COVID-19 pandemic.

Another source of core funding came from Germany's Federal Ministry for Economic Cooperation and Development (GIZ) with a grant to support the staff salary of one Technical Midwife Advisor during the 2014–2017 triennium.[31] This support enabled the ICM to provide technical assistance to Zimbabwe, Tanzania, Rwanda and Uganda in the form of competency-based education workshops. The GIZ grant also supported review of the ICM *Global Standards for Midwifery Education* and provided salary support for a resource mobilisation consultant to help the ICM review its fundraising activities.

Johnson and Johnson (J&J), a Premier Sponsor of ICM's Triennial Congresses since 1999, provided the ICM with an 18-month operational support grant in 2017. It was used to support ICM's communications activities during the 2017 ICM Triennial Congress in Toronto, Canada (daily newsletter, Wi-Fi capability, etc.); to develop a new website with advanced security features; and partially support a communications person at the ICM Headquarters. In addition, the grant provided partial salary support for a Midwife Advisor to the J&J/ICM Young Midwife Leaders Programme 2017–2018.[32]

In 2020 the Swedish International Development Agency (SIDA) provided €3,077,110 to the ICM, after several discussions with ICM leaders and the Secretariat about the capability of the ICM to carry out its core activities. This funding supported implementation of the 2021–2023 Triennial Strategy from August 2020 through to December 2023.[33] It also supported the ICM Secretariat and Board in focusing on building the ICM's capacity to build a strong infrastructure and become a more sustainable organisation.

Project Funding

Another important source of ICM income came in the form of grants and administrative overhead from specific projects, primarily at country levels. However, such funds could not be counted on each year. Grant writing required a lot of time and skills from Headquarters' staff and Board of Management members, but the benefits when grants were awarded contributed to ICM's financial solvency. (Refer to Chapter 10 and Annex D for list of partners and projects.) In addition, management and/or overhead costs were built into each grant proposal when allowed by the funder. However, when large grants ended, the activities of Confederation were severely curtailed, especially if not planned for in advance.[34]

Special Funds

A relatively small but important source of ICM income came in the form of donations for specific activities and awards. Individual donations across the years have been welcomed and allowed prosperous MAs to contribute to various ICM funds as described below. Individual midwife donations have been sporadic throughout the years, including Dorothea Lang's[35] generous donation of $38,000, some of which was used to gather the archival material for the ICM's Centennial celebration in 2022. All fundraising efforts required a lot of headquarters' time to solicit additional funds on a yearly basis.

A more recent effort to raise money for the ICM has been the inclusion of fund-raising as part of 5 May International Day of the Midwife (Chapter 10). These efforts by MAs have resulted in increased donations from HRC midwives to support LRC midwives to conferences, Council and workshops. When charity status was lost in 2000 with the move of the ICM's Headquarters to The Hague, the ICM needed to rely more heavily on grants to supplement Capitation Fees for selected LRC MAs and Congress registrations. In December 2019 the ICM Board approved the establishment of the WithWomen Charity that was formally launched at the 2021 Congress alongside the ICM Decade of the Midwife campaign.[36] The 2020 ICM Council approved this development for activities in keeping with the aims and objectives of the Confederation so that individuals and groups might once again donate to the ICM with tax relief in their own countries.

FINANCIAL SUPPORT FOR MEMBER ASSOCIATIONS AND MIDWIVES

In recognition of the highs and lows of finances at HQ over the years, as described briefly below, one way that the ICM and many of its wealthier MAs worked to meet the needs of sister MAs was to provide financial support in a variety of ways. A few examples of financial support discussed below reinforced ICM's long-held goal of representing and supporting all of the world's midwives.

Support for Council and Congress Participation

Capitation Assistance Fund: A special account was opened in 1989 at the request of the ICM Executive Committee to enable MAs to contribute to the payment of fees for other MAs unable to meet their fees. In addition, members with financial difficulties could apply directly for financial assistance by writing to the ICM Secretary General explaining their financial position as outlined in the ICM's Bye Law 32 and Bye Law 33 to have their Capitation Fee paid from this special account.[37] Payment of yearly capitation fees was a Constitutional requirement for maintaining membership in the ICM, including participating in ICM Council meetings.

Congress Interpretation Fund: The Congress Interpretation Fund was created in 1996 as one strategy to encourage participation of midwives from all over the world, knowing that the ICM was dedicated to offering educational sessions whenever possible in the three official languages of English, French and Spanish. The Terms of Reference (TORs) adopted in 1996 noted that the purpose was 'to subsidise the acquisition of additional translating/interpretation services for Congress plenary sessions in addition to those provided in English, French and Spanish.'[38] This Fund was used for countries like Japan with large contingencies of midwives attending the Congress needing translation (resulting in significant registration fees received).

Sponsor a Midwife Fund and Safe Motherhood Fund: The Sponsor a Midwife (SAM) Programme was initiated in 1990 by the Midwives Association of British Columbia, Canada (MABC) in preparation for the ICM Congress and pre-

Congress workshop in 1993. Carol Hird, incoming ICM Vice President (1987–1990), issued a call[39] to all the ICM MAs to raise funds for financial support of midwives from LRCs to enable their attendance at the 1993 Pre-Congress Workshop in Vancouver, British Columbia, that would focus on the quality of midwifery practice.[40] This call following the 1990 Congress asked members to donate to the Safe Motherhood Fund (SMF) through the Sponsor a Midwife (SAM) Programme. The result of that call was a total of $102,370 (Canadian) donated, with the majority raised from the ICM MAs. A total of 44 midwives were sponsored to attend the Pre-Congress Workshop and/or the ICM Council and Congress in 1993.[41]

The SAM programme's purpose 'was the support of individual midwives in resource poor countries where maternal mortality and morbidity rates are highest, by educating/upgrading of skills of midwives and/or their involvement in midwifery activities that promote Safe Motherhood.'[42] Midwives could be nominated by ICM MAs or by the ICM collaborative partners such as FIGO or the WHO. The midwife being sponsored had to meet certain criteria including having leadership potential, the ability to transform information into action, demonstrated commitment to the Aims of the Confederation, and, if sponsored to Congress, they had to present a paper. Though preference was given to midwives from LRC MAs, the individual did not have to be a member of an association in membership with the ICM. Sponsorship included travel, shared accommodation and daily meals plus other expenses including congress registration fees, visa or any inoculations required by the host country. The Secretary General kept a running list of sponsored midwives each triennium as the intent was, in principle, that an individual should not be sponsored to more than one consecutive ICM Congress or Workshop.

The ICM Safe Motherhood Fund (SMF) also had its roots during the 1993 ICM Congress in Vancouver, British Columbia. Dr Barbara Kwast issued an impassioned plea to midwives attending the 23rd Congress, and a total of £4,000 was collected.[43] In addition, ICM President Carol Hird at that time pushed to have a substantial portion of the profit from the ICM Congress transferred to ICM HQ, formally initiating the ICM Safe Motherhood Fund.[44] The general purpose of the ICM Safe Motherhood Fund in 1999 reflected the same purpose as the original TORs in 1996.[45] The fund-raising activity targeted mainly ICM's MAs, titled

'Sponsor a Midwife' or SAM programme, that was established in 1990 in addition to funds raised from the International Day of the Midwife (IDM) activities and collections taken at ICM workshops, conferences and congresses (See text box). In 1999, Council voted to integrate the Sponsor of Midwife programme into the Safe Motherhood Fund.[46]

> *Joan Walker relates one of her favourite memories as Secretary General that occurred during the 1993 ICM Vancouver Congress following the call for donations from the midwives present. She was handed the collected funds and quickly took them to her hotel room. The funds were then spread across her bed. Ruth Bennett, Sr Anne Thompson (Treasurer) and friend Pauline Phillips-Turner spent hours sorting into piles by each currency received; e.g. dollars, francs, krona, pounds sterling, yen and then converting the amounts to pounds sterling for a report to Congress. She then had to figure out how to transport them back to London and change every currency into pounds sterling for depositing in the ICM bank account!*

At subsequent Congresses, Dorothea Lang[47], a long-time ICM representative for the Americas from the USA and at the United Nations in New York City, issued the call for financial donations of at least 'one lunch' for the SMF during several ICM Triennial Congresses. With the help of Australian midwives and their red hats (Akubrras) held out for donations, many dollars continued to be raised for this important cause.[48] Refer to Chapter 7 detailing awards which were also a means of financially supporting midwives whilst recognising their successes and abilities in country.

RECURRING EXPENDITURES

Throughout its history, the ICM's recurring expenditures were related to maintenance of an ICM Headquarters, including space/rent/insurance; office supplies and equipment including postage, telephone and newsletter; audit and accountancy fees and the costs of staffing the Secretariat (refer to Chapter 3 for details for IMU). Other recurring costs included travel, lodging and food for Board in-person meetings, representation travel if not reimbursed by requesting agency and agreed project activities that involved staff, workshops and reports.

Though fund-raising efforts often resulted in additional income, the Board had to learn to wait until project monies arrived before spending them and/or beginning projects. In addition, once the ICM Secretariat moved to the Netherlands in 2000, the Board learned that project personnel needed to be placed on short-term contracts and not on full-time staff that were difficult to make redundant under Dutch NGO law if the person did not work out or funds were no longer available for that staff position.

FINANCIAL UPS AND DOWNS

The ICM's struggle for financial stability was similar to riding a roller coaster in some decades. A few examples of the ups and downs follow, though some of their impact was discussed earlier related to the Constitutional changes.

1970s: With the record stating that the ICM finances were very weak in the mid-1950s, in 1958 the ICM General Officers made a decision to focus on looking ahead to international collaboration as they included a positive decision to work with the International Federation of Gynecology and Obstetrics (FIGO). At the same time, the WHO had requested ICM's assistance in a worldwide collection of data on midwifery training and practice, and in 1960 ICM agreed to being a part of the ICM/FIGO joint study group (Chapter 16). The relationship with FIGO and the WHO led to support of joint ICM activities with those agencies, with some funding coming from each of those partners until a large grant from USAID was received in the early 1970s.

1980s: The ICM Executive Committee met in Paris in 1980[49] under a shadow of financial losses as there was a deficit of £931 for 1979 in spite of the USAID project monies covering 90 per cent of the cost of the Secretariat, including the Victoria Street office in London. This meant that the ICM needed its own premises and minimal staff. Outstanding rent to end the lease was £8,000 to the end of 1982, therefore the ICM had to find an alternate location by 1981 – which was an attic on Lower Belgrave Street, London (See Annex H Location of ICM HQs).

The ICM did recover slowly with the encouragement, leadership and management skills of Margaret Peters who, during a 1983 Executive Committee meeting in West Germany,[50] urged members to address issues facing the ICM 'coolly and logically to come to a considered solution to problems, and to consider the task ahead as a stage in ICM's maturity and to see the meeting as a coming of age leading to vigorous adulthood.'[51] A Board of Management resolution put to members of the Executive and adopted unanimously acknowledged that:

> 'The ICM is a valuable organisation with important aims to which we should all subscribe … This objective can be achieved, but only with the willing, professional commitment and strong financial support by all members of the Confederation.'[52]

Careful monitoring of income and expenses over several years was rewarded. The Treasurer's Report for 1987–1990 stated, 'Council will be pleased to note the continuing improved financial position of the Confederation allowing more work to be done to fulfil the object of advancing education in midwifery and spreading the knowledge of the art and science of midwifery.'[53]

1990s: With finances showing an improvement, the Board of Management and Secretariat did not rest on their laurels but continued to be financially astute, using newer technology in communications, using basic accommodation when attending meetings, being selective in representation and personally contributing in various ways, such as use of air miles. The result was to build up finances to benefit the ICM, which was quite successful.

2000s: The end of year statement of finances in February 2001 noted a number of items showing excess costs over budget. The SG (ten Hoope-Bender) noted that some of the apparent overspend, such as BoM expenses, were historically due to problems of being able to accurately detail actuals vs budgets in the past that were based on Board members' use of airline miles and volunteer work to keep down expenses. Other sources of overspend were costs of flights spent on representation that needed to be curtailed unless funded by the agency who invited the ICM.[54] Despite the 2002 Treasurer's report highlighting the financial stability of the ICM during the past three years and the Boards' efforts to control expenditures during 2002–2003[55], the ICM closed its books for the year 2003 with a deficit exceeding €100,000. This was due to unexpected costs associated primarily with legal review and drafting of the ICM Constitution to comply with Dutch law, recruitment of a new Secretary General and unrealised project income.[56] Other unanticipated costs included higher than expected costs for the Vienna Congress, the Council-directed unplanned Executive Committee meeting in 2003 (for constitution review) and a membership fee that did not correspond to the inflation rate. This situation caused the auditors to note that the ICM's continued existence was dependent upon its ability to increase structural income (member fees as well as other sources of temporary income from sponsors and donors) while reducing fixed expenditures (staff, travel, in-person meetings, etc.).

The Mid-Triennium Executive Meeting and Symposium in Trinidad resulted in a major loss of €32,000. The Recovery Budget of 2004 had projected a loss of €40,000. The actual deficit of €10,000 was covered with unexpected income of €22,400 arriving at ICM's HQs from Jhpiego's Maternal Newborn Health project in 2004. However, it became apparent that there were too many full-time staff at HQ at a time when income was falling. A financial recovery plan was implemented by the SG Kathy Herschderfer and the BoM in 2004. This followed multiple withdrawals from the organisation's Reserves fund to meet financial obligations of the ICM and its activities during the prior couple of years. The major goal of this plan was to restore the General Reserves deficiency over the next two years and gradually build up reserves to a stable minimum level by 2008 which would cover any unexpected events or financial problems.[57] This plan included short-term actions including an intense review of key staff needed to run the organisation; reducing representation costs; limiting in-person BoM meetings with the use of teleconferences and informing members of the need for an increase in membership fees.[58] Two staff positions (librarian and business manager) were removed and the Secretary General, the Communications Officer and the Programme Manager were agreed as essential full-time HQ staff.[59] The BoM donated about a quarter of their travel expenses, representation was reduced to priority partners only, and Thematic funding from the Dutch government was increased.[60] After much debate and discussion, the 2005 Council delegates agreed to a membership fee increase of 15 per cent for 2006.[61]

The financial recovery budget that started in 2004 demonstrated improvement through 2008, though 2007 was problematic as the Dutch government Thematic fund had ceased. Nearly every MA paid their yearly fees and even though there was an expected overspend, fewer projects than expected and very little project income, the General reserves were building. Financial advisors suggested an amount of €100,000 in General Reserves as this amount would keep the core business of the ICM going for 5–6 months without any additional funding. The Treasurer, Franka

Cadée, recommended this amount for 2009 that was agreed. It was also noted that 2008–2011 would depend on Congress income of €200,000 per year.[62]

2010: The recommended 30 per cent of budget for robust solvency in 2010 would have meant €600,000. There was only €393,859 in the account in 2010, though a healthy increase from €71,294 in 2007. The balance of funds/Reserves as of 31 December 2010 was €722,338 of which €11,466 were restricted.[63] However, there was a loss of 12 per cent or €72,397 in unpaid membership fees over the triennium, including 29/109 (3 per cent) MAs in 2010.[64]

The 2011–2014 triennium saw a different financial picture to that of the last one as the ICM remained focused on the recovery plan launched in Brisbane (2005) and continued in Glasgow (2008). The Treasurer, Marian van Huis, reported that the ICM was financially stable and more donors were contributing to its activities.[65] The General Reserves policy to maintain at least 30 per cent in that account to ensure solvency was exceeded in 2013 when the fund held 33.5 per cent of ICM's funds.[66] The loss of unpaid MAs' Capitation fees continued and instability of ICM's Headquarters' staffing were highlighted with the reassurance that the ICM finances were still sound.[67] Discussion during the 2011 Council included suggestions for helping those MAs unable to pay member fees through 'twinning' and introducing the idea that MAs look to donors in their own regions for such assistance. The ICM leadership reinforced the potential pitfalls of depending on donor income, though the Board had received unrestricted funds from the Swedish and Dutch governments and were in negotiations with the German government at the time.[68]

As noted in the 2014–2017 Triennial Report, ICM's General reserves had remained stable. However, it was also noted that the ICM was not in a position to invest in its own infrastructure or operations and remained dependent on donor organisations and Triennial Congresses. The number of donors increased from seven at the beginning of 2014 to ten in 2016, with an increase in donor funding from €1.3 million to €2.1 million by end of 2016. General reserve funds in 2016 dropped to 22.1 per cent due to an increase in project-related costs. The ICM Board developed a resource mobilisation strategy 2015–2017, addressed barriers and developed a new strategy to achieve ICM's strategic goals.[69]

The ICM's General Reserves took a nosedive during the 2017–2020 Triennium with a downturn from €455,069 in 2017 to €99,860 at the end of

2019.[70] This overspend was related to late approval and late receipt of funds for some grants while activities continued; delays in execution of some projects meaning delay in funds received; a projected income of €1 million more than the amount received; the ICM's decision to run Regional Conferences from HQ with two of the three at a loss; less than expected Congress funds from Toronto (€47,228 total compared to €204,442 from Prague, Czech Republic, Congress) and a global pandemic that forced the ICM to delay its 2020 Congress in Bali while several costs still had to be covered in anticipation of the Congress. Once again, the ICM was in the position of using General Reserves to cover core costs, a situation that leaders and MAs understood could not continue.

2020: The ICM entered the last two years of its first 100 years with the need to cut core costs, raise more funds from external donors and begin another financial recovery plan. Many partners are supporting the ICM and the leadership is seeking new ways to keep the ICM financially viable. It is hoped that the 2019 development of the ICM WithWoman Charity that was launched during the 2021 Congress will encourage individual midwives and other stakeholders to continue to invest in midwives for healthy women, newborns and families.

SUMMARY

The history of the ICM has been and continues to be affected by concerns for the financial viability of the organisation (Chapter 18). A brief overview of these concerns along with the generosity of individual midwives, Member Associations and partner organisations were discussed in this chapter. The fact that the ICM has survived, strengthened and been successful in supporting its members and midwives to provide quality care for women and childbearing families during the past 100 years is a testament, in part, to its devoted leaders, Secretariat and wise financial advisors.

100 Years of the International Confederation of Midwives

1 ICM. (SA/ICM/H/&/10). Wellcome Collection. *Correspondence Margaret Peters November 1981–September 1988.*
2 ICM. *Interorganizational Relationships: Guidelines.* Chiswick, London: ICM, 1996. ICM Position Statement. *Collaboration and Partnerships for Healthy Women and Infants.* The Hague: ICM, 2008.
3 HQ staff were only ICM individuals paid for their service. All elected Board members and ICM nominated midwives for representation volunteered their time and efforts. When travel and lodging was required of Board members, these costs were covered.
4 ICM. 'Membership of ICM.' *Board of Management Agenda Item 20* (October 1995), p 1. This agenda item referred to the financial crisis in 1981 that led to a 1982 constitutional change to ensure the Confederation met the requirements of the Charity Commissioners and to gain all the taxation benefits which would assist in the survival of the Confederation. This was in anticipation of applying for Registered Charity Status in the UK that was awarded in 1983 (Registered Charity No. 326297).
5 ICM. *Meeting of Foundation for the Support and Management of the ICM, October 2001, The Hague.* The Hague: ICM, F-Min 10/01.11: Finance 11.6 The initiation of a Finance Advisory committee (FAC), p 24.
6 ICM. *ICM Triennial Report 2017–2020.* www.internationalmidwives.org.
7 ICM. *ICM Council Meeting Minutes, Toronto, Canada, June 13, 2017.* The Hague: ICM, 2017, p 8.
8 *Communications* 6, 1932, p 17. The 1925 and 1928 Regulations of the IMU stated, 'Each affiliated union is obliged to pay yearly at last 5 dollars as a contribution to the international union if it has at most 200 members, and one dollar more for each five hundred members more.'
9 ICM. *Triennial Report 2008–2011.* The Hague: ICM, Financial Summary 2008–2011, p 24.
10 *Communications* 6, 1932, p 17.
11 ICM. *ICM Council Meeting Minutes, Kobe, October 1990.* Capitation Fees 1991–1993.
12 ICM. *ICM Council Meeting Minutes Manila, Philippines, 1999*, p 19. ICM Treasurer proposed using the UN Index of Human Development for determining LDC category for capitation fees and it was agreed. This proposal was first adopted by the ICM Board of Management during their meeting November 1998 in London (Agenda Item 12.3, p 8).
13 ICM. *Board of Management Agenda Item 20* (October 1995). 'Membership of ICM', pp 2–3.
14 ICM. *International Confederation of Midwives Constitution* 1999, Article 9: Suspension of Rights, p 3.
15 ICM. *Annual Report 1999 and 2000*, p 3. 'Among the many decisions taken by Council were also: adoption of a membership fee category for "least developed countries"'.
16 ICM. (SA/ICM/R/4). Wellcome Collection. *Marjorie Bayes' Draft History of ICM, 1st 50 years.*
17 ICM. (SA/ICM/R/4). Wellcome Collection. *Marjorie Bayes' Draft History of ICM, 1st 50 years.* Miss Bayes noted that membership had almost doubled since 1954, and Brazil, Greece, Iceland and Turkey were accepted into membership making 31 national associations from 27 countries.
18 ICM. *Triennial Report 1993–1996.* Chiswick, London: ICM, p 2 lists Member Associations by Region. ICM. *ICM Council Meeting Minutes, Oslo, Norway, 21–23 May 1996.* Agenda Item 44.2, May 1996, pp 1–4. These numbers were lower than the Triennial Report list most likely as those MAs who had not paid dues were not listed.
19 ICM. *Annual Report 1999.* Chiswick, London: ICM, p 1.
20 ICM. *Annual Report 2008.* The Hague: ICM.
21 ICM. *President's Report, Press Release.* 2011. Numbers prepared by ICM HQ staff.
22 ICM. *ICM Triennial Report 2014–2017.* The Hague: ICM, 2014. Triennial Financial Report 2014–2016, p 60.
23 ICM. *ICM Triennial Report 2017–2020.* Electronic copy on: www.internationalmidwives.org.
24 ICM. *ICM Council Meeting Minutes August 1987, The Hague.* London: ICM, 1987. Minute 87/14 'A substantial donation over the agreed amount was given to ICM by the congress organizers.' p 4.
25 ICM. ICM Council Meeting Minutes, Kobe, Japan, 2–4 October 1990. Agenda Item 11: Margaret Brain's Report of the Treasurer and Receipt of Audited Accounts 1987–1990, p 3 item 2.1 noted that in addition to the agreed Congress Capitation fee of £24,996 the donated from profits £16,145 to the ICM.
26 ICM. *Minutes of the ICM Executive Committee, 11 January 1995, Entebbe, Uganda.* MIN.95/13/1: 23rd Vancouver Congress, May 1993. Noted that very large profit split 50/50 between ICM and MABC. The Treasurer's Report covering May 1993–December 1994 reported £77,940 as ICM's share of Congress surplus. In addition, it reported £15,000 was transferred to seed the Oslo Congress as was done with the Vancouver Congress.
27 ICM. *ICM Triennial Report 1993–1996.* Chiswick, London: ICM, p 6.
28 Though many MAs viewed UK charity status as positive, the fact was that ICM had few activities that would eliminate the VAT and result in a refund to the ICM. Personal note from J Walker, former Secretary General.
29 One of the strong reasons for moving the ICM HQ from London to The Hague was the promise of core funding that began in 2000. In 2005 and 2006, for example, ICM received 160,000 Euros per year, of which 35,000 euros in 2006 were held over to 2007 budget. ICM. *Triennial Council Meeting Minutes 28–31 May 2008.* 'Agenda item 4: Finance, Treasurer's Report' 4.1.
30 The SIDA project began 1 June 2010. In 2013, the Swedish International Development Cooperation Agency (SIDA) continued to support the global work of ICM to achieve its strategic objectives and to strengthen midwifery through regional development. This included supporting headquarters operations. [Frances Day-Stirk personal papers]
31 ICM. *ICM Triennial Report 2014–2017.* The Hague: ICM, p 33.

32 ICM. *ICM Triennial Report 2017–2020*. The Hague: ICM, p 22.
33 Email from ICM Chief Executive Sally Pairman to Joyce Thompson, 19 April 2021.
34 ICM. Pamphlet: *International Confederation of Midwives*. London: ICM secretariat, 1981, p 11.
35 Dorothea Lang was an ardent supporter of many ICM activities, including serving years as one of the Americas' Regional Representatives and appointed ICM representative to the United Nations in New York City.
36 ICM. Board Minutes 2019. Email from Chief Executive Sally Pairman to Joyce Thompson, 19 April 2021.
37 MA Brain. *Report of the Treasurer and Receipt of Audited Accounts 1987–1990*, #1.2, p. 2, 7 July 1990. ICM Council Meeting 1990, Agenda Item 11.
38 ICM. *Draft Record of the International Confederation of Midwives Council Meeting Oslo, Norway, 21–23 May 1996*. London: ICM, 1996. Agenda 96.18, p 11. Congress Interpretation Fund: Terms of Reference.
39 Telephone call with Petra ten Hoope-Bender, 12-10-2019.
40 WHO. *Midwifery Practice: Measuring, Developing and Mobilizing Quality Care*. Geneva: WHO Division of Family Health, Pub. #WHO/FHE/MSM/94.12, 1994.
41 ICM. *Triennial Report 1993–1996*. Chiswick, London: ICM, 1996, p 5.
42 Pamphlet announcing, 'Sponsor a Midwife to the 27th Triennial Congress in Vienna, April 2002!' describes the history of the SAM programme. [Personal papers of Joyce Thompson]
43 ICM. *Triennial Report 1993–1996*. Chiswick, London: ICM, 1996, p 5.
44 ICM. *Draft Record of the International Confederation of Midwives Council Meeting Oslo, Norway, 21–23 May 1996*. Chiswick, London: ICM; Agenda 96.19, p 12. Safe Motherhood Fund Terms of Reference. 'After the Immediate Past President, Carol Hird, had presented the final report of the Vancouver Sponsor a Midwife Programme, a resolution that the funds remaining from this Programme be used for future Sponsor a Midwife projects was carried unanimously.' Terms of Reference carried unanimously.
45 ICM. *Safe Motherhood Fund of the International Confederation of Midwives: Terms of Reference*. London: ICM, 1999.
46 ICM. *ICM Council Meeting Minutes Manila, Philippines, 1999*, p 23.
47 Dorothea Lang, a US midwife, knew first-hand the struggle of many country midwives' work, based on her background of being born to missionary parents in Japan, and fighting the political battles needed with the US government that resulted in the Maternal-Infant Care (MIC) projects in New York City that provided needed midwifery care for low income women and families.
48 Personal experiences of authors contributing money to the 'red hat' activities in Congresses 1990–2000.
49 ICM. (SA/ICM/C/1/18). Wellcome Collection. *1975–1989 Executive Committee*.
50 ICM. (SA/ICM/C/1/18). Wellcome Collection. *1975–1989 Executive Committee*.
51 ICM. (SA/ICM/H/&/10). Wellcome Collection. *Correspondence Margaret Peters November 1981–September 1988*.
52 ICM. (SA/ICM/C/1/18). Wellcome Collection. *1975–1989 Executive Committee*.
53 ICM. *ICM Council Meeting Minutes, Kobe, Japan, October 2–4, 1990*. Agenda Item 11: Report of the Treasurer and Receipt of Audited Accounts 1987–1990 p 1.
54 ICM. *Meeting of the Board of Management [Foundation for the Support and Management of the ICM], The Hague 4th February 2001*. The Hague: ICM, F-Min. 02.01/5: Finance, p 7.
55 ICM. *ICM Council Meeting Minutes, Vienna, April 2002*. Agenda 02.20.2; Treasurer's Report, p 9.
56 Franka Cadée, ICM Treasurer. *Letter to all Member Associations, 25 August 2004*, describing financial difficulties from 2003, p 2. ICM. *ICM Council Meeting Minutes, Brisbane, Australia, 18–21 July 2005*. Agenda 05.20.1 Treasurer's report 2002–2005, pp 8–10.
57 Kathy Herschderfer letter to Joyce Thompson and Franka Cadée, 8 June 2004, *ICM Financial Recovery Plan (draft)*, April 2004, p 1.
58 Franka Cadée, ICM Treasurer. *Letter to all Member Associations, 25 August 2004*, describing financial difficulties from 2003 and need for an inflation correction to member dues in 2005.
59 Franka Cadée, ICM Treasurer. *Letter to all Member Associations, 25 August 2004*, describing financial difficulties from 2003 and need for an inflation correction to member dues in 2005.
60 *ICM Council Meeting Minutes, Brisbane, Australia, 18–21 July 2005*. Agenda 05.20.1 Treasurer's report 2002–2005, p 9.
61 *ICM Council Meeting Minutes, Brisbane, Australia, 18–21 July 2005*. Agenda 05.20.3 Fee Structure 2006–2008, p 13.
62 ICM. *ICM Council Meeting Minutes, Glasgow, Scotland, 28–31 May 2008*. Agenda 4: Finance, pp 5–7.
63 ICM. *ICM Council Meeting Minutes, Durban, South Africa, June 2011*. Agenda 7 Finance p 15.
64 ICM. *ICM Council Meeting Minutes, Durban, South Africa, December 2011*. The Hague: ICM, p.15.
65 ICM. *Triennial Report 2011–2014*. The Hague: ICM, Financial Summary, p 25.
66 ICM. *ICM Financial Report 2013*, p 8.
67 ICM. *ICM Council Meeting Minutes, Prague, 2014*. The Hague: ICM, p 13.
68 ICM. *ICM Council Meeting Minutes, Prague, 2014*. The Hague: ICM, p 14.
69 ICM. *Triennial Report 2014–2017*. The Hague: ICM, 2016. Triennial Financial Report 2014–2016, p 60.
70 ICM. *Triennial Report 2017–2020*. The Hague: ICM, 2020, p 36.

Chapter 7: *Support of ICM Business by the Secretariat*

Joan Walker recalls when she was asked in the summer of 1990 to help in the office for two days each week. The pressure of work in preparing for the Congress in Japan was at a time when Secretary General Marie Goubran was finding it far from easy healthwise to keep abreast of all that was required to be fulfilled. Joan was able to increase her time to either three or four days as required to achieve the work under Marie's guidance. Marie devoted herself to ICM working from home with Joan visiting her most days to report on the work and to be advised on the next day's work. Only six weeks before the Congress did Marie's Consultants stipulate that she was not to travel to Japan. Joan was asked to attend in order to ensure that all the documentation needed for the Executive and Council meetings would be on-site with Margaret Brain, the Treasurer, stepping in to undertake some of Marie's duties for these meetings.

INTRODUCTION

With the global remit and lofty aims of the ICM agreed by Member Associations (MAs), a well-supported headquarters (HQ) and staff would be expected to assist the activities needed to carry out the aims. This was not the case through most of the past 100 years, beginning in 1922 as Sr Anne Thompson, former ICM Treasurer, summarised.

> 'The administrative complexities caused by the constantly changing presidency
> and the lack of a fixed secretariat were an ongoing problem for the organisation,
> only partly solved by the constant presence of Professor Daels.'[1]

The increasing demands from an increasing number of MAs beginning in the 1980s and the increased visibility of the ICM globally requiring representation and collaborative efforts with UN agencies and other health partners continued to tax the limited staff of the ICM Secretariat.

Some of the Secretariat's challenges in carrying out activities mandated by the ICM Council during times with a positive financial environment (member dues, positive Congress income and donor funds) and during times of near bankruptcy are included. A focus on the communication strategies is included as these were/are essential to the work of the Confederation. The constants in the ICM's story since 1954 have been a 'static/permanent' location of headquarters and the employment of incredible staff led by wise and trusted Secretary Generals/Executive Officers.

ICM SECRETARIAT (HEADQUARTERS/HEAD OFFICE)
Geographical Locations

The re-establishment of the ICM in 1954 was accompanied by a dedicated office space with a part-time Secretary for the first time (Chapter 4). It also established the vital and long-time link between the ICM and the Royal College of Midwives (RCM) in the UK. Not only did the RCM provide physical space for ICM Headquarters' business, but it loaned one of its staff, Miss Marjorie Bayes, to take on the part-time position as ICM Secretary (then Secretary General), a tour of duty that lasted for the next 20 years.

The decision that the ICM needed an 'official' space to store its records and carry out its business was made during the 1954 ICM Council meeting in London.[2] The initial importance of siting the ICM Headquarters in the UK was reinforced when the Charity Commissioners accepted the application of the ICM for charity status in 1983.[3] This had important tax implications as the organisation was recognised as a non-profit one and did not have to pay certain taxes.[4]

The ICM Headquarters (HQ) space over time ran the gamut from a desk in the basement of a MA office (RCM), to an old, converted warehouse with flexible office spaces (Barley Mow, London, UK), to several hundred square feet with several enclosed offices for staff in modern high-rise buildings (The Hague, the Netherlands). The various locations of the ICM HQ are listed in Annex H. Initially the need for more space, especially with the advent of technology, computers, fax machines and photocopiers all requiring room to be housed. In addition, each move beyond the RCM contributed to the ICM's need for a clear identity as a global organisation. Financial restraints were also of primary concern in later years resulted in the move from a London suburb to the Netherlands with guaranteed Dutch government core funding. The discussion of a possible move of the office to Geneva to be closer to the WHO and UN agencies was again considered by the ICM Board during the 2017–2019 Triennium, with no final decision made at that time due to the high costs of Geneva real estate.[5]

Leadership of the Secretariat

The assigned work and activities of the ICM Secretariat was the responsibility of the contracted Secretary General/Chief Executive. Each was hired and evaluated annually by the ICM Board of Management/Board. The SG/CE had the responsibility to hire and supervise staff needed to assist in carrying out the work of the Confederation as directed by the ICM Council and in support of the work of the ICM Board. Table 7.1 below lists the names of the ICM Secretary Generals/Executive Officers and their years of service.

Table 7.1
ICM Secretary Generals & Chief Executive Officers 1922[6]–2022

Name	Country	Title	Years
Professor Frans Daels (OB/GYN)	Belgium	Executive Secretary[7]	1922–1939
Mme Mossé	France	President IMU 1939 and Congress/Secretariat	1939–1949[8]
Marjorie Bayes	UK	Secretary Executive Secretary[9] Volunteer – Part-time	1954–1975[10]
F Margaret Hardy	UK	Executive Secretary (PT)	1975–2/1980[11]
Elizabeth Leedham	UK	Executive Secretary (PT)	6/1980–1981[12]
Frances Cowper-Smith	UK (Canada)	Executive Secretary (PT)[13]	1981–1986[14]
Marie Goubran	UK	Executive Secretary (PT)[15]	1987–1990[16]
Joan Walker	UK	Secretary General[17] (PT-FT)[18]	1990[19]–1998[20]
Petra ten-Hoope Bender	Netherlands	Secretary General	1998–2003[21]
Della Sherratt (interim 3 months)	UK	Secretary General	2001[22]
Kathy Herschderfer	Netherlands	Secretary General	12/2003[23]–03/2008
Agneta Bridges	UK	Secretary General	03/2008–10/2008[24] (interim) 10/2008–02/2013

100 Years of the International Confederation of Midwives

Judith Brown (interim)	Australia	Chief Executive (interim)	03/2013–07/2013[25]
Frances Ganges	USA	Chief Executive	03/2013–02/2017
Sally Pairman	New Zealand	Chief Executive	01/2017[26]–

The Work of the Secretariat

'I was the Secretary General and carried expense money to Uganda for the ICM meeting. I was taken to the bank with escorts who were on the lookout for any attempt of a hold up. The bank manager hid us away from prying eyes whilst currency exchange was made over a considerable amount of time.'

Joan Walker, ICM SG, 1990s

The essential work of the ICM HQ staff early on revolved around organising and supporting Triennial Congresses along with Council, Board and other meetings; collecting member dues and managing finances; arranging for study visits of which there were many in the 1950s–1970s; responding to member queries and putting together a newsletter.[27]

The work of the Secretariat increased dramatically when, in 1969, the ICM became partners with the WHO and FIGO[28] that resulted in publication of the second Maternity Care in the World in 1976 (Chapter 12). As a result of these partnerships, the name of the Confederation became known in many countries of the world. Many associations and governments were involved in the WHO's request for ICM to gather midwifery information and in the ICM/FIGO project on training of midwives in family planning in low resource countries.[29]

The work of the SG/CE was often not commensurate with the time spent or remuneration as illustrated when in December 1982 Frances Cowper-Smith, then Secretary General, informed the Director of the Board of Management that she had too much work but could not do longer hours as there was no money to pay her.[30] Shortly before she left her post as Secretary General, Frances Cowper-Smith sent a letter to the Board of Management in July 1986 saying, 'too much work at Headquarters for 1 part-time person. I honestly cannot see anyone being willing to work full-time here, in complete isolation from the rest of the living world; it'd be a fairly rapid route to insanity, I imagine.'[31] However, the SG position was successfully filled in a part-time capacity by Marie Goubran in 1987–1990, with many other willing SG/CEs to follow. At the beginning of 1991, the ICM Board and Council agreed that the Secretary General post needed to be full-time. Joan Walker[32] became the first full-time Secretary General, and all successive leaders of the Secretariat have been full-time employees of the ICM. In 1991, whether it was the fact that the Confederation had a full-time Secretary General together with part-time secretaries who were fluent in French and Spanish or more members, the work appeared to increase exponentially as illustrated below.

A Day in the Life of the SG in the 1990s: Joan Walker
'Initially the staffing was me and a part-time secretary. The work in the office could never be described as isolated or on a route to insanity. Yes, with only screens dividing the various companies at Barley Mow (Chiswick, London, UK), there was a level of noise, but everyone respected each other's space to keep this to a minimum. No two days were the same. The work focused on several priorities simultaneously: working with and caring for the Member Associations; minutes, emails and phone calls with the Board of Management, the Executive Committee and Council; preparing for Congresses each Triennium; collecting material and writing the ICM newsletter before an editor was appointed to take over this role, and writing the international section for Midwifery; arranging for Regional Representatives or representatives to the United Nations' Offices to attend meetings on behalf of the Confederation and following up to secure a report after the meetings.'[33]

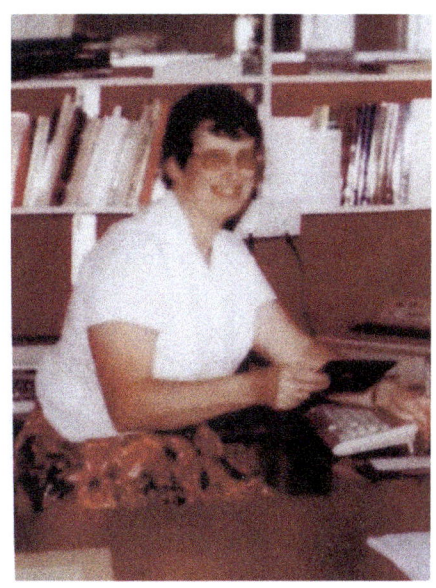

Secretary General Joan Walker in office in Chiswick (1990s) – ICM Archives at Wellcome Collection

The Secretary General would also attend meetings on behalf of the Confederation, some of which were UK based and others worldwide, and give lectures on International Midwifery at a local school. In addition, the SG was expected to keep files of all meetings and reports. Before a bookkeeper was employed by the ICM, the Secretary General undertook all financial duties from the paying of rent for the accommodation, payroll for employed staff, fees from members and the subsequent queries from the associations about these when differences crept in.

To add variety to the day it was not unusual to have midwives appearing at the office door with or without prior notice, possibly a midwife from a member association visiting the UK who would drop in for a social visit, or a midwife from the UK seeking to work in the library as part of a research project being undertaken. Some midwives undertaking projects seemed to have the impression that by contacting the Confederation with details of their project this would be miraculously done for them. They were sadly disappointed.

During 1990–1999, the staffing increased to two part-time secretaries, and part-time Librarian, newsletter editor, project worker and bookkeeper. The work of the Secretariat was facilitated in the 21st century with the introduction of new methods of communication and internet services.

Ongoing Work

As membership continued to increase over the years, the Secretariat staff increased slightly with more funded projects added into the mix of responsibilities. In addition, there were many volunteers over the years who contributed significantly to the daily work. This level of activity at the Secretariat continued in the 21st century. As noted by Frances Ganges (Chief Executive, 2013–2017): 'Regularly midwives reach out to the ICM Headquarters for support: an educator with a struggling pre-service programme; a researcher implementing a survey; a campaigner working to raise the profile of midwifery; an association engaging in the development of midwifery regulation; and numerous others preparing for the 30th Triennial Congress.'[34] She went on to add that each day the Secretariat team responded to countless emails, phone calls and requests from individuals and organisations around the world.

The organisation of activities within the Secretariat was reviewed and changed over the years, beginning with Petra ten Hoope-Bender and the move to the Netherlands. She revised staff policies and position descriptions and developed a Governance review document to track Board and staff activities each triennium. The more recent effort to streamline the activities occurred during the 2017–2020 triennium when the ICM President, Franka Cadée, wrote: 'We have started to redress the balance of our core work, which is to support the growth of our Midwives Associations, with our development work through the engagement of our partners.'[35] The current CE, Sally Pairman, provides a snapshot of her day in 2021.

100 Years of the International Confederation of Midwives

A Day in the Life of the CE in 2021: Sally Pairman

'As ICM's Chief Executive in 2021 my working life is significantly impacted by the COVID-19 pandemic. Instead of working side by side with Head Office Team Members in our open plan office in the centre of The Hague, we have all have spent the last 18 months working from home. What for me used to be a life of constant travel and face-to-face meetings is now a life of Zoom meetings, webinars and two-dimensional interactions. It really is life in front of a screen, and at all hours of the day and night to connect in many time zones. Technology has brought increased opportunities for collaboration but also increased expectations of constant availability and immediate response times. But despite this, I and the ICM staff found new ways to strengthen connections with our members, our partners and each other. Even though President, Franka Cadée, is based in the Netherlands, we have not been able to meet in person until recently and we, too, have used WhatsApp and Zoom for our very frequent communications.

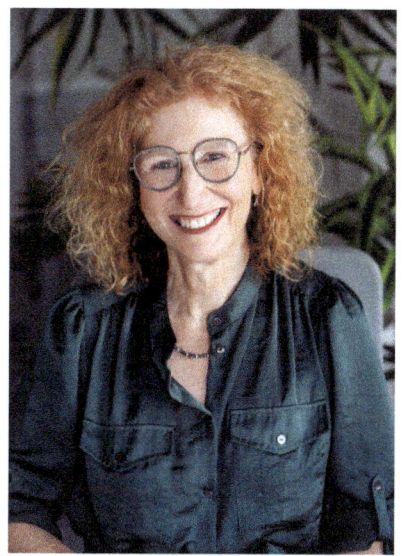

Chief Executive Sally Pairman (2022) – Courtesy of Sally Pairman.

'Technology keeps our Head Office Team connected and informed, with daily "check ins" via WhatsApp and twice-weekly Zoom meetings including using the break-out room functionality for "speed friending" as one way of giving us time to chat with each other informally in the absence of sharing an office together. This has become even more important as our team has grown this year – we are now a team of 21, all from different cultures and language groups and working across the globe and navigating many different time zones.

'Some things have not changed. As the CE I daily juggle activities across governance, operations, projects, partner collaborations, events, resource mobilisation, advocacy and communications, member associations and midwifery. The work is diverse and challenging – projects, campaigns and partnerships focused on strengthening our associations, raising the profile of midwives globally and deepening the research and evidence that supports midwife-led continuity of care (including this year's State of the World's Midwifery 2021). From big picture to sometimes small, emails arrive with constant regularity and expectation – requiring a triage approach for prioritisation. Social media has added another dimension to our work, and specialist communications and advocacy staff are a lifesaver!

'I am in regular communication with our members, partners, donors as well as policymakers and institutional leaders to ensure they have the information they need to inform decision-making. There is more – letters of condolence written to the many member associations who have lost midwives to COVID or to violence against women. With all that the Secretariat achieves, there is always more to do.'[36]

Staffing the Secretariat

The staffing of the ICM Secretariat was targeted towards expected activities and responsibilities, though available finances limited staff at times and at other times expanded staff available to do the work of the Confederation. When project funding was available, the Secretariat employed additional staff to carry out the project. One example was the UNFPA/ICM project, 'Investing in Midwives', with a remote headquarters and additional ICM staff in Ghana and Gabon. Staffing over the last 50 years ranged from one part-time Secretary General until 1991 to 9–10 full-time equivalent (FTE) staff in the early 2000s. The growth and restructuring of the Head Office in 2021 to include 21 staff members is the result of recognition from donors, including SIDA and the Gates Foundation, for the first time in many decades, that the ICM needs operational support in addition to programmatic funding.

COMMUNICATION WITH MEMBER ASSOCIATIONS

Little is known about the means of communications in the development stages of the Confederation, though Dr Frans Daels did his best to create a journal and record meetings of the IMU. After World War II, the authors found evidence of cables being sent to governments/Ministers of Health of the different countries with whom the Confederation was seeking to work. Quite often a duplicate copy was sent in the diplomatic bag from London, UK, as the cable system was either not trusted or unreliable in reaching the intended destination. Messages using this means meant a trip to the local post office which was the relay office. As communication technologies evolved, the ICM expanded its ability to communicate with it is members and partners throughout the world, essential to the work and success of the ICM.

Phone, Facsimile and Courier

1950s: Although undersea cables had been laid between countries from 1858 onwards with over two minutes to relay each character, it was not until the 1930s with the advent of the Telex system in the UK that things began to change. The public system opened up in 1954. The Telex depended on a telephone system and the recipient having a teleprinter. This system operated at around 60 words per minute in transmission and was expensive. Not everyone had a telephone, including some businesses, meaning a trip to the post office, though return messages were delivered by hand to the office address. It is not known when the Confederation had its first telephone, but indications are that there possibly was one by the 1954 Triennial Congress.

1970s: Time lapses/delays in sending and receiving messages related to the work of the ICM were many. When the ICM was working on the USAID project throughout the 1970s there are numerous citations of postal mail taking several weeks to reach countries. Thus, electronic means were the choice of communication, but these also were fraught with problems. Trying to select participants for the ICM workshops in countries meant working through the governments.[37] Once messages were with the Ministry of Health of the intended government there was always a further delay, sometimes with the Minister of Health not having the final say in the choice of participants for a workshop[38] or trying to identify midwives who met the intended criteria. These midwives were often far away from the seat of government. Therefore, on occasions to save time and effort on their part, the government would simply select one of its health ministry team (often not a midwife) which defeated achieving the improvements for maternity health care in that country.

The next time lapse was in messages coming back to the Confederation headquarters (HQ), with subsequent delays in returning details to the country once airline tickets were purchased to bring the identified midwife to the meeting or workshop. These proceedings realistically took between four to six weeks. A letter, dated 30 June 1973 to Marjorie Bayes (Secretary General of the ICM) from Dr Gingold, based in France, indicates that they had spoken on the telephone but also that a recorded postal delivery letter was being sent. This gives an indication that trips to the post office to relay messages were still a necessity.[39]

Working with the International Federation of Gynecology and Obstetrics

(FIGO) beginning in the 1970s resulted in numerous references to FIGO duplicating the ICM messages and sending to its member associations in countries as a back-up to work with governments in the respective countries.

1980s: It was not until the 1980s when Fax machines became more widely available that communications with the ICM MAs became easier. Even then the machines tended to be in government offices or in a few of the larger MA offices, especially in low resource countries (LRC) where most of the ICM country work was taking place. Telephones were becoming more common, but again, only in larger towns and cities of countries and certainly not in rural or remote settings where many LRC midwives were working.

Early in 1988 the ICM Headquarters obtained its first computer, quite a primitive affair, operated by two floppy discs: the first to start up the machine, which had to remain in during usage of the machine and the second was the one to save all work onto. Should work not be saved and the computer failed for any reason there was no hope of recovering any material, which Joan Walker recalls as happening to her when first working in the office. It was a case of starting from the beginning again! Work still needed to be printed out before it could either be sent by postal mail or sent via the fax machine to MAs.

1990s: During the 1990s ICM HQ upgraded its electronic systems. A personal laptop computer for office use, was purchased in 1994 that allowed for travel use by the Secretary General.[40] A more modern desktop computer was added and meant that where the recipient (MA) had the means to receive, emails could be sent. However, in the early days larger documents as attachments did not always get to the intended destination or even the email itself would disappear into cyberspace.

> *In 1991 Joan Walker, recalls a trip into central London from the office in Chiswick to purchase a mobile phone, these being a fairly new invention with the first call in the United Kingdom having been made in 1985. Stores selling them were few and far between. Once purchased Joan was able to be in contact with the office when travelling, although even then connection points were limited to major towns and cities.*

Another aspect of communications with members during the 1990s was preparing materials for meetings, particularly papers for the Triennial International Council meetings. The papers were typed and printed from the computer, then came the onerous task of photocopying them on the small photocopier which did not collate, double-side or staple as do photocopiers of today. Collation was usually done in a meeting room near the office which had a large table but had to be booked in advance and bookings for meetings took precedence so was time limited as to when it could be used. Pamphlets were also created explaining the aims of the Confederation, main activities and benefits of membership.[41]

An upgraded telephone by 1994 (see text below) meant that conference calls could be made enabling the BoM to discuss matters with the Secretary General. This certainly complemented meetings in moving business along and was less expensive than bringing the Board members together in between their quarterly meetings.

2000s: Throughout the 2000s technology completely changed all means of communications on a worldwide scale. Cable and telegram services and, to a degree, postal mail services were being demoted into history as email and social media communications led the way. One of the discussion items during the March 2005 Executive Committee meeting was the possibility of sending all Council papers electronically. However, it still needed to be recognised that not all countries enjoyed the same widespread availability and/or use of technology. However, during the 2014 Prague Congress, live web access to plenary sessions was available for a small fee to midwives who could not attend in person.[42] As Judith Brown, former ICM Director, noted:

> 'Midwives should celebrate the fact that communication has progressed so much. It's wonderful to have the world of midwifery made so more available and so interconnected through so many choices of personal communication. It has helped the ICM to grow over the last decade.'[43]

During the 2017–2020 triennium, the ICM Headquarters added new systems to better manage records and data. New systems and approaches for project and time management were developed and implemented in collaboration with the pro bono work of the lawyers, financial managers, Human Resource people and others who were members of the Finance and Risk Committee (FARC). The

ICM employed experienced project managers, not necessarily midwives, and finance managers dedicated to large projects to ensure they were delivered on time and on budget. With the support from an evaluation expert provided by the Gates Foundation more robust approaches to monitoring and evaluation across all projects were implemented.[44]

Newsletters

A very important method of communication with the ICM MAs was the production of a newsletter beginning in 1989. Its distribution was limited, however, as only one copy was sent to the MA headquarters/President, and it was often kept there and not shared with individual members of that association. This resulted in complaints from some midwives belonging to an ICM MAs who discovered there was an ICM Newsletter or that they could pay for an individual subscription. Once the newsletter was produced in electronic format beginning in 2009[45] it became more accessible to anyone who signed up to receive a copy.

The first issue of the newsletter was created and produced at ICM Headquarters in 1989, carrying the title Newsletter: International Confederation of Midwives. Marie Goubran was the first editor, and the eight-page document was filled with brief reports from member associations, the ICM Regions and its partners as well as notices of upcoming meetings of interest to midwives and a list of publications sent to the ICM HQ. The inside of the first page was a list of the Officers: Board of Management and Regional Representatives. This format continued until 2008 when the newsletter was produced electronically. In 1990[46], the newsletter contained brief resumes of elected Board of Management members and regional representatives in addition to other items. As each new election of midwives took place during Triennial Council meetings, those individuals were introduced to the larger membership through the newsletter. When the first International Day of the Midwife (IDM) was inaugurated in 1991[47], a brief summary of the ICM activities was included in the newsletter. The June 1992 Newsletter added a member association 'Action page' at the end, requesting input on various activities and projects.[48] In 1994, the first page began with a report of activities from the Board of Management[49] that offered members ongoing updates of Council directives and BoM activities.

With the July 1994 issue, the name of the newsletter was changed to International Midwifery Matters (IMM) with Volume 7, No 2.[50] By this time the document averaged 16 pages beginning with the editor's summary of activities to date along with news from MAs and regions, upcoming meetings and pages of publications of interest to midwives. The SG was still putting the newsletter together, printing it at HQ and sending it out to MAs.

When Elizabeth Duff joined the Headquarters staff in 1998 as the part-time (0.4 FTE) Editor, IMM was in Volume 11. The production process was such that everything was keyed in and printed in the ICM office and then photocopied. ICM office staff put the newsletter in envelopes for each MA and ICM partners and took the bundles to the franking machine in the Barley Mow reception area until the ICM had its own franking machine. There were rarely if ever any photos or images included. The content of IMM included reports from the Board and Regional representatives, news items and a list of any publications received at the ICM office. There were no articles. During 1998, the Editor continued to produce IMM on a quarterly basis, while developing ideas and researching costs for an enhanced style of publication, in effect moving from a newsletter to a small journal style. The new publication launched in January 1999, entitled International Midwifery (IM) and subtitled Journal of the International Confederation of Midwives. IM was printed by Albany Press, based just outside London in Hertfordshire. They also mailed out the copies. Photos of ICM activities were included.

The first issue of IM still contained reports; e.g. the ICM Francophone Congress (with a photo of Ruth Brauen) in both English and French; a conference of the Czech Association of Midwives and an 'international event' held by the Queensland branch of the Australian College of Midwives. It also carried an article by a Sara Nam, a midwife working in Afghanistan for MERLIN (Medical Emergency Relief International). In addition, there were two 'News' pages, one about the ICM and member associations, and one of 'worldwide news' of interest to midwives. The plan was to publish six issues a year, which continued until the end of 2005 when budget constraints caused a return to quarterly frequency.

An International Editorial Group (IEG) was proposed to the Board of Management by the IM editor in July 2000 with the proposed tasks to be fulfilled by the Regional Representatives. The BoM agreed that all Regional Representatives be given the option to join the IEG.[51] The IEG was set up during the Vienna Congress in 2002 with Penny Held, Europe; Christina Mudokwenyu-Rawdon, Africa; Pauline Glover, Asia-pacific and Mary Ann Shah, Americas. Members of the editorial group wrote leading articles in alternate issues, with

Board meeting reports in the others.

When the ICM newsletter was converted to an electronic format in 2009, the name had changed to ICM Newsletter. The content of the newsletter included summaries of Board and Council meetings, notes from elected officers, articles and updates submitted, results of ICM surveys of MAs, news from members and a list of Conferences and Events. The page numbers decreased as the number of issues increased. The list of publications received in the office no longer existed, in part because ICM HQ no longer had a library available for use by individual midwives. The electronic ICM newsletter reached more than 2,000 active subscribers by 2014.[52]

THE *INTERNATIONAL JOURNAL OF CHILDBIRTH*[53]

The genesis of the International Journal of Childbirth (IJCB) was conceived by Professor Soo Downe (University of Central Lancashire), an internationally respected midwife with a particular interest on the nature of normal birth and Associate Professor Denis Walsh (University of Nottingham, Division of Midwifery), a highly respected midwife and childbirth researcher. The goal was to provide a journal with a global focus that published peer reviewed articles on childbearing and birth. As Professors Downe and Walsh developed their concept, they also began seeking out organisations that might be interested in sponsoring the journal. The ICM was interested in identifying the IJCB as their official journal. However, ICM was unable to provide full support for the publication of the journal. During 2010 negotiations began between the ICM and Springer publishing company in the United States.[54] In 2011 Springer Publications agreed to publish the journal for the ICM.[55] At this time, Professor Kerri Schuiling, a midwife educator and researcher from the US, was brought on as a founding co-editor with Professor Walsh, and Professor Downe became the journal's Deputy Editor. The IJCB published its first issue in 2011 and cost $50 per year for ICM members.

The agreement between ICM and IJCB was maintained until 2016 at which time ICM leadership felt they could no longer continue to provide partial support for publishing the journal. Springer Publishing then took over the entirety of publishing the journal while keeping its international focus on birth and childbearing. At that time, the editorship of the journal also changed with the resignations of founding co-editors (Downe, Schuiling and Walsh) and Michelle

Murray, PhD, RNC-OB of Albuquerque, New Mexico, USA, became the next editor.

The journal retains its global focus and continues to solicit peer-reviewed articles for publication that cross-cut all professions involved with childbirth, including midwifery, maternal-foetal medicine, physiology, anthropology, traditional birth attendants, doulas and so forth. The journal is a quarterly publication and is listed in the Web of Science Emerging Sources Citation Index.

THE ICM WEBSITES

The World Wide Web (Web) originally conceived in 1989 and developed to meet the demand for automated information-sharing between scientists in universities and institutes around the world was opened to the public at large. In early 2000, Joyce Thompson (ICM Director 1999–2005) suggested that ICM should have its own website. She talked with Kim Updegrove, then a Nurse-Midwifery faculty member at Yale University, who agreed to create the site, named www.intlmidwives.org. By August 2000, the site had been fleshed out with links to ICM's mission, goals, vision statements, events, job postings, as well as online resources published by the American College of Nurse Midwives, Family Care International, the United Nations and other organisations. Among the events highlighted was the ICM's 26th Triennial Congress, in Vienna, 14–19 April 2002.[56]

Unfortunately, registration of the domain name lapsed in 2002, due to an administrative oversight at the ICM HQ. Worse was to come as the domain name was purchased immediately by a Russian entity that filled the pages with pornography and demanded a ransom to return the name to the ICM. Overnight ICM's web presence and promotion of the upcoming Vienna Congress disappeared and the ICM's commitment to protect and empower women had been replaced by vile examples of the exploitation of women. With no recourse, the ICM leadership promptly paid the ransom, re-registered the domain name, and deployed a modified page that automatically redirected to www.internationalmidwives.org which remains the organisation's web address in 2022.

An important lesson had been learned about the promise and perils of the ever-expanding use of the internet. Since this time the website was further developed in 2008[57] and again in February 2013[58] and more recently in 2018[59] to accommodate the growing importance of digital advocacy, the need to encourage better engagement with MAs by providing regular updates on activities and a special membership section, and reflect the ICM corporate identity.[60] The website was widely used in promoting the ICM, its activities and it now included the capacity for the registration, booking and communication with the thousands of midwives who attend each Triennial Congress. The website was again updated in 2018 following its crash in late 2017.

REPRESENTATION OF THE ICM

> 'Increasing prominence has placed additional responsibilities on the Board to ensure that whenever and wherever midwifery is under discussion or being considered internationally, the Confederation is appropriately represented by knowledgeable midwives.'[61]

One important strategy to support the business of the ICM but also to increase its visibility and the voices of midwives throughout the world was its willingness to represent the ICM at a variety of meetings of partners and potential partners over the years, including increasing numbers of donors. As representation requests increased the opportunity for a number of MAs to showcase their support of the ICM and its documents across the globe also increased.

The ICM Constitution and Council early on designated the Secretary General as the person to represent ICM at these invited meetings whenever possible.[62] Marjorie Bayes, ICM General Secretary 1954–1975, was the primary representative to other global organisations during her years of service, especially those in London and Geneva. As the number of invitations for the ICM attendance at global meetings of UN agencies, donors, NGOs and other agencies concerned with the welfare of mothers and babies grew, the need to expand the ICM representatives was evident. As noted in the 1990–1993 Triennial Report, 107 meetings were attended by ICM representatives 1990–1992, with the ICM SG attending 31 (29 per cent), including funerals of former ICM staff.[63] Other meetings were attended by members of the ICM Board/Executive, selected staff (Programme Manager) and MA midwives living close to the geographic location of the meeting with the expertise needed to speak about the ICM and the issues being discussed.

The majority of meetings attended by the ICM representatives were those held by long-term partners – the WHO, UNICEF, UNFPA, FIGO, IPA and ICN. Given that this representation activity went beyond the SG and Board, a policy on representation was agreed by the ICM Board in 2001.[64] This policy defined the expectations/responsibilities of the ICM and its representative in addition to criteria for selecting an individual midwife. These criteria included membership in an ICM MA and having basic/extensive knowledge of the Confederation and expertise in the content being discussed. The representative was also required to advocate for ICM and contribute to the meeting as appropriate. Reports were required and most were sent to the ICM HQ. Though representation continued into the 21st century at key partner meetings, the 2020 ICM Council agreed to stop naming individuals to the WHO and other UN offices across the globe as it was apparent many of the midwives selected were not interested and/or prepared to be an effective representative of the ICM.[65]

SUMMARY

Support for the ongoing business of ICM has been carried out from the ICM Headquarters by staff of the Secretariat in addition to Board members and selected representatives from MAs. This was no small task in any decade. The importance of communication is highlighted and has made great strides forward in the 21st century with the advent of new electronic platforms as noted in the 2017–2020 Triennial Report: '... new technology has allowed ICM to hold virtual videoconferencing Board meetings, working groups, and meetings with advisory groups, Member Associations and partners.' These virtual platforms have proved their worth in 2020/2021 with the need to hold the Council meeting virtually in June 2020 and postpone the Triennial Congress in Bali due to the Coronavirus pandemic, becoming a virtual ICM Triennial Congress in 2021.

The structure of the organisation with volunteer officers and MAs required understanding of the role and responsibilities of the ICM Secretariat as well as support for disseminating ICM publications and activities to their own members. These responsibilities have increased, and communication has improved greatly as communication technologies advanced.

100 Years of the International Confederation of Midwives

1. Sr Anne Thompson. A Birthday for Midwives. Seventy-five Years of International Collaboration. ICM: Chiswick, London, 1994, p 4. Professor Daels was the individual who functioned as Secretary of the IMU from 1922 to 1939.
2. ICM. (SA/ICM/R/4). Wellcome Collection. Marjorie Bayes' History of ICM 1st 50 years (2 of 3). Miss Bayes noted that the during the 1954 Congress the executive of 39 delegates representing 22 member countries met.
3. ICM. (SA/ICM/C/1/18, 1975-1989). Wellcome Collection. Executive Meeting minutes 21, 22, 23 March 1980. Minutes noted that the registration of ICM as a charity had failed, though 'further consideration was necessary'.
4. ICM. (SA/ICM/C.1/18/2). Wellcome Collection. Executive Committee Minutes 12–18 September 1981. During the discussion of a new constitution, some members were concerned that adoption of it would potentially cause ICM to lose it Charitable status worth £700–800 per year.
5. Note 29 April 2021 to Joyce Thompson from Ingela Wiklund, ICM Treasurer 2016–2020.
6. The person in charge of keeping IMU meetings on track and minutes recorded and filed from 1922 through 1940s was generally the person elected/nominated to chair the next meeting of the IMU, later referred to as the 'President'. The early individuals were physicians until Dr Daels in the mid-1930s suggested it was time for a midwife to be in the lead. This did not happen until the last pre-WWII congress in Paris 199 when he officially resigned his post as Secretary General. This meant that important papers were transferred from one country to the next and may have contributed to the loss of records during WWI and WWII, especially those held by Dr Daels in Ghent.
7. ICM. A Birthday for Midwives – Seventy-Five Years of International Collaboration. Chiswick, London: ICM, p 4.
8. ICM. A Birthday for Midwives – Seventy-Five Years of International Collaboration, p.4. Miss Edith Pye was president-elect and Mme Mossé President and host of the 1939 pre-War congress in Paris and appeared to retain the secretariat position through the 'silent' period of WWII. Mme Mossé also hosted one of the meetings to discuss re-establishing the IMU in 1949 and hoped the Secretariat would be based in France.
9. ICM. (SA/ICM/R/4). Wellcome Collection. Marjorie Bayes' History of ICM 1st 50 years (2 of 3). '1955 March pre-fix title of Executive added to secretary', p 2.
10. ICM. (SA/ICM/C1/18/2). Wellcome Collection. Minutes of Executive Committee 18th September, Brighton, UK. This document stated, '1954 move of secretariat from France to England when [ICM] became worldwide organization. Running costs subsidized by the Royal College of Midwives.' ICM. Triennial Report 1990–1993. 'Minute of Appreciation for Marjorie Bayes.' ICM: London, p 4. The report noted that Miss Bayes served from 1954–1975 as Executive Secretary of the ICM. (SA/ICM/C/1/18/1). Wellcome Collection. Executive Committee, Secretaries report, Helsinki, Finland, 10–13 March 1974, noted 'resignation of M Bayes as of 31st December 1975'. ICM. (SA/ICM/C1/18). Wellcome Collection. Executive Committee 21st June 1975, noted 'Miss Bayes tendered resignation from end of June 1975, an amendment from the March 1974 minutes'.
11. ICM. Triennial Report 1990–1993. 'Minute of Appreciation for Margaret Hardy.' ICM: London, p 4. The report noted that Miss Hardy served as ICM Executive Secretary from 1975–1980. Doris Haire. Letter 20 August 1975, congratulating Margaret Hardy on Appointment as ICM. F Margaret Hardy wrote to R Forestier of ONSSF in Paris (27 November 1979), 'I regret that I shall not be present at the Executive Committee meeting [planned for March 1980] as I shall be retiring from the post of Executive Secretary on 7th February 1980'. ICM. (SA/ICM/C/2/2). Wellcome Collection. Executive Committee correspondence noted the Miss Hardy resigned on 5 February 1980.
12. ICM. (SA/ICM/C/1/18). Wellcome Collection. Minutes of Executive Committee 21, 22, 23 March 1980, Hotel Westminster, Paris, France. This document noted that Miss Hardy resigned on 5 February 1980, Miss Leedham then acting Executive Secretary as 'No applications for Executive Secretary position coming vacant'. ICM. (SA/ICM/Q/7). Wellcome Collection. Recruitment. Miss Leedham paid daily rate for her last months of services (not employed).
13. ICM. (SA/ICM/Q/7). Wellcome Collection. Recruitment. Frances Cowper-Smith was paid £70 per day (considered a notional sum in lieu of benefits, superannuation/sick pay.
14. ICM. Triennial Report 1993–1996. Chiswick, London: ICM, 1996, p 4. Minute of Appreciation for Frances Cowper-Smith who died 26 December 1993. The report noted that Vale Frances Cowper-Smith served as ICM Executive Secretary 1981–1986. ICM. (SA/ICM/C/1/18/1). Wellcome Collection. Executive Committee, Secretaries report, Helsinki, Finland, 10–13 March 1974. Notes recorded that Assistant secretary, Mr Smith, Financial adviser (since 1972) present at meeting advised 1/3 of salary be paid by ICM.
15. The ICM Board decided that a full-time Secretary General was warranted, but Marie Goubran declined to move from part-time status due to her other responsibilities.
16. Marie Goubran's term of office as ICM Secretary General ended with her untimely death in December 1990.
17. ICM. ICM Council Meeting Minutes, 1990, p 10. The term 'Executive Secretary' was changed to 'Secretary General' by accord of the 1990 ICM Council. ICM. Report of Board of Management & Accounts for year ended 31 December 1990, p 5. Joan Walker was named acting ICM Secretary General during late 1990 during the last stages of illness of Marie Goubran who passed away on 3 December 1990.
18. ICM. Newsletter 4 (1), March 1991. p 1 'Press Release' noted that Miss Joan Walker appointed at the Secretary General as of 4 March 1991.

100 Years of the International Confederation of Midwives

19 ICM. ICM Council Meeting Minutes, 1990. Agenda item 90/24, p 13. ICM Council 1990 agreed that 'ICM both needs and can afford a fulltime Secretary General for the next Triennium.' Joan Walker was originally hired part-time upon death of Marie Goubran in December 1990, and employed full-time once search completed by the Board of Management. This position was funded by the Ford Foundation. Carol Hird and Margaret Peters. ICM Press Release, 1991. 'The President and Board of the International Confederation of Midwives are pleased to announce the appointment of Miss Joan Walker as Secretary General of the Confederation. Miss Walker takes up her appointment on 4 March 1991.'

20 Joan Walker. Letter of resignation dated 20 Jun 1997 to Margaret Peters and Joyce Thompson. Resignation to take effect 31 March 1998. [Personal papers of Joyce Thompson]

21 Petra ten Hoope-Bender. Email to ICM Board of 5/7/2003. 'I am writing to tell you that I plan to leave my post as Secretary General of ICM by the autumn of this year. I will then have served the organization for five years and feel that it is time for me to move on.'

22 Della Sherratt was appointed by the ICM Board of Management to cover the three-month sabbatical of Petra ten Hoope-Bender commencing 13 January 2001 following the death of Petra's husband.

23 Joyce Thompson. Director's Notes. International Midwifery 16(5), September/October 2003, p 51. 'I am pleased to announce that Kathy Herschderfer, a midwife from the Netherlands and currently co-chair of the ICM Research Standing Committee, was offered the position [sic: Secretary General]. Kathy has accepted and will begin her tenure on December 1, 2003.'

24 Bridget Lynch. Letter to Agneta Bridges dated September 27, 2009. In this letter, the ICM President noted that Dutch law had converted Agneta's Interim status to Permanent as of 1 October 2008 (six-month probationary period). The Board upheld her status during their June 2009 meeting. [Frances Day-Stirk personal papers]

25 Judith Brown was appointed interim ICM Chief Executive following the resignation of Agneta Bridges so that an international search for the next Chief Executive could be conducted. ICM. ICM Consultancy Agreement: Interim Secretary General, 18 March 2013. [Frances Day-Stirk Personal papers]

26 ICM. ICM Employment contract for Chief Executive. Sally Pairman signed 6 November 2016. Personal papers FDS.

27 ICM. The Constitution of the International Confederation of Midwives. September 1981, pp 1–2.

28 ICM. (SA/ICM/L/1/15). Wellcome Collection. ICM/USAID Project Final Report 1980. In 1972 through a grant from USAID the ICM commenced its project on midwifery and the promotion of Family Planning launched through Working Parties organised for developing countries in various regions of the world.

29 ICM. (SA/ICM/L/1/10). Wellcome Collection. USAID Project Activities and Progress Reports 1972–1978.

30 ICM. (SA/ICM/H7-10, 1 of 3). Wellcome Collection. Correspondence Margaret Peters November 1981–September 1988.

31 ICM. (SA/ICM/H7-10, 3 of 3). Wellcome Collection. Minutes of Board of Management Meetings.

32 Joan Walker. Personal memories. 'It was in one of these small spaces [Barley Mow] I became far more aware of what the Confederation was and did than I had ever picked up from the five International Congresses than I had attended, when I was asked to give some help to the Secretary General [Goubran] in the run-up to the 22nd International Congress to take place in Kobe Japan.'

33 Personal recollection of Joan Walker, Secretary General 1991–1998. Written in 2020.

34 Frances Ganges. Chief Executive report to the 30th ICM Congress, p 31, in the ICM Triennial Report 2011–2014.

35 ICM. Triennial Report 2017–2020. Message from the President, p 4.

36 Sally Pairman. Written description of her current role as the Chief Executive of the ICM.

37 The ICM/USAID Project targeted Low Resource Country midwives where communication networks relied mostly on governments, especially Ministries of Health.

38 Barbara Patterson correspondence March 1975–December 77; 23 June handwritten letter Belinda Brohier in Khartoum to Barbara. Wellcome Institute Library SA/ICM/L 3/1/1.

39 Dr Gingold's letter. Wellcome Institute Library document SA/ICM/.

40 Sr Anne Thompson, ICM Treasurer, to Director Margaret Peters and Deputy Director Joyce Thompson. 5 August 1994.

41 ICM. The International Confederation of Midwives: Healthy Women, Health Babies, Health Nations. ICM: London, 1993. In 1995, this pamphlet was expanded to include the structure of the ICM and ways to purchase ICM reports and postcards that were created for sale.

42 ICM 30th Triennial Congress, Prague, Czech Republic. Newsletter September 2013, p 5.

43 Judith Brown interview. 20 April 2019, p 2.

44 ICM. Triennial Report 2017–2020. The Hague: ICM, p 15.

45 ICM. ICM Newsletter, 1 (Autumn/Winter) 2009.

46 ICM. Newsletter 3(3), December 1990, p 1. This Newsletter contained an insert with the Obituary of Mrs E Marie Goubran, who died on the 13 December 1990.

47 ICM. Newsletter 4(2), July 1991, p 2. This issue of the Newsletter also contained the obituary for Miss Marjorie Bayes, p 2.

48 ICM. Newsletter 5(2), June 1992.

49 ICM. Newsletter 7(1) March 1994, p 1.

50 ICM. International Midwifery Matters, 7 (2), July 1994. Joan Walker was Secretary General and Editor.

51 ICM. Minutes of a Meeting of the Board of Management, July 20–22, 2000. Min 07.3, p 2.
52 ICM. Triennial Report 2011–2014, p 19.
53 Kerri Durnell Schuiling. Personal notes to Joyce Thompson 1-28-2021.
54 ICM. Triennial Report 2008–2011. The Hague: ICM, p 14.
55 Flyer from Springer Publishing Company announcing the new International Journal of Childbirth, co-edited by Denis Walsh and Kerri D Schuiling. The flyer was prepared for the 2002 Congress and encouraged subscriptions of $40 per year for ICM members signing up at the Congress and otherwise $50 per year.
56 The website as it existed on 18 August 2000 is accessible in the Internet Archive: https://web.archive.org/web/20010405055545/http://www.intlmidwives.org/
57 Email from ICM to Member Associations. 8 February 2008. 'At last our new ICM website is here.' Thus, an updated website was launched in 2008, and again in 2018 when it crashed and had to be re-created. The 2018 re-creation led to the loss of some of the key education and regulation tools.
58 ICM. Annual Report 2013. The Hague: ICM, 18 April 2014, p 3: 'The New Year saw the launch of the newly rebranded, updated website'. ICM. ICM Council Meeting Minutes, Prague, 2014, p 9.
59 Sally Pairman, ICM Chief Executive, notes to Joyce Thompson, 13 July 2021.
60 ICM. Triennial Report 2011–2014, p 19.
61 ICM. ICM Triennial Report 1990–1993. Representation, p 7.
62 1975–1989. Executive Committee Meeting 1–4 September, Jerusalem, Israel, 1978. Wellcome Institute Library document SA/ICM/C/1/18. Resolutions prepared for council #6: 'That, whenever possible, the Executive Secretary should represent the Confederation at meetings or consultations with other bodies or organizations. Where this is not possible representation should be at the discretion of the executive secretary after consultation with the General Officers.'
63 ICM. ICM Triennial Report 1990–1993. Annex II, pp 23–30.
64 ICM. Board of Management meeting minutes, 6 April 2001. 'Representation of ICM at International Meetings.'
65 ICM. ICM Council Meeting Minutes 2020 (virtual). Agenda item 4.3, p 4. Approval of the removal of article 12.2.6 of the ICM Articles of Association (Constitution) and Article 12.2.vi of the ICM Byelaws (discontinuation of UN representatives).

Section II: ICM: A Catalyst for Global Respect for Midwives and Women
Chapter 8: *ICM Vision, Mission and Strategic Directions*

'ICM will work toward achieving the following vision that empowers both women and midwives to be fully respected as persons who are also productive members of all societies.'[1]

INTRODUCTION

The ICM's story of growth and development continued from 1954 onward with activities framed by its dual aims/objects.[2] The organisation continued its growth and expansion globally, including the adoption of the ICM's Mission Statement in 1993 and Vision Statements in 1996. The ICM leaders sought outside consultation, such as the Strategy Day[3] facilitated by Geoff Ribbens in 1997 and the 'Meeting of the Minds'[4] in 2001 to become more intentional about strategic planning efforts as described later in this chapter. But why were these statements important to the organisation?

In the mid-1990s, the ICM leadership came from a variety of administrative, academic and leadership positions outside and within midwifery associations.[5] These individuals agreed the need for and importance of having statements of Vision and Mission agreed by the Member Associations (MAs) and shared with the outside world. The ICM's global influence was growing and strengthened with involvement in the Safe Motherhood Initiatives beginning in 1987 (Chapters 9, 15). Some of these leaders were present during the 1994 International Conference on Population Development (ICPD) that had influenced their thinking about women's sexual and reproductive rights and the ICM Deputy Director (Joyce Thompson) had delivered the ICM's Statement to the 4th World Conference on Women in 1995.[6] Women's rights as human rights became a much stronger rallying cry for midwives across the world as reflected in the ICM's position statements and revised core documents. The adoption of a clearly stated Vision and Mission were viewed as vital to the ICM's work with midwives and women.

The historical development of the ICM's *Vision*, *Mission* and *Strategic Directions* over several triennia is the primary foci of this chapter, demonstrating, in part, the maturation of the organisation. Content includes examples of how the organisation evolved over time in terms of its governance and management, and the difficulties encountered in achieving the strategic guidelines as they were developed, but which, as experience progressed, enabled the organisation to design successful activities that kept the Vision and Mission of the organisation alive.

VISION STATEMENTS

Given the understanding that a *Vision* statement describes the big picture of how things should be and a *Mission* statement describes how it plans to achieve the *Vision*, the market or sector to which it is directed (e.g. midwives and women), as well as the organisation's basic philosophical premises,[7] the ICM Board of Management (BoM) began drafting statements of Vision and Mission in 1995. They were influenced, in part, by the work of futurist Joel Barker[8] and work completed by the American College of Nurse-Midwives (ACNM) during their 'Listen to Women' campaign in the early 1990s (Chapter 14).

> 'Vision without action is merely a dream.
> Action without vision just passes the time.
> Vision with action can change the world!'
>
> Joel A Barker

The first ICM *Vision* statement was agreed by the ICM Executive Committee and adopted by the ICM Council in 1996[9], stating simply: **'Empowering Women ... Empowering Midwives'**. Based on this overall vision, the 1996 ICM Council agreed the complementary *Vision for the Future of Midwifery* and *Vision for Women and Their* Health[10], recognising that midwives and women share many of the same concerns. Excerpts from these two vision statements were based on the 1993 ICM Constitutional Aims and the 1993 *ICM Code of Ethics*[11], then incorporated into other Core ICM documents over the years. The two complementary vision statements are presented below to lay the foundation for how they influenced the development of later ICM core documents and position statements expressing the ICM MAs' ongoing commitment to empower women and midwives throughout the world.

100 Years of the International Confederation of Midwives

The Vision for Women and Their Health
ICM Envisions a world where:

- Women are respected and treated as persons in their own right in all societies Women stand as equal partners with men in the world order
- Women are recognised as crucial to the health of any nation
- Women and their families are part of a health care system with high quality care and easy access when needed
- Women have the right to choose from among safe options for care throughout their lives, including state-of-the-art care from competent providers who truly care about the woman and her health
- Women are educated and empowered to delight in a strong sense of self, to trust their bodies, to plan their pregnancies, and to make wise choices in their health care arena
- Women experience a reasonable standard of living, including a clean and safe environment, healthy food, and a reasonable place to live
- No woman has to fear for her life or the life of her baby when she is pregnant
- Women believe that birth is normal and prefer to avoid unnecessary interventions

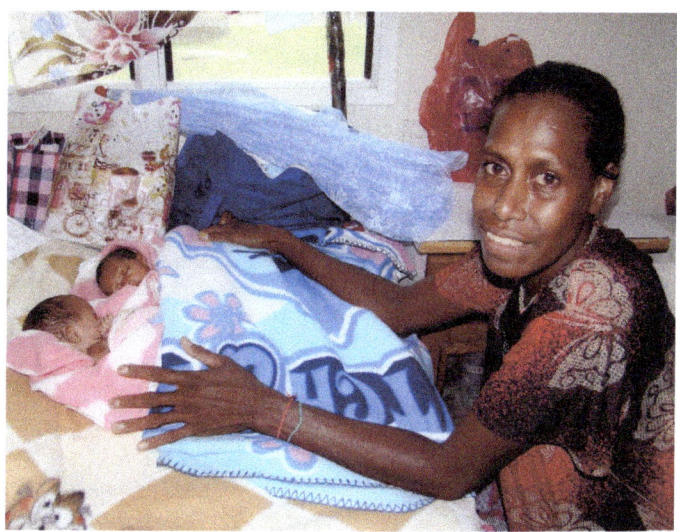

Solomon Islands' mother with twins – Courtesy of Karen Guilliland

The Vision for the Future of Midwifery
ICM envisions the following about the future of midwifery in the world:

- Midwives provide care in all settings and for all women who need midwifery care
- Midwives are well-qualified and remain competent and caring throughout their careers
- Midwives are autonomous health care providers who value team work in providing the total needs of women and their families
- Midwives are recognised for their activities of self-governance, including standards of practice, core competencies, codes of ethics, ongoing quality assessment and valid credentialling systems
- Midwifery education is available through a variety of routes and based on core competencies related to the needs of the country/area where the midwife is prepared
- Midwives are, and have to stay, responsible for their own training and education
- All qualified midwives are able to practice in keeping with their educational preparation and experience
- Midwives are recognised as the experts in the care of childbearing women and linchpins in any Safe Motherhood effort
- Midwives play a key role in determining the future of health care, including community-based primary health care for women and families
- Midwives are an integral part of any regulatory agency assigned the task of promulgating and enforcing rules and regulations governing midwifery practice
- Midwives are involved in research and policy work that validates and promotes midwifery care to the public
- Midwives believe that menstruation, pregnancy, birth and menopause are normal life events and rarely require medical intervention
- Midwives work with women to design a woman-responsive health care system

The Purpose statement introducing these two complementary Vision statements noted that: 'ICM will work toward achieving the following vision that empowers both women and midwives to be fully respected as persons who are also productive members of all societies.'[12] These vision statements were reviewed and reinforced by the ICM Council through 2007. Though neither complementary statement referred to the organisation as whole, together they offered a panorama of what the ICM was working towards during this time.

At the ICM Council in 2008, a new *Vision* statement was adopted that replaced the 1996 *Vision: Empowering Women ... Empowering Midwives* and the two complementary statements of vision, most likely in the interest of having only one statement.[13] In fact, a letter to the MAs prior to the 2008 ICM Council meeting noted that the Board worked with a consultant, 'in the development of effective, simple and powerful new Vision and Mission statements.'[14] The 2008 Vision statement[15] that continues to the present time reads:

> 'ICM envisions a world where every childbearing woman has access to a midwife's care for herself and her newborn.'

The new Vision statement was adopted after much discussion and debate on whether 'childbearing' should remain defining the women to be served or whether 'childbearing' should be eliminated, noting that every woman should have access to a midwife's care, whether or not she bore children. This debate had surfaced periodically with the wording of the Aims and Objects of the ICM over the years (Chapter 5) and continued in discussions of the Mission statement below. The debate highlights the ongoing struggle within the ICM MAs as to whether midwives should concentrate only on 'mothers' and 'childbearing women' as recipients of their services or broaden their practise to include adolescents and 'women during their reproductive years'. Many of these debates reflected the societal status accorded women at the time, including views of women/midwives as helpers versus professional health workers and childbearing as an essential society-maintaining function of both women and men that was expected of women[16], even if having too many babies too close together killed the women, especially in low resource countries (LRC).

It would appear that there were at least two basic reasons for this debate about who should be the focus of midwifery services. First was the concern among many midwifery associations that if midwives needed to be competent in and offer services beyond childbearing, it could dilute the impact of what they perceived as their core childbearing role, especially as many midwives were stretched beyond their capacity to deliver childbearing care in many countries. Another reason for the debate was the fact that the majority of midwives in Europe concentrated on providing childbearing care while most midwives in LRC and a few high resource countries (HRC) (e.g. Sweden, USA) were providing full-scope midwifery care including sexual and reproductive health (SRH) services based on need (LRC) and demand (HRC) from the women themselves. For many midwives and midwifery associations, however, it took until the early 21st century for family planning and other sexual and reproductive health services to be seen as accepted midwifery practice in most countries although this had been taught throughout the 1970s at the ICM workshops funded by the USAID. This change was facilitated when the evidence-based ICM *Essential Competencies for Basic Midwifery Practice* were first adopted by the ICM Council in 2002[17] (Chapter 12). History will determine if this focus solely on women who are pregnant or birthing will affect the credibility and global influence of the ICM in the future.

MISSION STATEMENTS

In 1993, the first Mission Statement was adopted by the ICM Council.[18] It read[19]:

> 'The International Confederation of Midwives will advance worldwide the aims and aspirations of midwives in the attainment of improved outcomes for women in their childbearing years, their newborn and their families wherever they reside.'

This statement continued as the ICM's mission until 2008 when the terms 'autonomous', 'most appropriate caregiver' and 'keeping birth normal' were added (see below).

The MA's debates over the order of the dual aims (midwives or childbearing women first) of the Confederation continued with the mission statements over the years, along with the scope of midwifery practice as discussed above under Vision. The struggle over the scope of midwifery care that was evident in discussion of the ICM *Vision* statement in 2008 was the same as those prior to adoption of the revised *Mission* statement in that same year. In addition, many

ICM MAs expressed concern that the ICM was focusing more on meeting the needs of women and childbearing families in the world than on meeting the needs of its MAs (Chapter 10).

In keeping with changes in leadership, member viewpoints, and the second wave of Feminism, the *Mission* statement was reviewed and revised again in 2008 and continued the same through 2022. The ICM Mission statement as of the time of this writing reads[20]:

> 'To strengthen member associations and to advance the profession of midwifery globally by promoting autonomous midwives as the most appropriate caregivers for childbearing women and in keeping birth normal, in order to enhance the reproductive health of women, and the health of their newborn and their families.'

STRATEGY DOCUMENTS

Three Strategic Objectives were agreed at the 1993 Council meeting after adoption of the written Mission statement to carry out the work of the ICM during the triennium that followed.

These Objectives were:
1) address women's health globally
2) strengthen the midwifery profession
3) promote the Organisation internationally.

These Strategic Objectives led to discussion of the Board of Management's draft Plan of Action for the next triennium within the 1993 ICM Council, 'intended to drive activities of Associations'[21] in recognition that the ICM accomplishes its goals primarily through the work of its MAs. The Plan of Action with 12 goals was adopted 'in principle' by the 1993 ICM Council and served as a discussion item during Executive and Regional meetings during 1993–1996.[22]

The *Vision* statement of 1996 together with the *Mission* statement and the three original strategic objectives were used as the foundation for a new era of strategic planning[23] beginning with first Global Strategy document. The *Global Strategic Plan 1996–1999* agreed during the 1996 ICM Council had 12 specific Goals (not in any priority order) with the Objectives, Activities and Outcomes for each outlined.[24]

Two additional goals were adopted in 1999 to carry out the three Strategic

Objectives and used for the Global Strategy 1999–2002.[25] The specific goals were:
1. To work towards achievement of the Safe Motherhood goals;
2. To demonstrate the potential of midwifery actions to reduce maternal and perinatal mortality and morbidity rates;
3. To extend the knowledge of midwifery and influence of midwives throughout the world in venues where decision making takes place and policies made about the delivery of maternity care;
4. To work with communities and women's groups to develop their knowledge and awareness of how to attain health;
5. To strengthen midwifery education and ongoing education programmes, including the role of the midwife as an educator;
6. To develop mechanisms to support midwives so they can fully practise their skills;
7. To encourage and support midwifery research and the pursuit of quality in care of women in the reproductive years;
8. To classify and define midwifery activities;
9. To secure the financial viability of the ICM;
10. To increase the number of associations of midwives in membership in countries where no member associations exist at present;
11. To disseminate information and provide forums by which member associations and their membership can share and develop from the experience of others; and
12. To develop national codes of ethics based on the *International Code of Ethics for Midwives;*
13. To raise the awareness of midwifery and extend the influence of midwives in national and international forums where policies relating to reproductive health care are made;
14. To strengthen and support midwives' professional autonomy and develop mechanisms that enable midwifery education, regulation and practice to be designed and governed primarily by midwives so that midwives can fully practise their skills.

Need for Outside Consultant – 1997
Following the May 1996 Council meeting in Oslo, Norway, the ICM Board of Management agreed the need to have a one-day strategic planning session

facilitated by an outside consultant, Mr Geoff Ribbens, to set more realistic goals and strategic activities for the new millennium (1999–2002) with an emphasis on financial viability and stability. The planning day was held on 19 June 1997, in London.[26] Mr Ribbens led the Board in a SWOT[27] analysis of the ICM, including identification of ICM's many strengths along with its key weaknesses with suggested strategies to address each one. Of importance to the development of the ICM were the identified weaknesses needing to be overcome, such as:

1. Dominance of English-speaking midwives, especially from the developed world;
2. Professional demarcation of midwifery as 'women's' work and a woman's profession;
3. Tendency to speak and decide with 'hearts' rather than sound business decisions on significant budgetary items (e.g. geographic sites of Congresses, mid-triennium meetings);
4. Sometimes 'presume' to make decisions on behalf of sister midwives rather than listening and giving voice to the silent ones (language barriers);
5. Unequal expertise in elected Directors and other volunteers without needed financial skills;
6. Financial/resource instability due to dependence on Congress income and MAs fees;
7. Limitation of time for ICM activities, especially among individual Regional Representatives;
8. Insufficient knowledge of member association resources, etc. that could advance ICM goals/aims;
9. Changing demands on Headquarters outstrip resources and some member associations do not understand what is reasonable to expect from the Secretariat given existing resources;
10. Volunteer officers and directors and a structure than admits only midwifery associations that limits others from joining;
11. Multiple levels of midwives within some countries with varying expertise;
12. Varying risk-taking behaviours – high for promotion of Safe Motherhood activities but conservative financial management.

This list of weaknesses was challenging at best and discouraging at the very least for the leaders of the ICM, reflecting the need for help in moving the Confederation forward in a sustainable manner. Many of these weaknesses were overcome with time; others, especially in the financial and leadership areas, experienced a much slower improvement (Chapter 5).

Meeting of the Minds – 2001

Of vital importance to the future of ICM was Jhpiego's MNH programme support of the 'Meeting of Minds' in February 2001, bringing together 40 midwifery leaders from all regions of the world to help set the ICM's strategic directions for its future.[28] Six Strategic Objectives were agreed following days of discussion of the strengths and needs of the ICM as an organisation. The strategic objectives were:

1) Increase Partnership/Collaboration/Networking;
2) Inclusion of midwives in policymaking groups;
3) Promotion of the philosophy of midwifery care;
4) Initiate activities, including advocacy, to improve the status of the midwifery profession, nationally and internationally;
5) Strengthen and disseminate work on evidence-based midwifery care nationally and internationally; and
6) Improve the human resource situation and requirements for midwifery provision of services.[29]

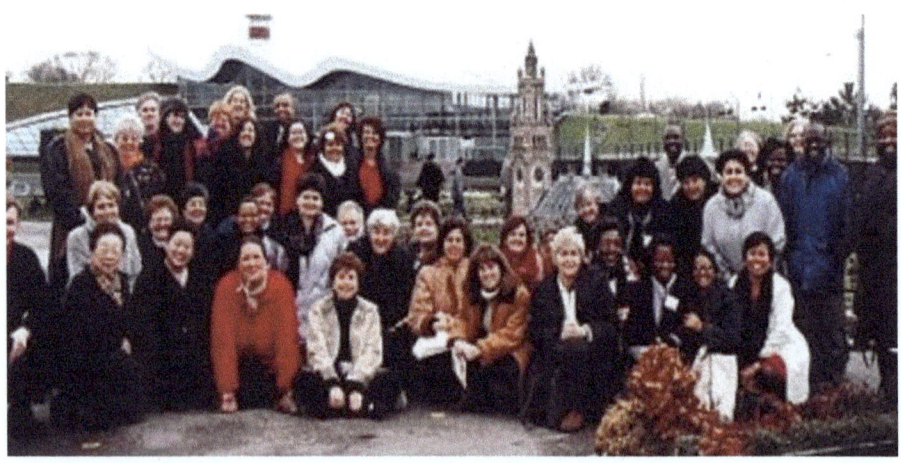

Participants at 'Meeting of the Minds' Technical Consultation of Midwifery Leaders 2001 – From ICM Minutes of the meeting

The Story Continues

The 2002 the ICM Council discussion of the *Global Strategy* document resulted in a slight rewording of the three original Strategic Objectives with three new goals added, including twinning of member associations. The Council directed the Board of Management to organise the now 15 specific goals by Strategic Objective, adopting 'in principle' the objectives and goals.[30]

The revised Global Strategy document was put to the ICM Council in 2005. It included a new goal 16 that read, 'continue to refine and strengthen the governance and management of ICM in order for it to achieve its aims and objectives'[31]. As noted in the introduction to the 2005–2008 Global Strategy document, the ICM reiterated that it accomplishes these goals primarily through its MAs and will:

1. **'Address women's health globally** with 4 goals focused on achievement of Safe Motherhood goals for all women using evidence-based midwifery practice, midwives influencing reproductive health policies, and working with women's groups;
2. **Strengthen the midwifery profession** with 6 goals focused on education, promoting professional autonomy, research, codes of ethics, midwifery human resource development and working collaboratively with other health workers to achieve optimal women's health globally; and
3. **Promote the organisation internationally** with 6 goals focused on securing financial viability for the ICM including increasing the number of MAs; strengthening governance and management of ICM to achieve its aims and objectives; facilitating sharing of members' experiences; and collaboration and consulting with international organisations, alliances and networks that share a common vision for the health of women and their families.'[32]

After much discussion during Council, the 2005–2008 *Global Strategy* document was agreed.[33]

The ICM Triennial Reports from 2008 onwards followed these three Strategic Objectives with the expansion of wording of goals for increased understanding by midwives and their partners.[34]

Strategic Planning during 2008 Council Meeting

In 2008 the ICM Board hired a management consultant, Thomas Lewinsky, to work with the ICM Council members in Glasgow. In addition to his assistance in helping MAs develop revised *Vision* and *Mission* statements in keeping with the realities of the day, he led the ICM MAs in the examination of strategic planning processes used until that time. Lewinsky reviewed the current structure of the ICM then made recommendations for an updated structure in accordance with new Dutch Articles of Association adopted in 2005. He recognised that the ICM did not have a clear strategic planning process which made accountability very difficult.[35]

Lewinsky proposed that the ICM needed to constantly review its purpose, operationalise its mission, set priorities for the organisation including 3–5 strategic objectives, use an effective transparent planning process through all levels, establish accountability of the Board and Secretariat to the Council, and, finally, the strategic plan should last 3–6 years.[36] Following much discussion, Council directed the Board to clarify the new governing structure focused on five strategic areas: 1) Review ICM partnerships and representation in global arena, 2) Establish a database of good practice, 3) Provide guidance on legislation issues, 4) Retain a strong presence in global areas and 5) Promote the midwifery profession and value of the midwife in keeping birth normal.[37] These strategic areas were then translated into the Strategic Directions as noted in Table 8.1 below.

New Approach in 2017

During the 2017 ICM Council, the Chair discussed the next triennium. The hallmarks were to remain, but the ICM was to move to an integrated model. The Board proposed an organising structure under the headings of Quality, Equity and Leadership:

- **Quality** meaning standardisation and sustainability.
- **Equity** meaning engagement (regions, collaboration) and member association programmes.
- **Leadership** meaning advocacy (approaching politics with one voice) and global partnerships as a strategy.[38]

The strategy was to look at areas within the ICM that needed to be focused on, and then decide how to demonstrate results. Thus, during the 2017–2020

triennium the ICM Board and Secretariat worked to accomplish the key strategic directions of Quality, Equity and Leadership focused:
- **Locally** with our Midwives Associations in countries.
- **Regionally** within the six ICM regions, through collaboration with all of our Member Associations.
- **Globally** on behalf of the more than 1 million midwives represented by our Member Associations.
- **Collaboratively** with our partners at local, regional and global levels.[39]

The Strategic Plan 2021–2023 shows the increasing maturity and inclusiveness of the position that the ICM now holds. It states, 'The strategic plan positions ICM as a partner, advocate, technical adviser, and knowledge base for midwives' associations and midwives around the world, allowing the organisation to grow and expand in tailored ways that will make the largest impact on the profession of midwifery, with broader impacts on gender equality human rights, diversity, and universal health coverage.'[40] In addition, the strategic planning process also aligned with the Year of the Midwife in 2020, and with plans to roll out the 'Decade of the Midwife' campaign with other partners in 2021.[41] This process allowed the ICM to focus and define the way forward through a holistic approach that will further enhance its impact and reach.

Strategic Directions Summarised

Below is a tabular snapshot of the Global Strategy that became Strategic Directions for the ICM since 2008 that continues to guide the work of the Confederation as determined by its Member Associations through policy directions agreed in the ICM Council Meetings.

Table 8.1
ICM Strategic Directions 2008–2022
ICM Strategic Directions with Objectives 2017–2023

Triennium	Strategic Directions
2008–2011[42] and 2011–2014[43]	1. Strengthen midwifery education and ongoing education programmes and the role of the midwife as an educator 2. Strengthen and support [enhance] midwives' professional autonomy to ensure midwifery education, regulation and practice is designed and governed specifically by midwives 3. Promote and support midwifery research that enhances and documents evidence-based midwifery practices 4. Raise awareness of midwifery and extend the influence of midwives in order to lobby and advocate for policy changes related to maternal, newborn and reproductive health care nationally and internationally 5. Enter into strategic collaborations with relevant international organisations, alliances and networks that share a common vision for the promotion of the health of women and their families
2014–2017[44]	1. Strengthen midwifery education, continuing education programmes and the role of the midwife as an educator 2. Enhance midwives' professional autonomy and ensure midwifery regulation, education and practice is designed and governed by midwives 3. Promote midwifery research that enhances and documents evidence-based midwifery practices 4. Advocate for midwifery and extend the influence of midwifery in policy development that drives service direction 5. Pursue strategic collaborations with relevant organisations and networks that share a common interest

2017–2020[45]	1. Quality 　a. Demand an enabling environment through which midwives can provide quality midwifery services 　b. Deliver global standards, resources and tools for education, regulation and associations to build the capacity, competency and professionalism of midwives 　c. Deliver as the experts on midwives and midwifery quality advice to stakeholders. 2. Equity 　a. Demand equitable access for midwives to midwifery education, regulation and continuing professional development 　b. Demand equitable access to midwife-led midwifery services for women 　c. Deliver equitable access to services and facilitate equitable opportunities for participation in ICM for Member Associations 3. Leadership 　a. Demand participation of midwives at the highest level of policy and decision-making at global, regional and local levels 　b. Deliver effective midwifery leadership and expertise
2021–2023[46]	**Goal: Position ICM as an expert in creating, advising, influencing and enabling the profession of midwifery globally.** *Strategic Priority 1:* Drive innovation and sustainability for the future of midwifery *Strategic Priority 2:* Develop, strengthen and support the rollout of a new professional framework for midwifery *Strategic Priority 3:* Foster a movement for midwifery, enabling and strengthening partnerships, advocacy and communications for midwifery, with women's voices at the centre The cross-cutting theme was **to promote gender equality** using a gender lens/perspective and giving it priority in each of the elements of the Strategic plan.

SUMMARY

It can be noted from Table 8.1 that the Global Strategy documents and Strategic Directions over the years relate directly back to the Aims and Objects in the Constitution and the Vision and Mission statements of the Confederation. The organisational loop is completed. The challenges and successes of carrying out these strategic directions are addressed in the chapters that follow, continuing the centennial story of the ICM.

100 Years of the International Confederation of Midwives

1. The Purpose statement introducing the 'Vision for Women and Their Health' and the 'Vision for the Future of Midwifery', 1996.
2. The term 'Objects' was used in most of the versions of the ICM Constitution from 1954 onward. More common use of an organisation's aim and objects is the term 'objectives'. The authors have chosen to use the term 'Objectives' reflective of today's common use in Constitutions.
3. ICM. *Strategic Planning Day, 19 June 1997*. London. [Personal papers of Joyce Thompson]
4. ICM & Maternal & Neonatal Health. *Meeting of the Minds: Technical Consultation of Midwifery Leaders. Workshop Report*. The Hague: ICM, 4–7 February 2001.
5. Triennial Reports for Board of Management elected officers 1993–1999 found in Wellcome Institute Library archives.
6. ICM. *Statement to the 4th World Conference on Women, Beijing, China, September 1995*. [Personal papers of Joyce Thompson]
7. UNFPA-LACRO Young Midwifery Leader Program. *Module 2 Module 9: Visioning & Strategic Planning*. Panama: UNFPA-LACRO, 2017.
8. Joel A Barker. *The Power of Vision* (video). 1991.
9. ICM. *Minutes of the ICM Council May 1996, Oslo, Norway*. The Vision for Women and for Midwifery were reinforced by the International Council in May 1999, Manila, Philippines. [Document in Executive Manual of 2002.] *Minutes of the International Confederation of Midwives Council Meeting … Vancouver, Canada … May 4, 5, 6, and 11, 1993*. MIN 93.36. Global Strategy: 1. 'Plan of action for next Triennium,' p 31. 'The mission statement and aims were as approved by the Executive Committee.' The rest of the *Global Strategy* document with the vision and goals was accepted in principle due to its complexity and referred out to members for comment in preparation for voting in 1996.
10. ICM. *Minutes of the International Confederation of Midwives Council Meeting … Vancouver, Canada…May 4, 5, 6, and 11, 1993*. MIN 93.36. Global Strategy: 1 'Plan of action for next Triennium.' p 31. *The Vision for Women and Their Health; The Vision for the Future of Midwifery*. The Hague: ICM, 1996. The formal Vision documents were officially adopted by the ICM Council in 1996 in Oslo, Norway, reviewed and reinforced by the International Council in May 1999, Manila, the Philippines.
    ICM. *The Vision for Women and Their Health; The Vision for the Future of Midwifery*. The Hague: ICM, 1993. These Vision statements were reviewed each triennium through 2007, when a proposal for eliminating them with a much shorter version following discussions with management consultant Thomas Lewinsky during the 2008 ICM Council. ICM. *ICM Council Meeting Minutes, Glasgow, Scotland, 2008*. The Hague: ICM, Agenda item 8.1.1. Governances, pp 15–16.
11. ICM. *International Code of Ethics for Midwives*. The Hague: ICM, 2020. The ICM *International Code of Ethics for Midwives* was first adopted in 1993 after regional consultations during 1990–1993. ICM. *Minutes of the International Confederation of Midwives Council Meeting … Vancouver, Canada. May 4,5,6,11, 1993*. MIN 93.22, p 19. The Code has been reviewed and reaffirmed by the ICM Council with minor changes every six years, with the most recent being 2020 (Chapter 11).
12. ICM. *Vision Statement* – 'Empowering Women … Empowering midwives', 1996, p 1 Statement of Purpose.
13. Management consultant Thomas Lewinsky led Council members in discussions of new vision and mission statements in keeping with the 2005 Dutch Constitution. ICM. *ICM Council Minutes, Glasgow, Scotland, 2008*. Agenda item 8.1.1. Governance, pp 15–16.
14. ICM. *Attention: For Member Association Consideration in Advance of ICM Council Meeting*. New ICM Vision and Mission Statements, 2007. Document in ICM Archives in Wellcome Collection.
15. ICM. *ICM Council Meeting Minutes, Glasgow, Scotland, 2008*. Agenda item 10.1.1.2, 2, 3, 4, 6, pp 21–23.
16. Margaret Peters. *Telephone Call with Joyce Thompson July 15, 2020*. Margaret reminded the authors that the history of midwifery is closely related to the history of women in each society; hence, the status of midwives that began as an important society-maintaining craft was slowly transformed into a respected profession moving toward equal status with medicine and nursing.
17. ICM. *ICM Council Minutes, Vienna Austria, April 2002*, Agenda 02.21.2 Essential competencies of basic midwifery practice, pp 12–13.
18. It was at this time that the Constitutional Aims were converted to a statement of mission.
19. ICM. *Minutes of the International Confederation of Midwives Council Meeting … Vancouver, Canada, … May 4, 5, 6, and 11, 1993*. MIN 93.36. Global Strategy: 1 Plan of action for next Triennium, p 31. ICM. *ICM Pamphlet, The International Confederation of Midwives*, 1999, p 1.
20. Downloaded from ICM Website 28 April 2020: www.internationalmidwives.org This mission statement was originally adopted during the ICM Council Meeting in 2008. ICM Triennial Reports of 2008, 2011, 2014, 2017 all have same Vision and Mission statements.
21. ICM. *Minutes of the International Confederation of Midwives Council Meeting … Vancouver, Canada…May 4, 5, 6, and 11, 1993*. MIN 93.36. Global Strategy: 1 'Plan of action for next Triennium,' p 31.

22 ICM. *Triennial Report 1993c1996*. ICM: London, 1996. Board of Management Report, p 3, lists the 12 goals set in 1993.
23 ICM. *Minutes of ICM Strategic Planning Day 19 June 1997*. [Personal papers of Joyce Thompson] 'During the Fall 1996 ICM Board of Management meeting, a decision was made to have a 1-day [facilitated] strategic planning session with Officers and members of the Board. The primary purpose of this planning session was to ... begin to set the goals and strategic activities for the new millennium, with an emphasis on financial viability and stability.' p 1.
24 ICM. *Global Strategic Plan 1996–1999*, pp 1–14. [Personal papers of Joyce Thompson]
25 ICM. *Global Strategic Plan 1996–1999*, pp 1–14. [Personal papers of Joyce Thompson]
26 ICM. *Strategic Planning Day, 19 June 1997*. London. [Personal papers of Joyce Thompson]
27 SWOT stands for an analysis of Strengths, Weaknesses, Opportunities and Threats.
28 ICM, Maternal & Neonatal Health, JHPIEGO Corporation. *Meeting of the Minds: Technical Consultation of Midwifery Leaders. 4–7 February 2001*. The Hague: Workshop Report, pp 13–16.
29 ICM. *Activities of the International Confederation of Midwives*. The Hague: ICM, 2001. Handout for public.
30 ICM. *ICM Council Meeting Minutes, Vienna, Austria, 2002*. Agenda item 02.21.1 Global Strategy, p 12.
31 ICM. *ICM Council Meeting Minutes, Brisbane, Australia, 18-21 July 2005*. Agenda item 05.21.1, pp 14–15. A new goal 16 was added following direction of the ICM Council in 2002 that related to governance and management.
32 ICM. *Global Strategy 2005–2008*. The Hague: ICM. [Joyce Thompson personal papers]
33 ICM. *ICM Council Meeting Minutes, Brisbane, Australia, 2005*. Agenda item 05.21.1, p 15.
34 ICM. *Triennial Report 2008–2011*. The Hague: ICM, 2011, pp 1–14; 18–22.
35 ICM. *ICM Council Meeting Minutes, Glasgow, Scotland, 2008*. Agenda item 8.1.2. Governance, pp 16–17.
36 ICM. *ICM Council Meeting Minutes, Glasgow, Scotland, 2008*. Agenda item 10.2 Strategic Planning Process, p 23.
37 ICM. *ICM Council Meeting Minutes, Glasgow, Scotland, 2008*. Agenda item 8.1.1. Governance, p 15.
38 ICM. *ICM Council Meeting Minutes, Toronto, Canada, 2017*. Open discussion, p 25.
39 ICM. *Triennial Report 2017–2020*. The Hague: ICM, p 4.
40 ICM. *Triennial Report 2017–2020*. The Hague: ICM, 2020. Can be downloaded from www.internationalmidwives.org
41 ICM. *Triennial Report 2017–2020*. The Hague: ICM, 2020. Can be downloaded from www.internationalmidwives.org
42 ICM. *Triennial Report 2008–2011*. The Hague: ICM pp 7, 11, 14, 18, 21.
43 ICM. *Triennial Report 2011–2014*. The Hague: ICM, 'Objectives', pp 12,14, 18, 19.
44 ICM. *Triennial Report 2014–2017*. The Hague: ICM, 2017, Strategic Directions, p 9.
45 ICM. *Triennial Report 2017–2020*. The Hague: ICM, 2020. Can be downloaded from www.internationalmidwives.org
46 ICM. *Triennial Report 2020–2023*. The Hague: ICM, 2020. Downloaded from www.internationalmidwives.org

Chapter 9: *Updating Midwives' Knowledge and Skills*

'I remember vividly the morning of the 1984 Triennial Congress in Sydney when I was called to the Registration Desk. There were several midwives from Iran who were standing there holding bags of Pistachio nuts they had brought with them. They asked if they could pay their registration fees with the nuts. They were desperate to attend the education sessions, coming from a country where midwives were undervalued and underpaid.'

Margaret Peters, ICM President

INTRODUCTION

Midwives since the 19th century have searched for ways to obtain updated knowledge and skills in order to provide the best care for mothers and babies. Meeting together was also valued as a time to share their 'stories' with one another and recharge their 'caring batteries' (Chapters 3 and 4), a key element of the ICM Congresses and workshops throughout the 20th and 21st centuries. IMU/ICM scientific congresses were the primary source of updated knowledge and skills for midwives and one of the most important ways that midwives continued their educational updates.

The content in this chapter addresses the ICM Congresses since 1954, Pre-Congress Workshops (PCWs) that began in 1987 with the global focus on promoting Safe Motherhood, Mid-Triennium Regional meetings with Symposia and selected country workshops supported by the ICM's global partners. Each of these gatherings addressed the needs/requests from Member Associations (MAs) and individual midwives to learn the most up-to-date information. In addition, information about midwifery education, practice and association development from a variety of country perspectives is included, complementing Regional Perspectives found in Chapter 13. A selection of these Congresses and educational efforts are highlighted for their significance to the growth and development of the ICM as an international organisation.

TRIENNIAL CONGRESSES: SCIENTIFIC MEETINGS

One decision mandated by the British-based ICM Constitution adopted during the 1954 Executive Committee meeting in London was that official ICM Congresses would occur every three years.[1] Since the mid-1950s, such Congresses have taken place in a variety of countries, often strengthening the national midwifery association that hosted the international gathering of midwives and showcasing the midwifery profession.[2] [Refer to Annex C: Table of Congresses and Themes 1954–2021.]

Locations of Congresses

By the time of the 1960 Congress in Rome the ICM finances were said to be more stable and 22 of 27 MAs were represented at the Executive Committee Meeting. This Congress was not without its mini-drama (see text box) and unique highlights.[3]

> *President Ellen Erup fractured her leg the day before the beginning of Congress and Vice-President Signora Luzzi, who was the President of the Italian Midwives Association, was terminally ill in hospital, passing away in November that year. The other Vice-President Madame Jay took up overseeing the Congress and is reported to have done this expertly.*

Several 'firsts' were claimed as the Union of Soviet Socialist Republics (USSR) sent a representative, revealing how far the name and reputation of the ICM reached. Another decision taken in 1960 was to revert to the pre-WWII practice of appointing the next President related to the next Congress rather than selecting a prominent midwife in the country currently hosting the Congress.[4] Group discussions were introduced during Congresses enabling the greater sharing of practice and experiences, with the crystallised opinions reported back to full Congress. A decision was made to add German as an official language for the 1963 Congress to enable a more inclusive participation. Another unique opportunity during the Rome Congress was an audience with Pope John for those interested.

Spain was the venue for the 1963 Triennial Congress, where on 29 June, the Madrid Spanish Midwives' Association presented the ICM with a gift of a Presidential Chain of Office.[5] This had been designed and made by Spanish craftspeople, made of silver links with a central blue enamel ICM badge. Since this time the names of Presidents have been engraved on the links with extra links added as required. During the 1966 Congress in Berlin, ICM President Frau Springborn recalled the city holding a very special niche in the annals of international midwifery as the very first international meeting for midwives was held here on 30 and 31 September 1900 under the chairmanship of Frau Olga Gebauer[6] (Chapter 3).

The ICM spread its wings beyond Europe by taking the 1969 triennial congress to Santiago, Chile. Three years later the 1972 Congress (see insert back cover) was held in the United States of America (USA). This location was significant in that midwifery had all but been obliterated in the USA during the course of the early 20th century.[7] The 1978 Congress was held in Israel and the 1984 Congress in Australia – the first in the Asia-Pacific Region. The 1999 ICM Congress was held in Manila, Philippines, the first in a low resource country. It required careful planning and many visits to Manila by the Director of ICM, Margaret Peters, during the lead-up three years from 1996 to assist in the programming needed for a successful Congress. The first ICM Congress held on the African continent was in Durban, South Africa, in 2011. (Annex C Lists Congress sites 1954–2021.)

Management of Triennial Congresses

Congresses were co-managed by the Host Association and the ICM Headquarters (HQ) following Guidelines for the Conduct of International Congresses in 1996.[8] The Host Association signed an 'Agreement to Host' contract that included the registration capitation fee that was to be returned to HQ along with the split of any profits among other items. A Congress Handbook facilitated this process and included the fact that the Host Association would select a congress organiser in the country to handle details in collaboration with the ICM HQ.[9] This often worked well until 2002 when the ICM Council voted that all future ICM Congresses were to be managed from HQ using a professional Congress organiser.[10]

Structure of Triennial Congresses

Congress usually began with an inter- or multi-faith celebration and an Opening Ceremony where flags of each nation in attendance were presented by that midwives' group wearing traditional dress until the early 2000s. Daily keynote speakers were generally global leaders in health and plenary speakers were international midwives, all of whom raised the profile of midwives internationally. Education sessions filled each day of the Congress. Time for social gatherings was set aside often involving a meal, with a much enjoyed 'cultural night' that included samples of food from the host country and dancing. From the 1990s onward, the number of exhibitors expanded in a trade display hall, offering midwives the opportunity to learn about the latest in treatment options for women and babies, published books of interest and time to test out the newest models for teaching. Johnson and Johnson International has been a Gold Sponsor of Congresses for many years.[11] These exhibitors also brought significant income into the ICM's bank account. The text below is one example of the excitement of midwives attending their first ICM Congress.

> *'We would have liked to tell you about the astute, dramatic, and eloquent presentation of Mme Jay of France, the contributions from the developing countries which are going to be increasingly important in the years to come, the lovely Concert Hall where we had our meetings, the reunion of old friends, the beauty of the native costumes, the wonderful social events, the lively entertainment, and above all, the smooth organization that made all this possible in one short week.'*
> **Ruth Coates and Marion Strachan of USA reporting on their first Congress attended in 1957 in Sweden.**

Each Congress in the last few decades was organised around a theme agreed by the ICM Board of Management/Board, with sub-themes for continuing education sessions. The Board of Management and Regional Representatives worked together with the Host Association to select international speakers of note from various countries and global partners with the intent of covering each Region so that midwives were exposed to a variety of viewpoints from many areas of the world. As will be noted in Chapter 10, the ICM Scientific Committee was established in 1990[12] to review and select oral and poster presentations that fit the themes of the Congress from the hundreds of abstracts received. The Research Standing Committee representative was added in 2002 as the number of research-based abstracts increased.[13] Most Congress Programmes can be accessed in the ICM archives at the Wellcome Institute Library in London with permission of the ICM.

The attendance at Congresses was high in countries with lots of midwives such as Japan and Australia or sites where midwives wished to visit, such as the United States, British Colombia and South Africa. European Congresses were generally well-attended due to the large number of midwives in many countries. The exception was the 1981 Congress in England that conflicted with other European meetings and held little interest at the time for British midwives who wanted the Congress in Asia[14], resulting in a significant financial loss that was covered by the Royal College of Midwives, as noted previously.

SAFE MOTHERHOOD PRE-CONGRESS WORKSHOPS

One of the important educational offerings for midwives from resource limited countries who would not otherwise be able to attend Council or Congresses was a series of PCWs on themes related to Safe Motherhood. The ICM organisationally became a vital partner in the global Safe Motherhood Initiatives (SMI) beginning in 1987, a sentinel event in the ICM's History as the connection with the WHO, other UN agencies and FIGO literally expanded the influence of the ICM and midwives across the globe. The ICM's involvement in the SMI began with collaborative pre-congress and other workshops/conferences addressing the various aspects of the SMI, including midwifery education, midwifery leadership and quality midwifery care.

The global Safe Motherhood Initiative was launched at the Nairobi Conference in February 1987.[15] The social injustice[16] reflected by the needless loss of women's lives during childbearing had been reflected upon and discussed at many earlier international meetings. The health organisations involved were especially concerned for childbearing women in low resource countries in sub-Sahara Africa, South-East Asia and Latin America. Part of the discussion during these meetings included the vital role that midwives could play in reducing the Maternal Mortality Rate (MMR) and the Neonatal Mortality Rate (NMR) along with morbidity rates among women and newborns. As noted by Joan Bentley (UK midwife working at WHO), most of the world's 'relatively well-educated and sophisticated midwives' represented in the ICM membership at that time worked primarily in well-equipped settings, leaving them unable 'to function effectively in poorly equipped rural health units with little or no managerial or technical support.'[17] She went on to note that many of these midwives also refused to work in such areas for personal reasons. This lack of understanding of the plight of midwives from low resource countries (LRCs) was slowly overcome as midwifery associations from these countries became ICM members.

The appointment of Barbara Kwast, a Dutch midwife and epidemiologist[18], as the WHO's Technical Advisor to the ICM in 1986, pushed the ICM into action. She worked very closely initially with Marie Goubran (ICM Secretary General) and Filippa Lugtenburg (ICM President) on efforts in 1987 to engage the ICM and midwives throughout the world in making pregnancy and birth safe for mothers and babies. Kwast continued to lead/support the ICM's SMI efforts for several years in workshops that linked midwifery education and practice efforts that made a difference in the health of childbearing women and newborns. Below is a brief overview of the Safe Motherhood workshops at the ICM triennial congresses from 1987 to 2005, followed by mid-triennium conferences, and selected SM country workshops. Each of these demonstrated the ICM's commitment and value in educating midwives, its MAs and global partners, and the workshops' value to the ICM's growth as an international organisation.

Purpose and Organisation of Pre-Congress Workshops

The overall purpose of holding ICM collaborative pre-congress workshops (PCWs), followed by mid-triennium conferences and workshops in Africa, India and Trinidad, was to share the magnitude of maternal and neonatal morbidity and mortality with midwives and provide them with the knowledge and tools needed to be active participants in efforts to make pregnancy and birth safer for all women and their newborns. These workshops fulfilled a large portion of the ICM's goal of providing educational updates for midwives. The WHO, UNICEF, UNFPA and FIGO along with midwives with extensive international experience provided much of the technical expertise required on the various Safe Motherhood topics.

Sadly, most of the midwives working with childbearing women facing alarming rates of death and disability lived in LRCs (99 per cent of maternal deaths occurred in non-industrialised countries in the 1980s). Many of these midwives were not part of an ICM MA, though through exposure to ICM workshops over time their country associations were organised and supported to become ICM members. Likewise, most LRC midwives required financial support to participate in the ICM workshops which was provided by several major donors such as UN agencies, USAID, the Rockefeller Foundation and several high resource country (HRC) MAs and individual midwives through the ICM Safe Motherhood Fund.[19]

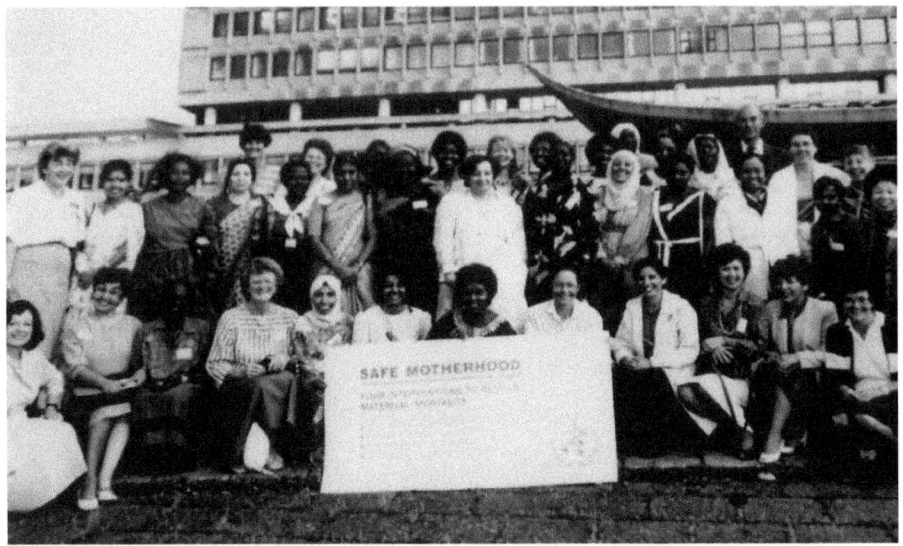

Safe Motherhood workshop in The Hague 1987 – ICM Archives at Wellcome Collection

The <u>organisation of each sponsored PCW</u> varied slightly from 1987 through to 2005. In 2002 the ICM Board adopted a manual detailing the distinct activities required in preparation for each workshop, during the workshop and after each workshop.[20] This manual pulled together successful aspects of the five prior PCWs, lessons learned, and gave future ICM Boards, staff and partners a guide to follow. The ICM SG kept a running list of participants in each workshop so that different countries and participants were targeted each triennium, spreading the knowledge and skills to as many midwives and countries as possible.[21]

<u>Elements of planning</u> each PCW included the definition, purpose, theme, duration, proposed venue, number of participants, sponsorship and fund-raising needed along with the ICM headquarters' (HQ) management of details, such as invitations, travel, lodging arrangements, briefing and selection of leaders. Designated individuals agreed by the ICM Board to lead the PCW worked on background papers and other materials to be used during the workshop including action plans and evaluation forms, inviting speakers with expertise matching the content chosen, and the plan for follow-up of action plans generally carried out by the ICM HQ staff. Simultaneously, ICM staff would work with collaborating partners on the selection of countries and midwife participants to be invited, the vetting process, budget and sponsorship needs along with confirming venue

details in the city and country of the next ICM Congress.

These collaborative efforts expanded the number of midwives involved in these activities beyond the ICM Board and staff and facilitated the development of important relationships with other international health organisations and NGOs who recognised the value of the ICM representing the world's midwives as a vital link in Safe Motherhood activities. Workshop methods included information sharing, small group work to address specific aspects, case studies and practice sessions using new content and practical skills, such as interviews of women experiencing violence. Evaluations were consistently very positive.

One of the greatest challenges to the ICM as an organisation with limited staff and methods of communication in the 1990s was gaining participants for the workshops. For example, prior to the time that electronic communication was somewhat functional at the ICM Headquarters, in all ICM MAs, and in LRCs without ICM MAs, the process of receiving nominations for midwives to attend the PCWs was very difficult. Following Board decisions on countries to be invited to nominate participants, the ICM Secretary General (the only staff member in the early 1990s) would send letters (and fax when available) to governments, the WHO and UNICEF country offices and ICM MAs. She also attempted to phone members (often without success due to lack of MA offices or working phones for the MA President), or because of a change in leadership without notifying the ICM HQ. Despite these barriers and challenges, the ICM and its collaborative partners were successful in providing up-to-date, evidence-based knowledge and skills for midwives in areas noted below in Table 9.1.

Table 9.1
Pre-Congress Collaborative Safe Motherhood Workshops

Year Date of Workshop	Place	Title Key Presenters/ or Authors of Background Papers	Responsible Partners & Representatives Sponsors	Number midwives & # countries
1987 21–22 August	Den Hague, Netherlands	**Women's Health & the Midwife: A Global Perspective** J Bentley, Dr J Mutambirwa & L Lorenzetti Action Statement	WHO – B Kwast ICM – M Peters, R Ashton, A Payne UNICEF	30 Invited 20 countries +ICM, WHO & UNICEF Secretariats FIGO & ICN Reps
1990 5–6 October	Kobe, Japan	**Midwifery Education: Action for Safe Motherhood** B Kwast & J Bentley: background paper Action Statement	WHO-B. Kwast ICM – H Schweitzer UNICEF G Maclean, A Kamara, V Tickner, & Dr Duangvadee Sungkhobol: Facilitators	40 Participants 19 countries + ICM, WHO, UNICF, ICN, FIGO, World Bank
1993 7–8 May	Vancouver, British Columbia	**Midwifery Practice: Measuring, Developing and Mobilizing Quality Care** Rosemary Jenkins: background paper Action Statement	WHO – B Kwast ICM – M Peters UNICEF RCM-ACNM UNFPA	38 participants 22 countries
1996 23–26 May	Oslo, Norway	**Strengthening Midwifery Within Safe Motherhood** J Thompson & V Ruth Bennett: background paper	ICM WHO UNICEF	38 invited 16 countries

1996[22] 23–26 May	Oslo, Norway	**Consultant/Adviser Workshop for Safe Motherhood**	Self-Pay workshop V Ruth Bennett	41 participants 15 countries
1999	Manila, Philippines	**Frontiers of Midwifery Care – STDs/HIV/AIDS in Safe Motherhood** Caroline Homer: Background paper	ICM – Ruth Ashton WHO – Sr Anne Thompson UNICEF UNFPA, UNAIDS – Sandra Anderson	50 participants 24 countries
2002 11–14 April	Vienna, Austria	**The Midwife's Role in Reducing Violence Against Adolescent Girls & Women: Promoting Safe Motherhood** Annotated bibliography of background information provided	ICM – Ruth Ashton WHO – Claudia Garcia Moreno UNICEF UNFPA – France Donnay FIGO	67 participants (45 sponsored, 22 self-pay) 32 countries[23]
2005 21–23 July	Brisbane, Australia	**Promoting the health of mothers and newborns during birth and the postnatal period** Frances Ganges (Independent consultant newborn health)	ICM – NT Moyo WHO – D Sherratt UNFPA POPPHI – D Armbruster Save the Children + many sponsors	43 Participants 29 countries

These PCWs had a definite <u>impact on the growth and development</u> of the ICM as an international NGO as they sought to update midwives' competencies to reduce maternal and newborn deaths and disabilities. Each of these workshops assisted the ICM in moving forward on setting global education and regulation standards and creating the tools that would strengthen its MAs and help them advocate for improved quality of care for women, childbearing families and newborns – key aims of the Confederation. An expected outcome of participation in these workshops and conferences was that the midwives who participated had an opportunity to update their practice competencies while also being supported by other midwives in the difficult tasks facing them to reduce the needless deaths of childbearing women and newborns. The workshops also strengthened the ICM's relationships with and support from UN agencies and major donors such as the Swedish International Development Cooperation Agency (SIDA) and the Dutch Ministry of Foreign Affairs. Details of each of these workshops can be found in the ICM published reports housed in the ICM archives at the Wellcome Institute Library in London and in the WHO archives for those published by the WHO.

MID-TRIENNIUM EXECUTIVE COMMITTEE MEETINGS WITH SYMPOSIA

The 1993 ICM Council members agreed that mid-triennium Executive Committee meetings should be held in developing countries whenever possible.[24] The reasons included increased support for midwives and midwifery associations in LRCs along with the opportunity to hold conferences or symposia for the midwives in those regions of the world where LRC midwives did not have the funds to travel to ICM Congresses and for whom continuing education courses/workshops were not available.[25] These conferences/symposia also offered the country MA the opportunity to host and therefore bring national notice to their efforts while strengthening their organisational capacity with the strong support of the ICM Secretariat.

The first such symposium titled 'Vision with Action – Midwives and Safe Motherhood',[26] was held in Entebbe, Uganda 13–15 January 1995. The two-day symposium, hosted by the Uganda Private Midwives Association, originally invited 40 midwives from African countries (32 invited were present). However, due to the great interest from other African midwives who were able to travel to Uganda, 62 observers were admitted who became active participants. Sr Anne Thompson (WHO, Geneva) gave an overview of the global Safe Motherhood Initiatives (SMI), and the rest of the speakers were from various African nations presenting activities ongoing in SMI, midwifery education, quality measures and political action needed to promote Safe Motherhood. Throughout the two days, African midwives described, discussed and debated the issues that were denying so many African women safe motherhood. This discussion also made real to the ICM Executive Committee members from HRCs the difficult situation that many African women and midwives face during childbearing as well as their newborns. English- and French-speaking African nations were represented, with

ICM regional representatives with those languages facilitating their participation.

The next mid-triennium Executive Committee meeting and Safe Motherhood workshop was held in New Delhi, India, February 1998.[27] The Australian College of Midwives Inc. volunteered to assist and support the logistics of hosting this meeting in a country without a midwifery association (the first time), supported by vote of the ICM Council members in May 1996.[28] The emphasis of this SM workshop was a shared commitment to improve the health of women and their babies by improving midwifery skills and better use/deployment of midwifery personnel.[29] India and other South-East Asian countries had a paucity of midwives and a high level of maternal and newborn deaths. The Safe Motherhood goal of halving the MMR by 2000 was not met in this region of the world, and midwives required support to make a difference in the health of women and their newborns. This support needed to come from the profession (skills update, including practise as well as advocacy skills) and from policymakers who needed to remove legal barriers to full-scope midwifery practice, especially midwives' use of life-saving skills.

The third and final mid-triennium Executive Committee meeting and workshop was held in Port-of-Spain, Trinidad in 2002. ICM Regional Conferences were to take the place of mid-triennium conferences that were attached to an Executive Committee meeting, and the Executive would continue to meet mid-triennium after 2002 when financially feasible.[30] Refer to Table 9.2.

Table 9.2
ICM Mid-Triennium Workshops/Symposia

Year	Place	Focus/Title	Responsible	Sponsors	# midwives present
1995 13–14 January	Lake Victoria, Uganda	'Vision with Action: Midwives & Safe Motherhood'	ICM V Ruth Bennett Joyce Thompson **67 Action Plans with follow-up**	ICM SM Fund DFID – UK WHO – Sr Anne Thompson MHD UNFPA	**35 invited** (24 Uganda & 11 from other sub-Saharan countries = 12 countries) **62 Observers**

100 Years of the International Confederation of Midwives

1998 17–18 February	New Delhi, India	Safe Motherhood Workshops 'Improving Women's Health Utilizing Persons with Midwifery Skills' 'Improving Women's Health with Midwifery Trained Personnel'	ICM/WHO ACMI Judi Brown Della Sherratt – UK Sr Anne Thompson (WHO)	ICM SM Fund WHO-Geneva WHO-SEARO UNICEF-New Delhi AUSAID DFID ICM MAs: Germany, Japan, RCM	**47 invited** (24 India) **17 countries** including two from Iran
2002	Port-of-Spain, Trinidad	PPH Prevention Bilingual workshop Young Midwifery Leaders Programme initiated	ICM Nester Moyo Judi Brown UNFPA-LACRO	ICM UNFPA-LACRO Jhpiego MNH	**425 midwives 35 countries** **Five YMLs Five countries** Germany, Malawi, Slovenia, South Arica, Trinidad

ICM-LED WORKSHOPS DURING CONGRESSES

Prior to each Triennial Congress, the ICM Board of Management would consider requests from MAs and decide on needed ICM activities and/or projects to be highlighted during planned concurrent Congress workshops. For example, when the ICM Code of Ethics for Midwives was adopted in 1993, a workshop was planned to talk about how MAs might use and/or develop a Code of Ethics themselves. This workshop was led by Joyce Thompson (Deputy Director) and Sr Anne Thompson (WHO).[31] Several education and research workshops were led during each Triennial Congress by members of ICM Standing Committees. For example, the ICM Research Standing Committee held four workshops during the ICM Congress in Brisbane in 2005 that included: 1) Developing a Research Agenda; 2) Scientific Writing for Midwives; 3) Evaluation Research in Developing and Developed countries and 4) Developing Guidelines for International Midwifery Research Collaboration.[32] The ICM staff and other midwife experts led workshops on use of ICM documents for advocacy, writing for publication, how to meet with political leaders, etc. In addition, ICM Partners such as the

J&J Paediatric Institute, White Ribbon Alliance and Jhpiego (POPPHI project) provided workshops for Congress participants. Midwives could choose which workshops to attend, and most ICM-led workshops were planned to avoid conflict with the scientific programme.

REGIONAL MEETINGS/CONFERENCES

It was expected that each ICM Region would host a regional meeting with educational sessions during each triennium, though that did not always happen. Europe and Asia-Pacific regions held the most Regional Conferences, in part because the stronger MAs provided or sought external funding from a variety of sources or, in the case of Europe, travel was much easier on the continent. The Americas and Africa regions had limited numbers of ICM MAs and used their annual meetings (Americas) or did not have the financial resources or capability of hosting such a conference (Africa). These meetings were very important to the region's midwives who were not able to attend Triennial Congresses for knowledge and skills updates. The meetings were essentially educational in nature with sponsored workshops on various topics, often led by ICM staff or donors such as UNFPA or Jhpiego MNH project. Time was set aside for updates from the ICM Board member(s) who were part of the MAs involved. The Regional Representative led open mic[33] sessions to hear the issues and concerns of regional MAs, often leading to draft position statements for consideration during the upcoming Triennial Council meetings.

Each ICM Region's MAs held meetings during the Triennial Council/ Congresses and planned for their Regional conference/workshops during that time. For example, the first Asia-Pacific Regional Conference was held in October 1985. It was a two-day meeting in Jakarta, Indonesia. ICM Regional Representatives were Pamela Hayes (Australia) and Cheiko Nohno (Japan). Six countries attended with Brunei sending two observers.[34] The first European regional workshop was held in Tubingen, West Germany in 1989 focusing on a basic introduction to research appreciation under the title, 'Research Needs Midwives – Midwives Need Research.'[35]

Most regional meetings were cost neutral when sufficient midwives attended (registration fees). However, occasionally the costs exceeded the income, and money was sought from HQ or donors to help the Host Association. At times, projected costs for a given meeting or conference were prohibitive and/or the political situation in a country was unstable, causing the proposed meeting to be cancelled.

Originally the ICM Regional Representatives assisted the host association in designing and implementing the regional meetings and managing the details of the Regional Conferences without financial support from ICM. During the 1990s each named Regional Representative was allocated £200 to fund an activity.[36] The Region would decide which MA would host the conference, and then a conference fee would be assessed to help support the meeting. From 2005 to 2017, the ICM left the management of these regional meetings to the Host association with support of the ICM Regional Representatives.

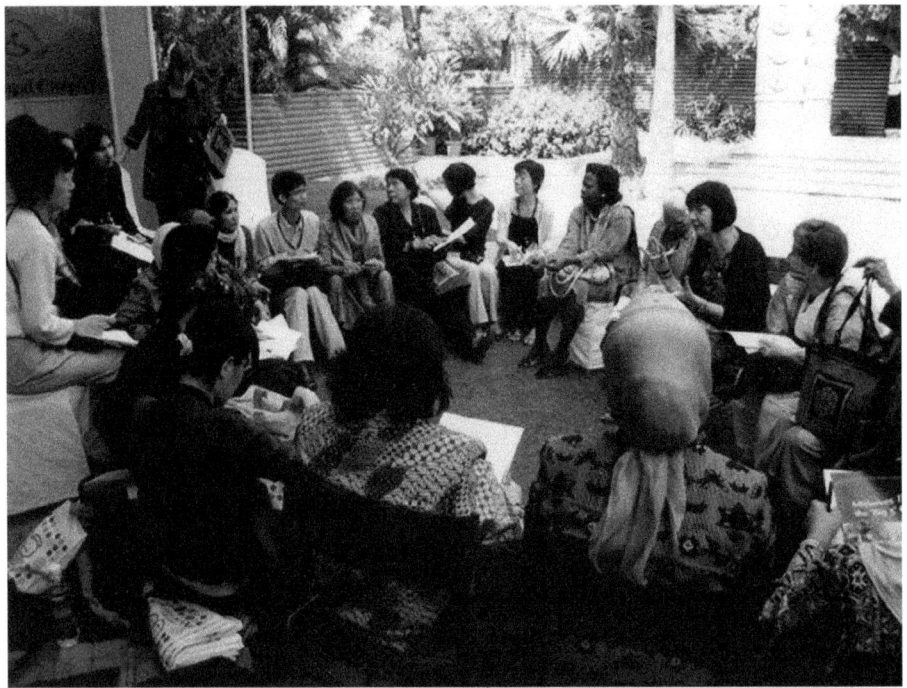

Asia-Pacific Regional Meeting, India 2009 – Courtesy of Karen Guilliland

Examples of more recent regional meetings include those held in July 2015 thousands of miles apart. They included one in the Americas (Suriname) and in one in Asia-Pacific (Japan) in 2015.[37] The Suriname Regional Conference was the 5th in the Americas and included presentations by the President of the ICM and inspirational closing remarks by the ICM's Global Goodwill Ambassador,

Her Excellency, Mrs Toyin Ojora Saraki. The theme of the conference, attended by approximately 200 midwives from MAs in the Caribbean, Latin and North America, was, 'Invest in healthy pregnancies; invest in midwives.' The Asia-Pacific regional conference had more than 3,200 delegates from 37 countries at the 11th Asia-Pacific meeting hosted by the three Japanese MAs. The conference theme was, 'Midwifery Care for Every Mother and her Newborn.' The conference was opened by Her Highness Imperial Princess of Japan.[38]

In 2017 the ICM Council voted to return the management of regional conferences to the ICM Headquarters using the contracted Professional Congress Organiser, P-CIN.[39] Collaboration with the Host Association continued. This decision was taken in an effort to control costs and implement sound management principles. Though the intent was good, sometimes the delay in decisions at HQ fostered delays in implementing the regional conference, such as happened in the Americas (Paraguay) in 2018. A revised Regional Conference handbook was adopted in 2021 to explain the joint responsibilities more clearly for MAs and P-CIN.

COUNTRY WORKSHOPS

There were several follow-up ICM/WHO Safe Motherhood sub-regional and country workshops after the 1987 collaborative Pre-Congress Workshop in The Hague, carried out primarily by the ICM HQ and WHO staff as they followed up on participants' plans of action.[40] Three examples follow.

Burkina Faso

Two ICM/WHO Regional Change Management workshops followed the 1987 Pre-Congress workshop: one for English-speaking African countries and one for French-speaking African countries. The Francophone workshop, held in Burkina Faso 12–19 January 1990, was led by Joan Bentley (WHO & ICM consultant), Barbara Kwast (WHO/MCH) and Eddie Bokoum (WHO Regional Office, Mali). This workshop was supported by the Burkina Faso Midwives Association, the Rockefeller Foundation and MotherCare, with midwives from Burkina Faso, Benin, Guinea, Mali, Mauritania, Niger, Senegal and Togo present.[41]

Ghana

From 16 to 21 January 1989 a sub-regional workshop for West Africa was held in Ghana, based on the Action Statement from the 1987 ICM Congress in The

Hague calling for the expansion of the midwives' role in maternal care from support to leadership in Safe Motherhood efforts. It was acknowledged at the time that 'midwives are rarely prepared or properly placed to take up such a role'.[42] The theme was 'Enhancing National Midwifery Services', co-sponsored by the ICM, WHO, the Rockefeller Foundation and the Ghana Registered Midwives Association.[43] The organisers took a country team approach to this workshop that included 25 midwives, medical officers, obstetricians and hospital administrators or health planners from The Gambia, Ghana, Liberia, Nigeria and Sierra Leone.

The goal of the workshop was to produce a firm plan of action within the constraints of existing health services in each country. The final detailed implementation plans were based on problems identified, solutions proposed, specific objectives and strategic activities as well as monitoring and evaluation plan. The four common issues identified included: 1) Insufficient professionally trained midwives with unsatisfactory distribution, especially to rural areas; 2) Inadequate number of midwife trainers well prepared with life-saving skills and low standards of midwifery practice; 3) Poor antenatal services with poor attendance (low value of prenatal care) and 4) Poor referral systems and processes including lack of emergency services and transport to reach needed care.[44]

Zimbabwe

The 2001 Safe Motherhood workshop in Harare, Zimbabwe, focused on Safe Motherhood as a basic human right for every woman,[45] the first rights-based conference for the ICM and African midwives. It was attended by 38 sponsored midwives (12 from Zimbabwe) from 19 sub-Saharan African countries. This workshop was especially important to the women (and midwives) of Africa, many of whom experienced very few rights within their society and their homes. Reproductive rights were the focus of the discussions, using the WHO manual, Advancing Safe Motherhood Through Human Rights and its Reproductive Rights Framework,[46] along with selected case studies from African adolescent girls and women. The keynote address was given by TL Ngwenya, Deputy Director of the Musasa Project, an NGO dedicated to combat domestic violence. Khosi Xaba of IPAS South Africa led participants in discussions about how it felt to have one's basic rights denied with Karen Otsea of IPAS presenting information on women's lack of choice related to access to safe abortions. Unsafe abortions were the number one cause of maternal mortality in many areas of the world due to lack of availability of family planning services and safe abortion care. Midwives' role in postabortion care was highlighted, and action plans developed to use this new rights-based approach to midwifery care.

The Regional Conference followed the SM workshop with a theme of, 'Achieving Midwifery Partnerships with Women for Safe Motherhood.' ICM Director, Joyce Thompson, gave the keynote address titled, 'Safe Motherhood: A Call to Action for Women, Men, and especially Midwives.' The value of this Conference to the ICM was affirmation of its vision[47] that midwifery partnerships with women implies consultation with women, advocacy for women and empowerment of women as midwives offer high quality, woman-centred care.

Specific Country Efforts: 2005 and Beyond

The ways that the ICM's major funders supported ICM activities throughout the world shifted following the 2005 PCW workshop, focusing more on country-level activities. Refer to Annex D: Table of ICM Partners & Projects 1951–2022.

ICM EDUCATION FOR MIDWIFERY TEACHERS

In keeping with the ICM's commitment to updating midwives' knowledge and skills, specific workshops addressing teacher competencies and setting global standards for midwifery education were vital, vastly improving the autonomy of the profession and global status of the ICM.

Competency-Based Education Workshops

Once the ICM Council adopted the first iteration of the Essential Competencies for Basic Midwifery Practice in 2002 (Chapter 12), efforts to assist MAs understand how to teach to these competencies began.[48] Competency-Based Education (CBE) workshops began in the Americas region in 2013 using the updated Essential Competencies. These were Trainer of Trainers (TOT) workshops so that midwifery teachers and clinical preceptors from several countries would learn 'How' to teach to competencies and then teach others to use the competency-based teaching, learning and evaluation strategies. These CBE capacity-building workshops preparing CBE Master Teachers for the rest of the world continued.[49] ICM Staff Martha Bokosi, Nester Moyo and Janet Lewis were prepared by Joyce Thompson, Emmanuelle Herbert and Catherine Carr (Jhpiego) and then became part of the global team of ICM consultants in CBE. Two manuals by an ICM

Consultant (Joyce Thompson) were written for use by these CBE Master Teachers in Francophone and Anglophone Africa, Latin America, Haiti and elsewhere when requested by a MA and/or midwifery education programme director.

Strengthening Midwifery Education in French-speaking Africa

The Sanofi Espoir Foundation began partnering with ICM to update French-speaking African midwifery education programmes and teachers in keeping with the ICM Education Standards in 2016. For example, Emmanuelle Herbert (Canada), one of the ICM CBE Master Teachers, led several Trainer of Trainers (TOT) workshops for French-speaking midwifery teachers during 2016–2017 funded by Sanofi.[50]

Global Standards for Basic Midwifery Education with Guidelines

The ICM Global Standards for Midwifery Education with Guidelines was agreed by the ICM Board of Management in 2010, endorsed by the ICM Council in 2011 and revised in 2013 (Chapter 14). These standards and their accompanying Guidelines have been used in all regions of the world to assess current midwifery education curricula and/or in the design of new midwifery education programmes.

Midwifery Education Accreditation Programme (MEAP)

Adoption of the essential practice competencies and education standards provided the basis for the most recent ICM activity in accreditation of midwifery education programmes. The Midwifery Education Accreditation Programme (MEAP) has been in development since 2015, with financial support from the Bill and Melinda Gates Foundation.[51] MEAP was tested in three additional countries in 2020.[52] The ICM Education Standing Committee (ESC), working with the ICM Secretariat, finalised the MEAP in 2021 for use globally where needed. This programme continued to be field tested in 2021 and is available on the ICM website[53] to MAs and country educators/other stakeholders interested in strengthening midwifery education based on the ICM competencies and standards. The Gates Foundation grant supported the ICM in further development of the Midwifery Education Development Pathway (MEDPath), a virtual portal for sharing educational tools.

Additional education resources

Education resources since the 1990s for MAs and those responsible for midwifery education in a given geographic area include Position Statements reflected in Annex A and tools developed by ICM consultants for use by MAs. These included:

- ICM Curriculum Mapping Tool, 2011 (rev. 2013), that allowed midwifery educators to determine concordance of their midwifery curriculum with the ICM essential competencies;
- ICM Standard Equipment List for Competency-Based Skills Training in Midwifery Schools, 2012;
- ICM Curriculum Models for Midwifery Education, 2012, with four modules including one that provided a sample curriculum plan for a 3-year direct entry and an 18-month post-nursing programme and another module describing competency-based education;
- ICM Gap Analysis tool for the Education Standards developed for Africa in 2011 and expanded use in Latin America; and
- ICM Competency-Based Education (CBE) Manuals for CBE Master Teachers and Continuing Education (CE) Workshops developed in 2014 and used by ICM consultants in Latin America, Mexico, French- and English-speaking African nations, the Caribbean and South Asia, among other countries.

Many midwifery teachers and preceptors, especially in LRCs where midwifery was relatively new, have used one or more of these documents and found them very useful. In addition, ICM consultants were part of the team that developed the WHO's Midwifery Educator Core Competencies in 2013 that have been disseminated and available for use by midwifery educators throughout the world. These resources were used by the ICM and other midwifery education consultants to strengthen midwifery education in areas of world where needed, once again strengthening the autonomy of the midwifery profession globally and heightening the visibility/importance of the ICM. The ICM Glossary of Terms[54] is the only education resource on the ICM website in 2021, though contact information for the ICM Education Standing Committee (ESC) is available. 'An online learning platform (Moodle) has been established to support ICM's Consultancy Service and the delivery of online resources for Member Associations and to support ICM's MEDPath programme.'[55]

SUMMARY OF ICM's EDUCATIONAL EFFORTS

The desire of midwives across the globe to gather together, share practices and stories of their work in a variety of arenas and locations has permeated the 100-year story of the ICM. One of the two aims of the ICM for a century is *to advance worldwide the goals and aspirations of midwives* by strengthening midwifery associations and midwives in order to provide high quality, evidence-based midwifery care. The content in this chapter focused specifically on the essential mandate of the ICM to provide many pathways to advancing midwifery knowledge and skills, including the provision of educational workshops, conferences and tools in efforts to meet this Constitutional aim. Midwives throughout the world have expressed very positive responses to each of these ICM educational efforts.

100 Years of the International Confederation of Midwives

1. ICM. The International Confederation of Midwives Constitution Agreed by Council on September 10th, 1954. Article IV: International Council, 2: 'Meetings of the Confederation and Council shall be held triennially, circumstances permitting. Council may meet more frequently.'
2. Katherine Kendall. Sixteenth International Confederation of Midwives Congress. Journal of Nurse-Midwifery XVIII:1, Spring 1973, p 25. Kendall wrote of the siting of the Congress in the United States, 'it was a truly historic occasion to have a Congress on Midwifery held in the United States since nurse-midwives or qualified midwives have had a difficult time establishing themselves as accepted members of the maternal health team in this country.' She went on to write, 'In this country it is hoped that the excellent response to the [ICM] Congress from the media, from the government and from professional organizations, will prove to be a turning point for nurse-midwifery, and nurse midwives will be able to take their place as fully accepted members of the health care team for mothers and infants.' p 27. ICM. ICM Congress report from Vancouver, British Columbia, May 1993, began with Government's announcement of the legal recognition of midwifery practice in British Columbia.
3. ICM. (SA/ICM/R/4/) Wellcome Collection. Marjorie Bayes' History of the ICM first 50 Years.
4. ICM. (SA/ICM/R/4/) Wellcome Collection. Marjorie Bayes' History of the ICM 50 fifty Years.
5. ICM. (SA/ICM/R/4/) Wellcome Collection. Marjorie Bayes' History of the ICM 50 fifty Years Marjorie Bayes.
6. ICM. (SA/ICM/H/7/1). Wellcome Collections. Introduction for programme Congress Berlin.
7. JB Litoff. The American Midwife Debate. A sourcebook on its modern origins. London: Greenwood Press, 1986.
8. ICM. Guidelines for the Conduct of International Congresses. Chiswick, London: ICM, 1996.
9. ICM. ICM Council Meeting Minutes, Kobe, Japan, 1990. Agenda Item 90/17: Congress Organizer, p. 7.
10. ICM. ICM Council Meeting Minutes, Vienna, Austria, 2002. The Hague: ICM, p 19.
11. Once Johnson and Johnson Commercial eliminated their support of artificial infant feeding, it became of Gold Sponsor of ICM Congresses in 2002.
12. ICM. ICM Council Meeting Minutes October 2nd–4th, 1990, Kobe, Japan. Minute 90/17.2. Central Scientific Committee for Triennial Congresses. Motion agreed including a financial provision for the Committee in 1993 budget and to have the Committee make decisions on abstracts for the 1996 Congress.
13. ICM. Minutes of the ICM Board of Management, February 2001. The Hague: ICM, Min 02/01/13: Research Standing Committee, p 4.
14. Interview with Karin Christiani, Director of Board of Management in 1981. 12 May 2021.
15. B Herz and AR Measham. The Safe Motherhood Initiative: Proposals for Action. Paper presented at the Safe Motherhood Conference, Nairobi, Kenya, 7 February 1987; The Safe Motherhood Initiative: A Call to Action, Concluding Statement of the International Safe Motherhood Conference, 10–13 February 1987, Nairobi, Kenya.
16. WHO. Safe motherhood Initiative Steering Committee Report. Geneva: WHO Division of Family Health, 1987; (Pub. #FHE/87.6), p 2.
17. Joan Bentley. Women's Health and the Midwife: A Global Perspective. Report of Collaborative Pre-Congress Workshop: The Hague, The Netherlands, 21–22 August 1987. Geneva: WHO (Pub. # WHO/MCH/87.5), p 5.
18. Barbara Kwast, a Dutch midwife, started working at the WHO's Maternal and Child Health department in 1986 as the designated Technical Officer for ICM, working closely with Marie Goubran, ICM Executive Secretary and ICM President Filippa Lugtenburg, also a Dutch midwife. (Interview by Petra ten-Hoope Bender, 2017).
19. ICM. Safe Motherhood Fund of the International Confederation of Midwives Terms of Reference. ICM Council Agenda Item, 1999.
20. ICM. Manual: The Collaborative Safe Motherhood Pre-Congress Workshop in Collaboration with Its Partners The Hague: ICM, 2002, Board Agenda Item 16, pp 1–30.
21. List of Pre-Congress Workshop Country Participants 1993, 1996, 1999, 2000. [Personal papers of Joyce Thompson]
22. The Board of Management was aware of an increased interest from high resource country midwives who wished to work in ICM projects in LRCs and understood that they needed background and support to be effective consultants. Thus, a self-pay workshop was held with time for interaction between participants in both workshops. Listening to the needs of LRC midwives was valuable for those wishing to serve as consultants in such areas of the world. This was the first and only self-pay pre-congress workshop in ICM history.
23. ICM. ICM Council Minutes, Brisbane, Australia, 18–21 July 2005. MIN 05.16.5 Pre-Congress workshops: Vienna and Brisbane, p 7.
24. ICM. Minutes of ICM Council Meeting May 4–6, 11, 1993. London: ICM, adopted May 1996 – Wellcome archives. ICM. ICM Manual for The Mid-Triennium Meetings: Regional Conference and Regional Workshop. 2002, p 5. The first Mid-Triennial Meeting was held in Entebbe, Uganda, January 1995. The next Mid-Triennial meetings included New Delhi, India in February 1998; and April 2004 in Trinidad and Tobago. According to Frances Day Stirk (January 2021 call), the Mid-Triennium meetings were suspended after Trinidad when the ICM Board agreed to focus on Regional Conferences.

25 This decision was very expensive for the ICM Executive Committee, an example of ICM Council voting with their 'hearts' to support sister midwives, a weakness identified by the Board during the 1997 Strategy Day with facilitator Geoff Ribbens. There were donors supporting some of the participants and activities, but not the costs of getting the Executive Committee to the site.
26 V Ruth Bennett & Joyce E Thompson. Proceedings of Symposium: Vision with Action – Midwifery and Safe Motherhood. London: ICM, 1995. (ISBN 0-904218 04 X).
27 ICM. Report of Workshop and Symposium, New Delhi, India, February 1998. London: ICM, 1998.
28 ICM. Draft Record of the International Confederation of Midwives Council Meeting, Oslo, Norway, 21–23 May 1996. London: ICM Archives, 1996, Record 96.19, p 8.
29 ICM. Report of Workshop and Symposium, New Delhi, India, February 1998. London: ICM, 1998, p 2.
30 ICM. Council Meeting Minutes 2005. Agenda 05.16.4, p 7. Mid-Triennium Executive Committee meetings with attached SM workshops were replaced by ICM Regional Conferences after 2002.
31 ICM. Ethics Workshop Notes and Report. Chiswick, London: ICM, 27 May 1996 [Personal papers of Joyce Thompson]
32 ICM. Board of Management Meeting, Agenda item 15.1. ICM Research Standing Committee Report 2 March 2005.
33 'Open mic' refers to meetings where anyone can speak to any issue they wish to raise; generally there is a topic but no agenda from the leader other than to hear what the members are thinking about given issues.
34 Karen Guilliland. ICM Asia Pacific Region History 1984 to 2020. Unpublished. Shared with authors April 2021.
35 RCM. Report of the Regional Representative, 1990, p 1.
36 ICM. (SA/ICM/C/1/21). Wellcome Collection. Executive Committee May 1993. The transference of monies to the Regional Representatives was discussed.
37 ICM. ICM Triennial Report 2014–2017. The Hague: ICM, 2016, p 57.
38 ICM. ICM Triennial Report 2014–2017. The Hague: ICM, 2016, p 58.
39 ICM. ICM Council Meeting Minutes Toronto, Canada, June 2017. Agenda Item 7.2 ICM Regional Conferences, pp 27, 30. This congress organiser was demonstrated excellence in managing the Prague Congress and was chosen to continue with other ICM meetings.
40 Ann Thomson, editor. ICM/WHO West African Sub-Regional Workshop 'Enhancing National Midwifery Services'. Midwifery 5 (1989), p 6.
41 Notes from Barbara Kwast, 14 January 2020.
42 ICM, WHO, Rockefeller Foundation, GRMA. Planning for Action by Midwives: Mobilising Midwifery Personal for Safe Motherhood. London: ICM, 1989. Preface p v.
43 ICM, WHO, Rockefeller Foundation, GRMA. Planning for Action by Midwives: Mobilising Midwifery Personal for Safe Motherhood. London: ICM, 1989. This booklet was the report of the workshop on 'Enhancing National Midwifery Services' held in Accra, Ghana, 16–21 January 1989.
44 ICM, WHO, Rockefeller Foundation, GRMA. Planning for Action by Midwives: Mobilising Midwifery Personal for Safe Motherhood. London: ICM, 1989. Outcomes, pp 15–16.
45 ICM: Report of the Safe Motherhood Workshop and Mid-Triennium Conference Held in Harare, Zimbabwe March 15–18, 2001. London: ICM, 2001 – report compiled by N Moyo, ICM Programme Manager.
46 WHO. WHO Manual: Advancing Safe Motherhood Through Human Rights. Geneva: WHO, 2001 (Pub. #WHO/RHR/01.5).
47 ICM. Empowering Women – Empowering Midwives: The Vision for Women and Their Health. London: ICM, adopted by the ICM Council, May 1996.
48 J Fullerton, J Thompson, P Johnson. Competency-based education: The essential basis of pre-service education for the professional midwifery workforce. Midwifery 2013. http://dx.doi.org/10.1016/j.midw.2013.07.006
49 JB Thompson, JT Fullerton, C Carr, P Elgueta, E Hebert, A Luyben. Global Workshops in Midwifery Competency-Based Educational Methodologies: Lessons Learned. International Journal of Childbirth 7 (1):2017, pp 4–17. http://dx.doi.org/10.1891/2156-5287.7.1.4
50 ICM. Triennial Report 2014–2017. The Hague: ICM, p 30. Contributions from the Sanofi Espoir Foundation to ICM began in 2014 offering Midwives for Life Awards. In 2016, the Foundation worked with ICM to strengthen midwifery education in 22 French-speaking African Countries. Emmanuelle Hebert, CAM member of the ICM Board, led CBE TOT workshops in Comoros, June 2015; Dubai, November 2016 and Cote d'Ivoire in 2017 (Personal message to Joyce Thompson).
51 The Gates Foundation's financial support through December 2022 was $4.8 million.
52 ICM. Triennial Report 2017–2020. The Hague: ICM, 2020, p 17.
53 https://www.internationalmidwives.org/icm-publications/meap.html
54 ICM. Glossary of Terms. The Hague: ICM, 2011; updated 2017.
55 ICM. Triennial Report 2017–2020. The Hague: ICM, 2020, p 15. Can be downloaded from www.internationalmidwives.org

Chapter 10: *Strengthening Member Associations*

'In-country midwives need the collective force of a strong association; i.e., an association that is able to reach its goals. Strengthening individual member associations enhances the ability of midwives worldwide to achieve the goal of improving the health of women and children.'

Nester Moyo, Zimbabwe, 2001

INTRODUCTION

The 'aims and objects'[1] of the ICM throughout history reinforce that the core business of the organisation has been to support the Member Associations (MAs) in strengthening midwives and midwifery practice globally in order to promote and maintain optimum reproductive health of childbearing women and their newborns. Many ICM leaders since 1922 have accepted this dual focus of ICM business. The ICM involvement in the global Safe Motherhood Initiatives beginning in the late 1980s tilted the balance toward childbearing women and in the early 21st century the balance tilted back toward emphasis on strengthening midwifery associations and the autonomy of midwives as an important part of meeting the needs of women. As Nester Moyo noted in the quote above, strong midwifery associations were vital to midwives' ability to save lives, especially in areas of the world where midwives were underpaid and undervalued.[2] The ICM needs strong associations in membership to contribute to its work globally, regionally and nationally. This work of the Confederation focused on MAs and services is addressed in this Chapter. Education provided by the ICM to the midwives of the world is addressed in Chapter 9.

THE WORK OF THE CONFEDERATION

The work of the Confederation was outlined in each Constitution of the Confederation. The list of ICM activities from 1981 further explained the activities expected of the ICM outlined in the Constitution of 1954,[3] repeated in similar form through 1996, when the new Mission and Vision statements led to the development of a Global Strategy document with goals and activities. The

2005 Dutch-based Articles of Association did not include such a list as the ICM Council was now agreeing activities based on the adopted Strategic Directions. However, the clarity of work to support MAs listed in the 1981 Constitution offers insight into nearly a century of activities carried out in the name of the Confederation. The list included:

- ✓ Publication of journals, monographs, pamphlets, reports of conferences, seminars, visits and other papers relevant to the aims of the Confederation. Such publications shall include a periodical newsletter issued at such intervals as the Confederation may determine;
- ✓ Arrangement of study groups, meetings, seminars and conferences which may be on a local, regional or worldwide basis and to encourage the international exchange of midwifery research, educational curricula and practice;
- ✓ Provision for the exchange of visits between members of associations, individual or in groups;
- ✓ Organisation of international visits to enable midwives and other persons to exchange views and to inform themselves on matters of common interest;
- ✓ Arranging international congresses of midwives which, as far as is practicable, shall be held triennially or at such other times as council shall determine and in such countries as the council may determine;
- ✓ Maintaining at the headquarters of the Confederation a centre for the dissemination and exchange of information on midwifery matters;
- ✓ Inviting at its discretion and on such conditions as it may decide other organisations or persons to participate in any of its activities;
- ✓ Authorising on such conditions as it may decide midwives to represent the Confederation in activities of other international and national organisations;
- ✓ Doing all such other lawful things as are necessary for the attainment of the object of the Confederation.[4]

Many of these activities were continued into the 21st century, such as publication of reports and newsletters, holding Congresses, building partnerships and increasing the visibility of midwives through representation at a variety of meetings. Study groups, exchange visits and maintaining a centre for dissemination and exchange of information at the ICM Headquarters were not continued beyond 2005 due to financial constraints and other, more pressing, Secretariat responsibilities. However, increased internet capability worldwide and use of the updated ICM Website to share key information and activities took the place of in-person visits to the ICM HQ to take advantage of global resources held there until the early 2000s.

MEMBER ASSOCIATION ISSUES ADDRESSED

As the membership in the ICM grew, so did the number of issues requiring action that were affecting those MAs. The central issues surrounding the provision of high-quality care for childbearing women and their newborns by well-prepared, competent midwives that began in the 1920s continued throughout the 100-year history of the Confederation. These issues began in the 1920s with European midwives discussing the safety and place of birth including use of Nitrous Oxide for pain in labour[5], along with ways to improve the status of midwives when other professions began offering childbearing services and other issues being addressed over the years as described below.

Council Agreed ICM Policy, Position, Statement and Core Documents (Annex A)

MA issues came from Regional Representatives' (Chapter 5) reports and open forums held during the ICM Council meetings where delegates presented their most pressing concerns. Many of these concerns, once shared with MAs from various parts of the world represented in Council meetings, resulted in ICM Position and Policy Statements, Core Documents and standards (Refer to Annex A for table of issues and resulting statements). MA issues/needs remained fairly similar during the ICM's 100-year history, such as addressing the autonomy of the profession, the need for evidence-based practice and quality education to promote the health of women and newborns, along with global concerns for the health of the planet and meeting global health goals.[6] As MAs from other areas of the world beyond Europe joined the ICM beginning in the 1950s (refer to MA charts in Annex G), issues of place of birth, safe birthing and newborn practices continued with growing concerns for promoting the health and rights of women, the education and regulation of autonomous midwives, and the safety of women and midwives themselves in the face of discrimination and violence took on a variety of perspectives.

Many of the Position Statements agreed prior to the 21st century were updated, usually on a 6-year cycle, and sometimes renamed, especially as the ICM MAs kept in tune with changing societal views of women and childbearing. In addition, names of some statements changed once the Vision and Mission statements were updated. As times and circumstances changed, such as civil wars, increased demand for well-qualified midwives, a renewed interest in human rights for all individuals, the ICM Council adopted new or revised statements and core documents.

In 2017, a Member Association Survey was conducted from the ICM HQ asking members' expectations of the ICM. The survey was circulated to 130 MAs, with 87 responses from 68 MAs located in 62 countries. Over 98 per cent of the associations joined the ICM to be a part of a global movement for midwives and 73 per cent rated the ICM's documents as the most significant and valuable ICM services received.[7]

Challenging Balance of Member Concerns

One of the most challenging aspects of meeting the needs of MAs in an increasing number of countries of the world was finding a balance between issues affecting midwives in one country or area of the world with issues potentially affecting all midwives and midwifery associations. For example, during the era of Safe Motherhood Initiatives (1987–2000+) with Pre-Congress workshops for low resource country (LRC) midwives (Chapter 9), some high resource country (HRC) midwives criticised ICM leadership for addressing the needs of LRC midwives in areas of the world where maternal and neonatal deaths were highest to the perceived detriment of the HRC MAs' needs. Of note was that most of the midwives working with childbearing women facing alarming rates of death and disability lived in resource limited countries (99 per cent of maternal deaths occurred in non-industrialised countries in the 1980–90s[8]). Many of these midwives were not part of an ICM MA, though through exposure to the ICM workshops over time their country associations were supported to become ICM members and many did. For example, the number of LRC MAs in Africa and South-East Asia increased from 1993 onwards, in part from their awareness of the value of the Confederation to them and their value to the ICM (Chapter 13). Likewise, most LRC midwives required financial support to participate in the ICM workshops. Thus, the ICM workshops beyond Triennial Congresses targeted midwives from LRCs whose access to ongoing education opportunities were very limited as were salaries. International partners and several HRC MAs and individual midwives provided much of the financial support and shared expertise needed, stifling most of the imbalance criticism (Refer to Chapter 6 on finances for details).

AWARDS FOR EXEMPLARY MIDWIVES

One way to provide recognition and strengthen midwives and associations came in the form of a variety of awards for exemplary midwives, most often chosen from LRC countries. These awards also allowed these exemplary midwives to attend the triennial Council and/or Congresses. Three examples of such awards follow.

Marie Goubran Memorial Leadership Award – 1991 (Annex I)

Marie Goubran, Secretary General of the ICM from 1987 to 1990, guided the Confederation through some very difficult times and raised its international profile considerably. After her untimely death in December 1990, in response to MAs requests, the ICM Board of Management in conjunction with the Goubran family, established the ICM Marie Goubran Memorial Award, 'in recognition of her dedication to midwifery and her efforts in uniting midwives from all over the world'[9]. The memorial award was agreed in 1991 in honour of Marie and in keeping with her leadership and passionate commitment for childbearing women and families all over the world.[10] The original purpose statement for the Marie Goubran Award was to assist in the furthering of midwifery education and practice in countries with special needs and limited funding opportunities through the provision of grants, scholarships and awards to midwives who demonstrated the potential to act as change agents in their region or country. A revised statement of purpose in 2004 noted that 'this memorial award was established to recognise midwives in countries with special

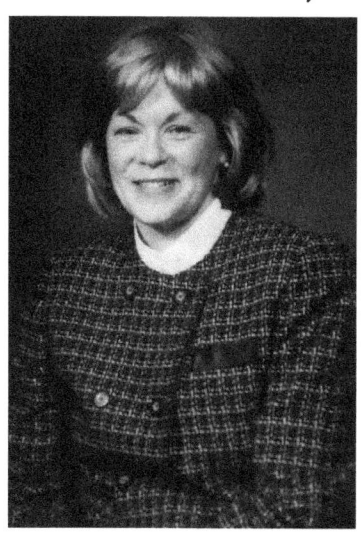

Executive Secretary Marie Goubran 1987–1990 – ICM Archives at Wellcome Collection

needs and limited funding opportunities who demonstrate similar leadership and commitment.'[11]

This award, marked by a certificate, originally was given every three years with nominees meeting leadership criteria in keeping with the ICM's aims and objects. The final selection of awardees was made by the ICM Board of Management (BoM) and initially a representative of the Goubran family based on written nominations from the individual's midwifery association or the midwife herself. Award winners were funded to attend the ICM Congress during which they received their award and funds for their proposed activities. Each awardee was expected to submit a detailed report to ICM Headquarters six months following receipt of the funds describing the activities carried out with the award money. The primary source of funds initially came from the Goubran family, and then it was open to donations from prior Secretary Generals, Board members, MAs and anyone else supporting the purpose of the award.[12] Johnson and Johnson International began supporting the fund in the early 2000s.[13] There was interest in also continuing in some way to support awardees in their leadership efforts, though nothing specific agreed.[14] However, one awardee, Nester Moyo, became a treasured member of the ICM Secretariat and developed many tools to strengthen midwifery associations throughout the world. In 2014 the Award was given to its first male midwife, Kingsley Musama, who was providing respectful maternity care to mothers in Zambia (Annex I has a list of Goubran Award winners).

Columbia University Award for Midwives and Their Associations – 2001

The Columbia University Award was established in 2001 to honour midwives who have demonstrated the potential to act as change agents in their country in the reduction of maternal and neonatal death and disability and who have the ability to support the strengthening of their midwifery association.[15] Unlike other awards, this award of $5,000 per one midwife per region was scheduled to be given every year. The award money was to be used to strengthen the activities of the midwives' association in accord with the proposed three-year programme addressing one of the following areas: Vision and strategy development; leadership development; advocacy or other things such as providing new IT support for the association headquarters or supporting efforts for the International Day of the Midwife celebrations. Annual reports are required with follow-up by the ICM

Secretariat. The nominations and proposals were selected by the ICM Board and a representative of Columbia University's Averting Maternal Death and Disability (AMDD) Programme.[16]

Saving Newborn Lives from Save the Children Award for Midwives – 2005

This award was first presented in 2005. The purpose of the award was, 'to bestow an award to midwives who have demonstrated achievements as change agents in improving newborn health at the community level through training and/or provision of services in Sub-Saharan Africa or Asia'[17]. Awards were given to one or two midwives each triennium who were experienced in newborn care. Each awardee received a plaque or certificate along with travel, accommodation, meals and registration fees to the Congress the year the award was received. The Board of Management and a representative of Save the Children USA make the final selection of awardees based on nominations and material received. A sixth-month report of newborn activities is required following receipt of the award, sent to the ICM Headquarters for review.

SUPPORT FOR COUNTRY ACTIVITIES
Working Parties

One of the ways that the ICM addressed the needs of midwives and its MAs, especially during the 1960s–1980s, was the use of Working Parties. During the early years of the ICM/FIGO Joint Study Project (Chapter 16) there was a recommendation that each continent should have a group of midwives and obstetricians meet to continue the discussions of the role of the midwife in maternity care and how to support the needs that were identified by region and country in the 1966 study.[18]

Members of the ICM/FIGO JSG meeting in London in 1972 agreed that the aim of continued study of midwifery training and practise in the world was, 'To continue the improvement of maternal and childcare, and the quality of maternal and child life through the inclusion of Family Planning among the services provided by midwives of all categories in their expanding role'[19]. A grant from the United States Aid for International Development (USAID) was used to convene Working Parties in developing countries over a period of five years to carry out the education mandates for midwives. From December 1972 through

to October 1975, nine Working Parties were convened: Anglophone East and West Africa, Francophone Central and West Africa, Central and South America, the Caribbean and East and West Asia.[20] Reports are available for:
1. ICM-FIGO Anglophone East Africa Working Party: Mrs Perpetua W Kanyoko, Regional Field Director.[21]
2. ICM-FIGO All India Working Party, Miss M Philip, Regional Field Director.[22]
3. ICM 'Cento' Countries Working Party, Turkey, included resource persons from Pakistan, Iran, Afghanistan and Turkey.[23]
4. ICM Anglophone Middle East Regional Seminar on Expanded Involvement of the Midwife in Reproductive Health.[24]

Projects with Collaborative Partners/Donors

ICM members and their midwives benefited from the ICM's efforts to establish long-term relationships with major donors (Chapters 15 and 16) that resulted in a variety of country and/or regional specific projects to support MAs and update the knowledge and skills of midwives to address specific identified needs. Following a stakeholders' meeting convened by the ICM in 2015, an increased number of international donors were interested in supporting ICM projects. Examples of more recent projects to support MAs are described briefly, continuing the ICM's story of the value of partnerships (Annex D has a complete list of ICM partners).

Johnson and Johnson International: Johnson and Johnson (J&J) corporation has been a long-time supporter of the ICM, beginning in the mid-1990s with small grants for specific activities at regional levels. J&J began as a Gold sponsor of ICM Triennial Congresses in 2002. They expanded their financial support with the sponsorship of the ICM's annual Education, Research, and Marie Goubran Agent of Change Awards in the early 21st century. In 2019 they supported two new ICM awards – the Touch Ambassador and the Midwives in Action awards with a financial prize. In 2018, J&J gave ICM an 18-month capacity development grant for resource mobilisation and planning for an ICM consultancy service co-funded by UNFPA for MAs in need of these education and regulation consultants.[25]

Johns Hopkins Programme for International Education of Gynecology and Obstetrics (Jhpiego): Jhpiego funds supported the field-testing of Essential Competencies (2000), the Meeting of the Minds in 2001, and through the Maternal

Newborn Health programme, funded midwives to attend the 2001 mid-triennium workshop in Zimbabwe. More recently, Jhpiego was involved in the production of the 'Helping Mothers Survive' training modules.[26]

Sanofi Espoir Foundation [France]: In 2013, the Foundation supported a small grants programme titled A Midwife for Every Mother and Baby and from 2015 to 2019 a programme for strengthening midwifery education in French-Speaking Africa. This programme included CBE workshops and mentoring midwifery educators.

Laerdal Global Health[27]: Laerdal Global Health funded 10,000 Happy Birthdays 2014–2017[28] in Malawi and Zambia using Jhpiego's Helping Mothers Survive Bleeding After Birth (HMS-BAB) and the American Academy of Paediatrics' Helping Babies Breathe (HBB). These skills workshops were held in all regions on the world. The ICM and Laerdal Global Health continued their partnership for midwives and midwifery associations with 50,000 Happy Birthdays 2018–2020, focusing on Rwanda, Ethiopia and Tanzania.

Bill & Melinda Gates Foundation: Continued ICM support that began in 2013 with a grant to support Expanding Quality Midwifery Services (2015–2017) included the development and testing of the ICM's Midwifery Education Accreditation Programme (MEAP) and in-country testing of ICM's Midwifery Services Framework (MSF). A grant for Strengthening Midwifery Services was awarded 2018–2021 with the intent of continued testing of the MSF and MEAP along with creation of MEDPath and ICM's Global Midwifery Competency Assessment Tool.

Direct Relief: In 2015, the ICM received funds from Direct Relief to distribute Midwives' Kits free of charge to midwifery associations, primarily in resource-poor and humanitarian settings. Direct Relief designed the first-ever Midwife Kit with ICM's technical expertise. Each kit contains the 59 essential items a midwife needs to perform 50-facility-based deliveries at a cost of $25 per safe birth.[29] During the pilot year of this joint project, Direct Relief delivered over 400 kits to midwives in four countries: Sierra Leone, Liberia, Philippines and Somaliland. In 2016, 199 midwife kits were provided to birthing clinics in Sierra Leone, Liberia, Malawi, Nepal, Haiti and Mexico and in 2017 an additional 250 kits went to clinics in Vietnam, Nepal, Togo, Liberia, Malia, Sierra Leone, Liberia and Haiti. A follow-on project was funded in 2019 to monitor the distribution of this essential midwifery equipment and continue the interactive mapping of midwifery services.[30]

Strengthening Midwifery Services (SMS) with UNFPA: ICM's partnership with UNFPA began with Pre-Congress Workshops in the 1990s and is one of ICM's long-term and strongest supporters (Chapter 15). In recent years, the ICM and UNFPA agreed an annual workplan. It now includes support for the development of ICM's Advocacy toolkit described below, Respectful Maternity Care workshops around the world, midwifery education and other consultant services.[31] All of these activities are strengthening MAs, especially in areas of greatest need.

Swedish International Development Agency (SIDA): the ICM's partnership with SIDA began in 2009 with funds to support ICM activities related to supporting midwives, especially in LRCs, to address MDGs 4 and 5.

White Ribbon Alliance: Supported Midwives' Voices, Midwives' Realities publication with the WHO and the ICM in 2016.

MacArthur Foundation: In 2016, the MacArthur Foundation supported Strengthening Midwifery Associations in Mexico (November 2016–May 2018) and an additional grant 2018–2020 was given to the ICM to raise the profile of midwifery through advocacy and multi-stakeholder collaboration.

New Venture Fund: The fund collaborated with UNFPA on Respectful Care by and for midwives and advocacy skills for midwives in 2017.

TOOLS TO STRENGTHEN MEMBER ASSOCIATIONS

The initial tools to strengthen Member Associations (MAs) since the rebirth of ICM in 1954 were in the form of Core Documents, Position and Policy Statements that could be used by MAs in advocacy campaigns with key stakeholders and policymakers concerned with the education, regulation and practice of midwives in their country/region. A series of Handbooks for Council meetings along with a timeline for sending out Council documents assured MAs of having the needed information prior to the Triennial Congresses. In addition, Congress handbooks[32] and a variety of small booklets explaining what the ICM was, how to become a member and an overview of its history[33] at various times were available to MAs without cost.

Other ICM tools and programmes meant to strengthen MAs are described briefly below. The adoption of global competencies and standards (Chapter 12) and these tools matched the ICM's focus on Education, Regulation and Association (ERA) activities during the first two decades of the 21st century. In addition, ICM initially established three official Standing Committees (research, education and professional practice) to support the work of the ICM and its MAs that grew to six in the early 2000s.

Midwifery Association Strengthening

<u>Twinning Member Associations:</u> The twinning concept of high resource country (HRC) MAs assisting low resource country (LRC) MAs to meet their obligations to the ICM took a variety of forms prior to the formal definition of the ICM Twinning Concept in 2006.[34] For example, the German Midwives' Association paid the 1989 and 1990 capitation fees for the midwifery association in Sierra Leone[35] so it could continue to benefit from ICM membership and attend the triennial Council meeting. The Royal College of Midwives, the American College of Nurse-Midwives, the Midwives Section of the Japanese Nursing Association and the Japanese Midwives Association were among others who provided funds for LRC midwives to participate in ICM Councils and Congresses as well as regional meetings. In addition, strong midwifery associations were helping with the development of new and/or the strengthening of midwifery associations in countries with small numbers of midwives or who did not have political support to develop and expand their associations. The International Day of the Midwife activities described below also give further insight into how MAs from HRCs began supporting others in LDC countries.

With funding from the Dutch Ministry of Foreign Affairs to support work to strengthen midwife capacity in the ICM regions, some of this resource was used for the ICM twinning programme. More recently, twinning of HRC MAs with LRC MAs has contributed to stronger associations during 2011–2014 in Sierra Leone (The Netherlands)[36], Papua New Guinea (Australia), Tanzania (Canada), Mali (Switzerland) and Vietnam (Japan).[37]

<u>Young Midwifery Leaders Programme (YML)</u>: During a 2001 international consultative meeting, convened by the ICM, 'The Meeting of the Minds', leadership development was identified as a key issue for the ICM to address with its MAs.[38] Participants noted that preparing for succession planning in midwifery associations is vital to the ongoing strength and success of any association. In addition, the ICM received repeated requests from MAs for leadership training.[39] During 2002–2003 Judi Brown, Deputy Director of the Board of Management (1999–2002, 2002–2005) brainstormed with Nester Moyo, the ICM

Programme Manager, the idea of creating midwifery leaders among relatively young midwives. The overall purpose of the YML programme was to establish a culture of leadership within the MAs, regionally and internationally, so that competent midwives and midwifery services would be available to address the sexual and reproductive health needs for all women and newborns in the region. The three-year programme was designed as a combination of virtual and face-to-face meetings with Nester Moyo as Coordinator, use of a series of self-study modules written by specialists on the various topics of leadership development, and exposure to selected ICM leaders.[40] The success of the programme was based on forming a dynamic mentor-mentee relationship.[41]

The first ICM Young Midwifery Leaders' (YML) Programme was launched in Trinidad, April 2004, with five mentor-mentee dyads.[42] The mentee-mentor dyads included Teja Zacksek (Slovenia) mentored by Valerie Fleming; Mumudelanji Keith Lopato (Malawi) mentored by Lennie A Kamwendo; Elgonda Eritzema Bekker (South Africa) mentored by Diana du Plessis; Suzanne Raetz (Germany) mentored by Jule Friedrich and Kathy-Ann Alphonso Lootawan (Trinidad) mentored by Emerald Leon-Williams.[43] The YML programme was funded initially by the MNH project of Jhpiego and ICM core funding; individual midwife donations helped to finance the last meeting of the YMLs in 2007. Other partners volunteered their expertise; for example, POLICY Project agreed to run a workshop in February 2005 on advocacy.[44]

The first ICM Young Midwifery Leaders (YML) Programme resulted in several important successes. For example, within the first year Keith Lopato met with the Malawi Minister of Health and the MOH Nursing Director, Dr Ann Phoya. Keith's opinion was sought during policymaking and problem-solving meetings relating to midwifery and nursing. Elgonda Bekker initiated a White Ribbon Alliance chapter in South Africa and a research group for midwives within her midwifery association. The Trinidad and Tobago midwifery association has been making good use of Kathy Ann Alphonso's leadership skills, including her offering a lactation management workshop for its members.[45]

Lack of funds ended the first round of the global YML programme in 2007. However, three UNFPA/ICM YML programmes were carried out in the Latin America, the Caribbean and Mexico between 2013 and 2019.[46] Collaboration with Johnson and Johnson resulted in a second global YML programme with 30 participants that was launched in 2016 during the Women Deliver Conference in Copenhagen.[47]

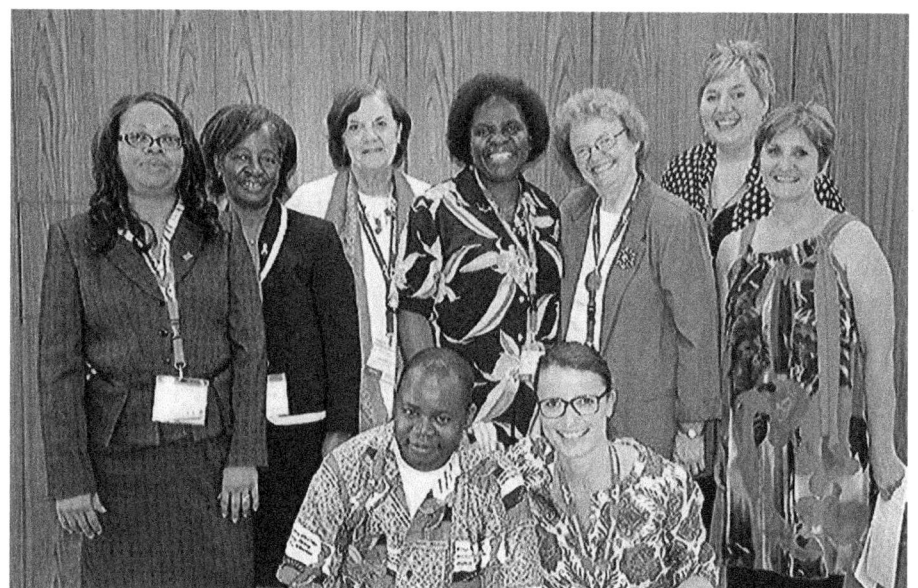

Young Midwifery Leaders and Mentors (2014), Left to right: Kathy Ann Alfonso Lotowan (Trinidad & Tobago); Lennie Kamwendo (Malawi); Judith Brown; Nester Moyo; Joyce Thompson; Elgonda Bekker (South Africa); Diana du Plessis (South Africa).
Front row: Mumudelanji Keith Lopato (Malawi); Suzanne Raetz (Germany). - Courtesy of Joyce Thompson

Member Association Capacity Assessment Tool (MACAT): Nester Moyo, the ICM Programme Director, developed the MACAT to assist MAs in capacity building noting that the ability to fulfil the roles and responsibilities required of midwives and their associations depended on the association's capacity/strength as an organisation. The final tool was based on Nester Moyo's 2002 'Proposal for Strengthening Midwives Associations' that included key things required of a strong midwifery association: 1) a representative membership; 2) leadership training and development; 3) organisational management skills; 4) vision and strategy development; 5) skills to identify its needs; 6) development of advocacy skills; 7) visible public support and 8) visibility.[48] Since 2003 the existing MACAT tool was used by MAs to assess midwifery association needs and develop strategic interventions needed.

In 2011, the MACAT underwent extensive review of the literature and focus groups to produce the next draft for review and adoption by the ICM Council. The revised MACAT has seven main sections, each representing an aspect of the association.[49]

A. Governance
B. Management practices and leadership
C. Financial resource management
D. Functions
E. Collaboration, partnership and networks
F. Visibility including media relations
G. Sustainability

<u>Midwifery Services Framework (MSF):</u> The MSF was developed by ICM staff and Board following a Midwifery Services Technical Advisory Meeting held 2–4 February 2009 in Geneva Switzerland, chaired by ICM President Bridget Lynch. The list of participants included a total of 25 representatives of the WHO, UNFPA, Jhpiego, ACNM, FIGO and individual consultants in addition to eight ICM staff.[50] The development began in 2009[51] with the financial support of the Gates Foundation. It was adopted by the ICM Council in 2017.

> 'The MSF is a mechanism for any country that wants to establish or strengthen its midwifery services within the context of its sexual, reproductive, maternal and newborn health services. The MSF also serves as a process for evaluating how the core components of ICM's current midwifery professional framework (education, regulation and association) are in place in a country, identifying gaps, prioritising actions, and establishing and implementing workstreams to address identified gaps.'[52]

It has been introduced in Lesotho, Bangladesh, Afghanistan and Kyrgyzstan. Training and orientation of MSF facilitators has been conducted and expressions of interest have been received from various stakeholders since that time.[53] From 2018 to 2020 the MSF was tested in three new countries with the financial support of the Bill and Melinda Gates Foundation.[54]

<u>ICM RESPECT Toolkit</u>[55]: In 2018, ICM began developing a series of workshops on Respectful Maternity Care (RMC) to present at regional conferences in Dubai, Paraguay and Namibia. At each workshop, there was an overwhelming call for more education and support to change the behaviour of health workers caring for women during pregnancy and birth. Many recent studies show that disrespect and abuse of women are common, ranging from verbal abuse and physical violence to

stigma and discrimination. This occurs in low- and high-income countries at an alarming rate and is contributing to women's declining access to essential antenatal or childbirth care. Supported by UNFPA, the ICM RESPECT toolkit provides step-by-step guidance on why and how to run a RMC workshop. In addition, the ICM Secretariat has added many videos, lesson plans, PowerPoint slides and reference documents with a facilitator guide on how to go through each step of a workshop. It is intended that these materials should be adapted for local use, and they are available in English, French and Spanish on the ICM website.

ICM Advocacy Toolkits: One of the important aspects of strengthening the ICM MAs during the past two decades has been addressing their need to understand, advocate for and participate in the development of health policies at national and regional levels that improve the reproductive health of women and men, and the health of newborns and infants. The POLICY Project and the USAID-funded Maternal and Neonatal Health (MNH) project led by Jhpiego took the lead in training midwives in advocacy and leadership following the 2001 'Meeting of the Minds'. They offered workshops in The Gambia (December 2001), Bangladesh (July 2002), and Argentina (February 2003) 'to introduce midwives to the practice of policy development and implementation and the role of advocacy in influencing the policy process.'[56] As a result of these workshops, POLICY Project and MNH developed a manual entitled, 'Networking for Policy change: An Advocacy Training Manual', as a result of lessons learnt.

A second advocacy toolkit based on the outcomes of the State of the World's Midwifery (SoWMy) Report of 2011 was developed by Family Care International (FCI). It was made available to the ICM and its MAs and updated following the 2014 SoWMy report. This advocacy tool was used by UNFPA consultants in the Caribbean, Mexico and Latin America with midwifery associations and individual midwives.

In 2020, a 16-page ICM advocacy toolkit was designed and made available to MAs with financial support from UNFPA as part of its annual workplan with the ICM for Strengthening Midwifery Services.[57] The toolkit is easy to understand and easy to use. It was put together to give midwives and midwifery associations the tools to advocate for increased resources for midwifery globally as well as locally. The toolkit can help midwives raise awareness and educate their communities about certain health issues; to advocate for increased rights and protections for their profession; to amplify the voices and needs of midwives in their country and globally to key leaders and policymakers. As an educational tool, this resource provides an introduction and guide to advocacy. It offers a clear overview of advocacy, based on the key questions: What? Where? Who? Why? and How? The toolkit contains advice on the best way to use it as well resources to use in advocacy efforts. It is suggested that if MAs wish to develop their own advocacy programme, the toolkit can help them consider the audience, messaging and advocacy activities that could strengthen MA advocacy efforts, impact and outcomes.[58]

ICM's Inaugural Global Goodwill Ambassador: An important step forward in the ICM's advocacy efforts was the selection of its first Global Goodwill Ambassador, Her Excellency Toyin Ojora-Saraki, First Lady of Kwara State, Nigeria, for a 6-year term 2014–2020.[59] She had dedicated over two decades to philanthropy and was the Founder and President of the Wellbeing Foundation Africa (WBFA) advocating internationally for maternal, newborn and child health and improved health systems across Africa. HE Ojora-Saraki is also a global advocate for the UN's Every Woman Every Child effort and sits on the Board of the Global Foundation for the Elimination of Domestic Violence, among other posts. In this role, HE Toyin Ojora-Saraki helped raise awareness and the influence of midwives and midwifery whilst lobbying and advocating for policy changes related to maternal, newborn and reproductive health care nationally and internationally. She was chosen especially for her ability to promote the ICM's strategic priorities in countries that bear the highest burden of maternal and newborn deaths in the early 21st century.[60]

ICM STANDING COMMITTEES (SC)

The dual aims of the Confederation are carried out in a variety of ways focused on responding to MAs' needs and issues. MAs were constantly asking the ICM for support and tools for starting new or strengthening existing basic midwifery education programmes. In addition, regulatory support was a top priority in many countries as midwives were being restricted in what they could do. Appointment of the ICM Standing Committees (SC) over the years has been one way to meet these MA needs and encourage MAs to take an active role in such committees. SC efforts resulted in the development of many guidelines and tools for use by MAs. Each committee includes members from all regions of the world so that midwives' voices from every country are heard and incorporated into documents

Professional Practice Committee (PPC)

The Professional Practice Committee was established in 1996 but did not survive beyond 2002[61] due to tremendous variations in midwifery practice across the globe resulting in lack of agreement on practice standards, and concern as to whether ICM should be involved in setting such standards. A Practice Standing Committee was discussed many times in ICM Council meetings, but as of 2022 such a committee has yet to be re-established. The three longer-time ICM Standing Committees, their history and their remits are briefly discussed below.

ICM Research Standing Committee (RSC) – 1996

The Research Standing Committee (RSC) was officially established with clear Terms of Reference during the ICM Council meeting in May 1996[62] based on the recommendation of the 1995 Executive Committee.[63] The ICM had adopted two prior Position Statements on the role of the midwife in research that reaffirmed MAs' belief that 'acceptable standards of midwifery practice, education and management are based on reliable and valid research and accurate evaluation of midwifery practices.'[64] The Purpose of the RSC was to strengthen the development of midwifery research within the Confederation by the provision of a venue within the structure of the organisation that supported the overall mission and aims of the Confederation.

Membership of the RSC began with a minimum of one midwife researcher from each ICM region who met during each Triennial Council and/or Congress and during Executive Committee meetings as needed. Initially, the RSC was convened by a member of the Board of Management, but as its network grew, the ICM-appointed co-chairs of the committee took over this role. Among the co-chairs of the RSC were Jane Sandall (UK), Holly Kennedy (USA), Kathy Herschderfer (Netherlands), Kerri Schuiling (USA) and Hora Soltani (UK).

The RSC provides ICM's MAs with up-to-date information on all aspects of midwifery practice, education and service. It plays a key role in the development of the ICM Triennial Congresses, including holding research workshops, and is the foundation of midwifery's Three Pillars of Education, Regulation and Associations (ERA) with ongoing research being the lifeblood of any vibrant profession.

2021 Roles of The Research Standing Committee:[65]
- Identifies midwifery research in progress and takes part in the discussions to develop the ICM research strategy.
- Creates communication networks among researchers working in reproductive health and midwifery.
- Maintains a database of researchers which acts as a source of information and support.
- Recommends to the ICM Board, Executive Committee and Council, activities, priorities, strategies and practices for midwifery research throughout the world.
- Reviews abstracts submitted for peer-review for ICM Congresses.
- Plans RSC involvement in each ICM congress and facilitates research workshops at these.
- Provides a resource of expert midwifery research workers for access by the ICM if required.

Membership on the RSC grew over the years as the numbers of international midwifery researchers grew. A research advisory network was established in May 2002[66] to maintain communication across international boundaries and support multi-centre and multinational research on issues of interest and importance to midwives, on sexual and reproductive health, and to the ICM as a whole. In preparation for the 2002 Congress, the Vienna Scientific Programme Committee asked that one of the RSC co-chairs assist and be co-opted onto this committee.[67] Following the Vienna Congress, the RSC was asked by the ICM Scientific Programme Committee to participate in the review of research papers submitted for presentation at future Triennial Congresses, and they agreed. In addition, the RSC created guidelines for the ethical conduct of research with individuals in a variety of cultures that were subsequently published.[68]

Education Standing Committee (ESC) – 2002
The ICM Education Standing Committee (ESC) had a rocky beginning. It was initially established in 2002 with Terms of Reference agreed by Council.[69] Its Purpose was to strengthen the consideration of education issues within the overall mission and aims of the Confederation using a core group of one midwifery educator from each ICM region. The ESC was expected to do its

work via electronic communication with one face-to-face meeting during each Triennial Congress.

There was a period of six years with limited or no activity until 2008. A workshop for midwifery educators was held during the Triennial Congress in Glasgow with 27 midwives engaged in education volunteering to participate in a new structure for the ESC. The re-established ESC began their agreed work in May 2009 with co-chairs Ans Luyben (Europe), Mary Barger (USA/Americas) and Susan McDonald (Asia-Pacific) with six sections with their own lead person, representing all regions of the ICM. The sections included 1) Programme planning, 2) Networking, 3) Initial and Higher education, 4) Competencies and Standards, 5) Practical Placements and 6) Safe Motherhood, with the co-chairs responsible for Strategic Planning.[70]

The ESC was strengthened with the ICM Council's endorsement of the *Global Standards for Midwifery Education* with *Guidelines* in 2011 that its members helped to develop (Chapter 12). The ESC took on the responsibility for monitoring the dissemination and use of the global standards. The emphasis of the 2011–2014 triennium focused on dissemination and support of the revised ICM *Essential Competencies for Basic Midwifery Practice* (2010) and standards. The ESC was now solidified and offered a variety of education workshops during Triennial Congresses. For example, the workshops in Durban 2011 included 1) Implementing Global Standards for Midwifery Education: how to go ahead; 2) How midwifery education can help to promote Safe Motherhood; 3) Practical placements in midwifery education and 4) Using simulation and IT technology in midwifery education. For the past several years, members of the ESC have participated in development of the Midwifery Education Accreditation Programme (MEAP) that is being field-testing in 2021–2022.

The ESC's current remit is to promote the international standardisation of midwifery education. It supports the development and expansion of high-quality undergraduate and post-graduate midwifery education programmes and oversees the production of the resources required to support this international standardisation and its effective implementation.

<u>2021 Terms of Reference</u>[71]
- Works with other ICM Standing Committees to define global education standards for midwifery.

- Identifies strategies for implementation of global education standards.
- Supports member associations and regulators to strengthen midwifery education in countries and jurisdictions.
- Provides a platform for sharing resources and midwifery education strategies.
- Develops a network of midwifery educators.
- Acts as a resource of expert midwifery educators for access and use by the ICM and partners.
- Focuses on strategic implications with regard to the development, implementation and evaluation of education activities.
- Facilitates specifically targeted education workshops at each Triennial Congress.
- Contributes to the process for decision and selection of any ICM education awardees.

ICM Regulation Standing Committee (RegSC) – 2008

The ICM Regulation Standing Committee (RegSC) was established in 2008.[72] Judi Brown, ICM Deputy Director and the ICM representative to the international nursing and regulatory meetings hosted by the International Council of Nurses, asked that membership of this RegSC include both those who are subject to regulation and those who implement regulatory frameworks. The goals of this SC focused on the development and support of regulatory systems that define midwifery practice accurately; that there is midwifery regulation in place with education and practice standards; that midwives are registered/licensed and that midwifery practice is accountable to the public/society.

The 2021 Terms of Reference state that the RegSC:
- Works with other ICM Standing Committees to define global regulation standards for midwifery.
- Identifies strategies for implementation of global regulation standards.
- Supports member associations and regulators to strengthen midwifery regulation in countries and jurisdictions.
- Provides a platform for sharing resources and midwifery regulation strategies.
- Develops a network of midwifery regulators.

- Acts as a resource of expert midwifery regulators for access and use by the ICM and partners.
- Focuses on strategic implications with regard to the development, implementation and evaluation of regulation activities.
- Facilitates specifically targeted regulation workshops at each Congress.
- Contributes to process for decision and selection of any ICM education awardees.[73]

This same committee, co-chaired by Sally Pairman (New Zealand) and Louise Silverton (UK), worked to establish Global Standards for Midwifery Regulation that were adopted by the ICM Council in 2011 and developed the Regulation Toolkit made available for MA use in 2016 (Chapter 12).

Recent ICM Standing Committees
There were two additional ICM Committees elevated to 'Standing' Committee status during the 2017–2020 triennium. Both groups were in existence for many decades as advisory to the ICM Board on finances and Congresses.[74] The Finance and Resource Committee (FiRe committee) advises the Board on the discharge of its fiduciary responsibilities in finance and resource management. The Scientific Professional and Programme Committee (SPPC) is responsible for planning and organising the Scientific Professional programme of the Triennial Congresses.

THE INTERNATIONAL DAY OF THE MIDWIFE (5 May)
Following the 1981 Congress in Brighton, England, the ICM began to take action to become a reasonably stable organisation, with increasing membership of midwifery associations across the world and the beginning of financial stability. While the task of consolidating its sustainability still had to continue, there was also a feeling that the Confederation should be undertaking more activities that would strengthen links, not only with other relevant global organisations but also with individual midwives who may not be a member of an ICM MA.

The idea of establishing a day when every midwife could celebrate achievements, connect with colleagues and promote the significance of the midwifery profession at the country level was first discussed at the 1984 Council meeting in Sydney, Australia.[75] More formal action was decided during the 1987 meeting in The Hague, the Netherlands, and the date of 5 May was proposed as a suitable day.[76] Shortly afterwards, enquiries were launched by the ICM Secretariat as to the necessary procedures for establishing an official International Day.

During the May 1989 meeting of the ICM Executive Committee in London, members were informed about the UN's criteria and procedures for the proclamation of an International Day. Any theme and actions would have to be 'universally applicable' and a member government of the UN would need to refer the request to the UN Economic and Social Council. All the ICM MAs were requested to volunteer to take forward an application via their own government. Meanwhile, all MAs and other midwives could still observe 5 May and the chosen theme for the whole of the next decade was 'Towards Safe Birth for All by the Year 2000'.[77]

With this theme in mind, the 1990 Council in Kobe, Japan, formally adopted the International Day of the Midwife (IDM) as an ICM activity to be observed officially on 5 May 1991.[78] IDM became an almost immediate success. The Executive Committee members in Madrid, Spain, December 1991, were told

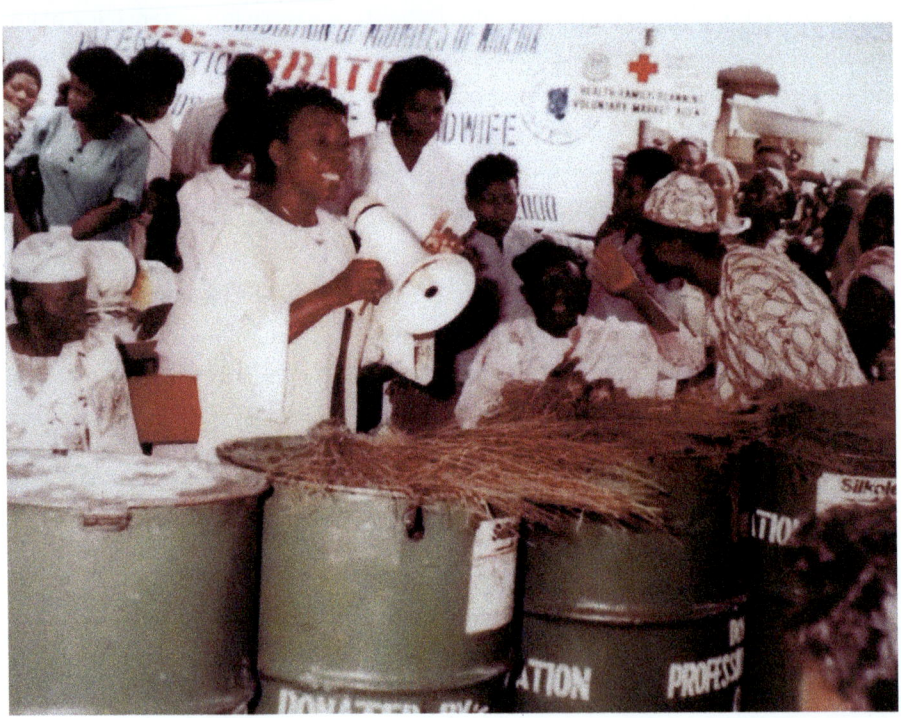

Midwives teaching the importance of Nutrition in the marketplace to mark the International Day of the Midwife – ICM Archives at Wellcome Collection

by the Board of Management that 'enterprising initiatives to mark the IDM' had been reported. For example, in the United Kingdom the RCM hired Westminster Abbey, London, for a service during which Ruth Ashton and Joan Walker read lessons to a very full Abbey. The RCM also raised money which was used to purchase a Land Rover which ICM past-Treasurer, Margaret Brain presented to Isha Daraby Kabia in Uganda. Another example was the gift of bicycles by the RCM as a means for the Ugandan midwives to have a wider access to support their communities. Church services were also held in Kingston, Jamaica and in South Australia, with the MA also securing a prime-time slot on national television.

The enthusiastic response to the IDM was renewed in 1992, and a new angle to activities had arisen. The Board noted that while IDM remains primarily a celebration of midwifery and a strategy for raising awareness, sensitising peoples and governments and putting midwifery on the public agenda, nevertheless midwives in many parts of the world turned their energies to organising events designed to raise funds to support the Safe Motherhood Initiative.

While considering plans for IDM 1993 – due to it falling in the week preceding the Vancouver Congress – the Board decided that it now seemed opportune to use IDM's potential for winning hearts and opening purses by formally incorporating an element of fund-raising into the celebrations. This growing enthusiasm was confirmed at the 1993 Council meeting in Vancouver, Canada, when the Board of Management submitted a paper entitled 'International Day of the Midwife: Evolution and Future Development'. This stated:

> 'The 5th May has been marked by an overwhelming and enormously varied response by midwives and their supporters worldwide ... news has reached HQ of festivities and celebrations which involved everyone from newborn babies to cabinet ministers and royalty. In 1991 the theme "Towards Safe Birth for all by the Year 2000" had fired imaginations and released creativity.'[79]

Many exciting IDMs have followed since 1993, with the Secretariat and Board providing themes and written documents to support MAs' celebrations in their countries. The results have added not only to the visibility of midwives and their practice but also to the ICM MAs' abilities to support midwives from countries with high levels of maternal and newborn deaths.

The 1999 the ICM Council adopted the triennial theme of 'Equity of access for all women to midwifery' and yearly sub-themes with: 2000 being 'Midwives support girls' and women's right to equal status in the community and to choice and control in reproductive health care'; 2001 being 'Midwives provide appropriate and holistic healthcare for women and families in challenging circumstances' and 2002 being 'Midwives work with women to ensure access to reproductive healthcare is seen as a human right'.[80] The IDM theme in 2005 was 'Midwives and Women-a partnership for health' to align with Millennium Development Goal (MDG) #3, the promotion of gender equity and the empowerment of women[81] and the 2007 theme was 'Midwives Reach Out to Women Wherever They Are'.[82]

The IDM theme in 2017 was 'Midwives, Mothers and Families – Partners for Life'. IDM activity in 2017 was headed up with the theme, 'I Believe in Partnership' and consisted of encouraging shared views and photos of partner activities on all ICM platforms. In 2019 the IDM theme had an even stronger message in keeping with global efforts to promote human rights, titled, 'Midwives: Defenders of Women's Rights' and was the most engaged/liked Twitter theme that year.[83] This support reflected the ICM's prior core documents and commitment to the important partnership between women and midwives. The 2021 theme was 'Follow the data: Invest in Midwives' corresponding to the release of the 2021 State of the World's Midwifery report[84] (Chapter 15).

SUMMARY

The content in this chapter highlighted many of the ways that ICM addressed the needs and issues of its MAs over the years. These included the production of documents, standards and position statements providing advocacy tools at the local level; workshops that addressed the needs of midwives at country or regional levels; programmes and projects to strengthen MAs; or expanding the capacity to meet MAs' needs through use of ICM Standing Committees. The International Day of the Midwife has served to highlight the role and accomplishments of midwives in all areas of the world. As noted at the beginning, the core business of the ICM is its MAs, and the ICM strives to balance the needs of midwives with the needs of women during their reproductive years and their newborns. The challenges of maintaining the balance between ICM's dual aims and the needs of MAs in a specific region of the world has kept ICM leadership focused and challenged for a century.

100 Years of the International Confederation of Midwives

1 The authors have used 'Objects' as the term used in the Constitution from 1954 to 2005 when the Dutch Association was agreed. Readers may be more familiar with the term 'Objectives' though both carry the same meaning.
2 Nester M Moyo. Strengthening Midwives Associations background document. 13 December 2001 p 1.
3 ICM. The International Confederation of Midwives Constitution Agreed by Council on September 10th, 1954. Article II, p 1. [Personal papers of Helen Varney Burst to be sent to the Wellcome Library ICM archives.]
4 ICM. The Constitution of the International Confederation of Midwives. September 1981, p 12.
5 ICM. (SA/ICM/R/4/) Wellcome Collection. Marjorie Bayes' History of the ICM first 50 Years, p 2. Ellen Erup letter of Miss Bayes, 5 July 1973. She noted that during the 1934 Congress Dr Minetts presented the new method of pain relief for labour using Nitrous Oxide and its air apparatus.
6 ICM. ICM Council Meeting Minutes, Vancouver, BC, 4–6, 11 May 1993. Appendix I, pp 1–12. ICM. ICM Council Meeting Minutes, Vienna, Austria, April 2002. Agenda 02.14: Regional Reports, pp 5–6.
7 ICM. ICM Council Meeting Minutes Toronto, Canada, 13 July 2017. Agenda 6.2 Feedback from Member Association Survey on Expectations of ICM.
8 Elizabeth Gilmore, 'Midwives of the world united – A report of the 20th congress of the International Confederation of Midwives, which took place in Sydney, September 1984.' Midwifery 1:3–6, 1984, p.3.
9 ICM. ICM Triennial Report 1990–1993. Chiswick, London: ICM, p 5. ICM. The Marie Goubran Memorial Award. Brochure written in conjunction with Alex Goubran, Marie's eldest son, May 1999 p 3.
10 ICM. Executive Committee Meeting 1991. Agenda item 7.1: Terms of Reference for Marie Goubran Memorial Fund. Marie was instrumental in getting ICM involved in the Safe Motherhood Initiatives in 1987 that many would agree moved the organisation out of the shadows and into the light globally!
11 ICM. Marie Goubran Memorial Fund Terms of Reference for the Award. June 2001. Terms of Reference Marie Goubran Secretary General Leadership Award. July 2004.
12 Kathy Herschderfer. Email to Alex Goubran, June 6, 2004, following dinner and discussion of the future of the Marie Goubran award. [Personal papers of Joyce Thompson]
13 ICM. Triennial Report 2014–2017. The Hague: ICM, 2014, p 36: The Marie Goubran Award.
14 Alex M Goubran. Email to Joyce Thompson June 7, 2004. [Personal papers of Joyce Thompson]
15 ICM. ICM Council Minutes Vienna, Austria, April 2002. Agenda item 18.
16 ICM. Columbia University Award for Midwives and Their Associations. The Hague: ICM, Terms of Reference for the Award, pp 1–2.
17 ICM. Save the Children Award for Midwives: Terms of Reference for the Award. 2002.
18 FIGO/ICM Joint Study Group. Maternity Care in the World: International Survey of Midwifery Practice and Training 2nd Edition. Great Britain: CM Printing Services, 1976, p vi. MG Candau. Maternity Care in the World: An International Survey of Midwifery Practice and Training. Oxford: Pergamon Press, 1966, 'The World Situation', p 18.
19 WHO. Maternity Care in the World. Report of a Joint Study Group of the International Federation of Gynaecology and Obstetrics and the International Confederation of Midwives. England: CM Printing Services, 1976, p x.
20 WHO. Maternity Care in the World. Report of a Joint Study Group of the International Federation of Gynaecology and Obstetrics and the International Confederation of Midwives. England: C.M. Printing Services, 1976, pp xi–xiii. ICM. Report of the 17th International Congress, Lausanne, Switzerland 21–28 June 1975, p 236.
21 Report of the Anglophone East Africa Working Party Nairobi, Kenya, 29th November–8th December 1973. London: ICM/FIGO Joint Study Group, p 1.
22 Report of All India Working Party, New Delhi, India, November 5th–12th 1976. London: Joint Study Group of the ICM/FIGO, p 6.
23 ICM 'Cento' Countries Working Part, Istanbul, Turkey, December 7th–14th, 1976. London: ICM, 1976.
24 ICM-FIGO Anglophone Middle East Regional Seminar, Khartoum, Sudan, November 12th–18th, 1977. London: ICM, 1977.
25 ICM. Triennial Report 2017–2020. The Hague: ICM, p 22.
26 Helping Mothers Survive (HMS) is a suite of programmes developed by Jhpiego, in line with the latest WHO guidelines and endorsed by global professional organisation such as ICM, FIGO, AAP, ICN and UNFPA.
27 ICM. Triennial Report 2017–2020. The Hague: ICM, p 18.
28 ICM. Triennial Report 2014–2017. The Hague: ICM, p 27.
29 ICM. Triennial Report 2014–2017. The Hague: ICM, p 51.
30 ICM. Triennial Report 2017–2020. The Hague: ICM, p 21.
31 ICM. Triennial Report 2017–2020. The Hague: ICM, p 20.
32 The first Congress Handbook was prepared by the Board of Management and Secretariat in 1999.
33 ICM Secretariat. The International Confederation of Midwives. London: ICM, 1981. This was a 17-page booklet with a forward and brief history of ICM by Marjorie Bayes, and additional content that included the 1972 Definition of the Midwife, key ICM activities and partners, the structure and Aim and Activities of the confederation, and a discussion of membership and its advantages.

34 ICM. Triennial Report 2008–2011. The Hague: ICM, p 11: Twinning.
35 ICM. ICM Council Meeting Minutes Kobe, Japan, October 1990. ICM Regional Representative Report on Anglophone African Countries for 1987–1990 Triennium, p 4.
36 ICM. Triennial Report 2008–2011. The Hague: ICM, back cover.
37 ICM. Triennial Report 2011–2014. The Hague: ICM, p 14.
38 International News. Midwifery 17:2, pp 158–159.
39 Nester Moyo. ICM promotes international leadership development for young midwives. International Midwifery 17:4 (July/August), 2004, p 44.
40 Nester Moyo. International Young Midwifery Leaders Programme. The Hague: ICM, November 2003.
41 JB Thompson, NT Moyo, JT Fullerton. Young Midwifery Leaders Programs: Capacity building for the future. International Journal of Childbirth 6(2), 2016, pp 58–67. http:/dx.doi.org/10.1891/2156-5287.6.2.58.
42 Nester Moyo. ICM promotes international leadership development for young midwives. International Midwifery 17:4 (July/August), 2004, pp 44–45.
43 ICM. Address List: YML Programme April 2004–March 2007. The Hague: ICM. [Personal papers of Joyce Thompson]
44 Nester Moyo. Programme Manager's Report May to September 2004. Executive Committee Agenda item 5.2, p 3.
45 Nester Moyo. Programme Manager's Report May to September 2004. Executive Committee Agenda item 5.2, p 2.
46 JB Thompson, NT Moyo, JT Fullerton. Young Midwifery Leaders Programs: Capacity building for the future. International Journal of Childbirth 6(2), 2016, pp 58–67. http:/dx.doi.org/10.1891/2156-5287.6.2.58.
47 ICM. Triennial Report 2014–2017. The Hague: ICM, 2017, p 28. Triennial report 2017–2020, p 21.
48 Nester Moyo. ICM Proposal: Strengthening Midwifery Association. April 2, 2002, pp 4–5. Board of Management Agenda 8.3. [Personal papers of Joyce Thompson]
49 ICM. ICM Minutes of Council 14–17 June 2011, Durban, South Africa. The Hague: ICM. 2011, p 21.
50 ICM. Report of ICM Midwifery Services Technical Advisory Meeting 2–4 February 2009. The Hague: ICM, List of Participants and details of deliberations. [Personal papers of Joyce Thompson]
51 ICM. Triennial Report 2008–2011. The Hague: ICM, p 13: Developing a Globally Midwifery Services Framework.
52 ICM. Triennial Report 2017–2020. The Hague: ICM, p 16.
53 ICM. ICM Minutes of Council 13–16 June 2017, Toronto, Canada. The Hague: ICM, 2017, p 18.
54 Downloaded from www.internationalmidwives.org on 17 March 2021.
55 Adapted from ICM website. Downloaded from www.internationalmidwives.org on 17 March 2021.
56 ICM/JHPIEGO/MNH/POLICY PROJECT. Advocacy and Leadership Workshops: Progress Report. Agenda 14.2, Executive Committee 2003.
57 ICM. Triennial Report 2017–2020. The Hague: ICM, 2020, p 20.
58 Downloaded and adapted from ICM website: www.internationalmidwives.org on 17 March 2021.
59 ICM. ICM Triennial Report 2011–2014. ICM's Inaugural Global Goodwill Ambassador, p 21.
60 ICM. ICM Triennial Report 2011–2014. ICM's Inaugural Global Goodwill Ambassador, p 21.
61 ICM. ICM Council Meeting Minutes, April 2002, Vienna, Austria. The Hague: ICM, 2002, p 31. Agenda 42.1 & 42.2 Professional Practice Standing Committee dissolved by vote of Council.
62 ICM. Draft Record of the ICM Council Meeting Oslo, Norway, 21–23 May 1996. Agenda 96.30 Research Standing Committee, p 16. Terms of Reference adopted unanimously.
63 ICM. (SA/ICM/C/1/22). Wellcome Collection. Meeting of the Executive Committee, Uganda 11 January 1995. Research Standing Committee Terms of Reference adopted by the ICM Executive Committee January 1995.
64 ICM. (SA/ICM/C/1/22). Wellcome Collection. Meeting of the Executive Committee, Uganda 11 January 1995. Research Standing Committee Terms of Reference, p 1. Adopted by the ICM Executive Committee January 1995.
65 Downloaded from www.internationalmidwives.org on 17 March 2021.
66 ICM. ICM Council Meeting Minutes Brisbane, Australia 18–21 July 2005. Agenda 17.1: Research Standing Committee Triennial Report 2002–2005, p 4 – Research Advisory Network.
67 ICM. Minutes of the ICM Board of Management, February 2001. The Hague: ICM, Min 02/01/13: Research Standing Committee, p 4.
68 HP Kennedy, MJ Renfrew, BC Madi, D Opoku, JB Thompson. The conduct of ethical research collaboration across international and culturally diverse communities. Midwifery. 22:2 (May 12), 2006, pp 100–7.
69 ICM. ICM Council Meeting Minutes, April 2002, Vienna, Austria. The Hague: ICM, 2002, p 32. Agenda 42.4: Education Standing committee.
70 Ans Luyben, Mary Barger, Susan McDonald. Triennial Report of Activities of the Education Standing committee (2008–2011), January 2011, pp 1–2. Re-establishing the Education Standing Committee.
71 Adapted from Terms of Reference of Education Standing Committee downloaded from www.internationalmidwives.org on 17 March 2021.

72 ICM. ICM Council Meeting Minutes, Brisbane, Australia 18–21 July 2005. Item: 21.4.3 Regulation Standing Committee Terms of Reference adopted, pp 18–19.
73 Downloaded from www.internationalmidwives.org on 18 March 2021.
74 ICM. ICM Triennial Report 2014–2017. ICM Standing Committees, p 9, reflects the addition of previous ICM committees to the level of Standing Committees. These included the Scientific Professional and Programme Committee (SPPC) and the Finance and Resource Committee (FiRe Committee).
75 ICM. ICM Council Meeting Minutes, Sydney, Australia, 1984.
76 ICM. ICM Council Meeting Minutes, The Hague, Netherlands, 18–20, 23, 25 August 1987. Minutes 87/20: International Midwives Day, p 8.
77 ICM. Executive Committee Meeting Minutes, London, May 1989. ICM. ICM Council Meeting Minutes, Kobe, Japan, October 2–4, 1990. Minute 87/20 International Midwives Day, p 4.
78 ICM. ICM Council Meeting Minutes, Kobe, Japan, October 2–4, 1990. Minute 87/20 International Midwives Day, p 4.
79 ICM Board of Management. International Day of the Midwife: Evolution and Future Development, May 1993. ICM. ICM Council Meeting Minutes, Vancouver, British Columbia, 4–6, 11 May 1993. MIN 93.23 International Day of the Midwife, pp 20–21.
80 ICM. ICM Council Meeting Minutes, Manila, Philippines, May 1999. Agenda 99.33 International Day of the Midwife, pp 33–34.
81 UNDP. Millennium Development Goals, 2000–2015. New York: United Nations, 2000.
82 ICM. International Midwifery. Journal of the ICM. 20:1 (March 2007), p 16.
83 ICM. Annual Report 2019. The Hague: ICM, 2019.
84 Downloaded from www.internationalmidwives.org on 5 July 2021.

Chapter 11: *ICM's Core Documents*

'Like the proverbial house built upon the sand the ICM has been buffeted by many storms mainly in the form of finance and war. Although severely shaken the house stood. Along came the need to extend the house but the sand was shifting as the environment changed. Wise leaders saw and predicted further and ongoing changes. Their response was not to demolish the house but to underpin it and put in a solid and deep base able to withstand changes and enable the house to be extended. These core and guidance documents are the ones forming the base on which the ICM has continued to grow and develop.'

Joan Walker's Reflections on the ICM

INTRODUCTION

Whether midwifery is a profession or a 'calling' (vocation) has been a long-standing debate throughout the history of midwifery in the world, though the early practitioners and today's midwives have always accepted their 'professional' status. Questions about the status of midwifery as a 'profession' often came from outside midwifery, whether to challenge the scope of practice by others who thought childbearing was their domain or the legitimacy of a predominantly women's work qualifying as a profession. Two basic questions in the 20th and 21st centuries that the ICM and its Member Associations (MAs) have faced are: 1) Is midwifery a profession (or a discipline) distinct from other health professions involved in providing services for women and childbearing families, and 2) What role does 'autonomy' play in cementing midwifery's status as a profession?

What is a Profession?

One dictionary definition of 'profession' defines this word, of Latin origin, as 'a calling requiring specialised knowledge and often long and intensive academic preparation.'[1] Other definitions, such as that used in Sweden, define a profession as an occupation with its own area of competence (which no others have), own education, regulation and research with an ethical code. The early 'learned' professions included medicine, law and theology. More recent use of the term 'profession' reflects a group that agrees that it has a body of specialised knowledge, will adhere to accepted standards of education and practice, acknowledges its ethical obligations, and has some form of credentialing that allows one to be recognised as a professional and paid for one's services.[2] In other words, not only does the midwifery profession require formal education that includes its unique or specialised aspects, a code of ethics, standards that guide midwifery behaviour and practice, and societal acceptance through regulation, it must be responsible for defining and maintaining these. Over time, the ICM developed the needed documents of a 'profession' in the format of position statements, core documents and standards.

> 'Midwifery is a brave and political tradition, standing for dignity as well as science.'
>
> Kate Gilmore, UNHCHR, June 2017

Why Autonomy?

Autonomy often comes into the discussion of 'profession' and 'responsibility'. In its simplest form, autonomy means 'self-governing' from the Greek auto (self) and nomos (governing). When the ICM published its Glossary of Terms in 2011 (updated in 2017), to assist members and those outside the profession in understanding the newly minted standards for education and regulation, 'autonomous midwifery profession' was defined as: 'A professional group of midwives granted legal authority to self-govern and self-regulate, thereby publicly holding midwives accountable for meeting professional standards in order to promote the safety of women and newborns in their care'[3].

The glossary also provided the definition of autonomous as: 'Self-governing, self-regulating; taking responsibility for one's decisions and actions and their outcomes'[4] as reinforcement of what it means to have midwifery considered a profession. Inherent in these definitions is the group's responsibility to clearly define who a midwife is and the scope of midwifery practice, along with an agreed code of moral behaviour and standards for education, regulation and practice. However, nowhere in these definitions does the ICM imply that midwives can function in isolation from other professions or international partners – the somewhat negative adolescent view that, 'I can do it myself!' Thus, to be self-regulating and responsible for midwifery affairs is congruent with respecting and working with other professional groups and partners as discussed throughout this book.

The evolution of the autonomy of the midwifery profession led by clear actions of the ICM since 1972 are discussed in this chapter, focusing on what has been defined as ICM core documents,[5] beginning in 1972 with the Definition of the Midwife. Content in Chapter 12 addresses the 21st century adoption of the ICM standards for midwifery education and regulation. Taken together, the content in these two chapters reinforce ICM's position that midwifery is an autonomous profession and its practitioners are professionals.

INTERNATIONAL DEFINITION OF THE MIDWIFE

Among the significant powers of the ICM Council delegates is agreeing the definition of:
- who is a midwife,
- what is the midwifery scope of practice and
- how should a midwife be educated and regulated.

There was consensus among ICM leaders and member associations that having an agreed international definition of who a midwife was and the midwifery scope of practice was a key milestone in ICM's organisational development. The brief historical evolution of the definition of the midwife adopted by ICM Councils over the years follows.

The Road to the First Joint ICM/FIGO/WHO International Definition of the Midwife – 1972

The first ICM Council-agreed definition of the midwife came from the collective views of the members of the WHO Expert Committee on 'The Midwife in Maternity Care'. As noted in Chapter 13, this group was charged with examining the status of midwives and midwifery practice in the world. The members agreed the need for a clear definition of the midwife in order to carry out their mandate and thus adopted the first International Definition of the Midwife in 1965.[6] The second International Definition of the Midwife came out of the ICM/FIGO Working Party on Midwifery Training in European Countries in 1969 discussed in Chapter 16.[7] The third International Definition of the Midwife came from the ICM/FIGO Joint Study Group (JSG)[8] who thought the earlier WHO definition was out of date. This 1972 draft definition was divided into two sections:

'A Midwife is a person who, having been regularly admitted to a midwifery education programme, duly recognised in the country in which it is located, has successfully completed the prescribed course of studies in midwifery and has acquired the requisite qualifications to be registered and/or legally licensed to practise midwifery.

Sphere of Practice:
'She must be able to give the necessary supervision, care and advice to women during pregnancy, labour and the post-partum period, to conduct deliveries on her own responsibility and to care for the newborn and the infant. This care includes preventative measure, the detection of abnormal conditions in mother and child, the procurement of medical assistance and the execution of emergency measures in the absence of medical help.

'She has an important task in health counselling and education, not only for patients but also within the family and community. The work should involve ante-natal education and preparation for parenthood and extends to certain areas of gynaecology, family planning and child care.

'She may practice in hospitals, clinics, health units, domiciliary conditions or any other service.'[9]

The JSG recommended that this amended 1972 International Definition of the Midwife be circulated to Governments, FIGO, ICM, WHO, IPPF and other international organisations. The process expected was that members of the JSG would take this definition and other recommendations from the 1966 study back to their professional associations for discussion and approval at their next meetings.[10] The ICM adopted this joint definition during its 1972 Council meeting[11] in Washington DC; FIGO adopted it during its international meeting in 1973[12] and the WHO soon after.[13] The reason that FIGO and WHO appeared at the bottom of the ICM definition until 2005 was that it was essentially drafted by representatives of both health professional groups and used by the WHO in their work globally. The ICM categorised this first formal definition of the midwife and scope of practice as one document under the title 'Position Statement'.[14]

The changes in the ICM International Definition of the Midwife over the next 50 years are documented in various Council meeting minutes. The Definition was reviewed and unchanged (minor wordsmithing of scope of practice) in 1990

100 Years of the International Confederation of Midwives

and once again endorsed by FIGO in 1991 and the WHO in 1992.[15] Changes thereafter are briefly described below.

Updated ICM Definition of the Midwife

In 2005, the ICM Council voted to eliminate reference to the gender of the midwife, using 'midwife' in place of 'she' throughout the definition.[16] After much discussion it was also agreed to not ask FIGO and the WHO to agree to the definition, but possibly endorse it without reference on the printed version of the revised ICM definition.[17] The importance of having an agreed international definition of the midwife without other attributions reflected ICM's ongoing efforts to promote the autonomy of the profession. The ICM Council reviewed and updated the Definition and Scope of Practice of the Midwife on several occasions[18], with the significant update in 2011 that created a definition that was consistent with the revised essential competencies and new education and regulation standards.[19]

The most recent review was in 2017 without changes. The current definition reads:

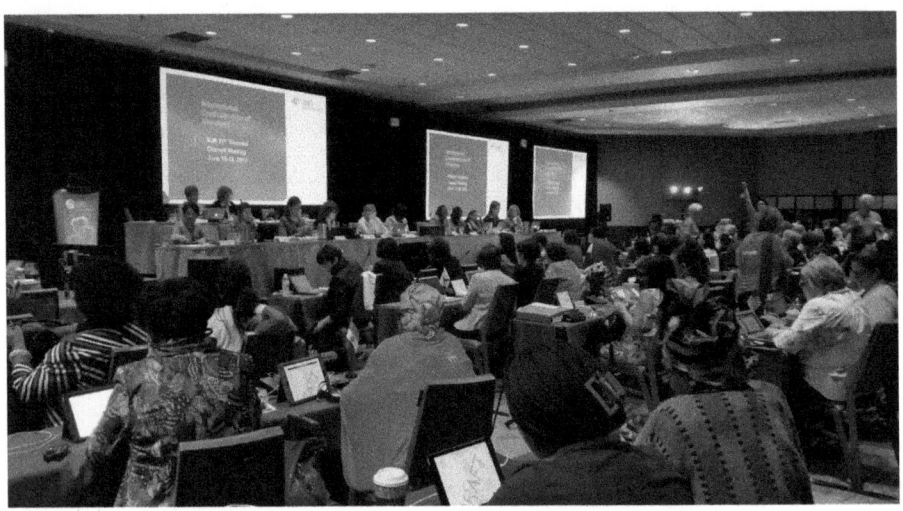

2017 ICM Council Meeting in Toronto – ICM Archives at Wellcome Collection

> 'A midwife is a person who has successfully completed a midwifery education programme that is based on the ICM Essential Competencies for Basic Midwifery Practice and the framework of the ICM Global Standards for Midwifery Education and is recognized in the country where it is located; who has acquired

the requisite qualifications to be registered and/or legally licensed to practice midwifery and use the title "midwife"; and who demonstrates competency in the practice of midwifery'.[20]

SCOPE OF MIDWIFERY PRACTICE

The scope of midwifery practice was defined in 1972 as Sphere of Practice, a part of the first *Definition of the Midwife* as noted earlier. There were many ICM Council discussions over the years related to key parts of the ICM scope of practice. Some of these debates centred on whether midwives should focus their practice solely on childbearing women or should include care for women in their reproductive years who were not pregnant. Many of these debates are chronicled in Chapter 8's discussion of the *Vision* and *Mission* statements over the years. An important sentence began the scope of practice in 2005, recognising the midwife as responsible and accountable professional working in partnership with women.[21]

The *Scope of Practice* was titled separately from the Definition of the Midwife in Durban, 2011, following the recommendation of the joint Education and Regulation task forces at that time.

The *Definition* and *Scope of Practice* were also considered Core Documents as of that time.[22] There were no changes with the review in 2017. Thus, the current 2021 ICM definition of the midwife's scope of practice reads:

'Scope of Practice

The midwife is recognised as a responsible and accountable professional who works in partnership with women to give the necessary support, care and advice during pregnancy, labour and the postpartum period, to conduct births on the midwife's own responsibility and to provide care for the newborn and the infant. This care includes preventative measures, the promotion of normal birth, the detection of complications in mother and child, the accessing of medical care or other appropriate assistance and the carrying out of emergency measures.

The midwife has an important task in health counselling and education, not only for the woman, but also within the family and the community. This work should involve antenatal education and preparation for parenthood and may extend to women's health, sexual or reproductive health[23] and child care.

A midwife may practise in any setting including the home, community, hospitals, clinics, or health units.'[24]

INTERNATIONAL CODE OF ETHICS FOR MIDWIVES (1993)

As noted in the introduction to this chapter, autonomous professions have a code of moral behaviour often called a code of ethics. The development of the first ICM *International Code of Ethics for Midwives* underwent a 6-year process of consultation prior to its unanimous acceptance by the 1993 ICM Council.[25] The discussion of the need for a code of ethics began in August 1987 when an abstract was accepted from Drs Henry and Joyce Thompson[26] that proposed a draft code of ethics for professional midwifery that they had written for presentation during the ICM Congress in The Hague. The Thompsons' intent was to familiarise the ICM Council with basic tenets of codes of ethics and, hopefully, begin the discussion as to whether the ICM should adopt a global code of moral behaviour for professional midwives.

The ICM Board accepted the Thompsons' abstract but limited attendance to the Executive Committee members for the half-day workshop. The workshop was divided into an introduction to ethical theory and moral development followed by a discussion of the need for an international code for midwives. 'Major concerns raised included how statements [of ethics] might be worded to reflect the diversity of midwifery practice throughout the world (as well as similarities), what national and local politics needed to be considered, and whether midwifery dilemmas in practice differ by region or locale.'[27] Given these concerns, no attempt was made to agree on language in 1987 though plans for follow-up were discussed.

In December 1991, the ICM Board requested a second ethics workshop for the ICM Executive Committee led by the Thompsons in Madrid, Spain. During this meeting, several drafts of the code of ethics were developed based on review and discussion of the values inherent in the ICM Definition of the Midwife, the Constitution's Aims and Objects, and accepted ICM position statements relevant to ethical conduct of the midwife. In the interest of providing a worldwide focus to the ICM code, the Executive Committee analysed seven MAs' codes received at the ICM HQ during 1991, highlighting the common ethical concerns of safety, competence, accountability, confidentiality, respect for human dignity, client involvement in decisions, appropriate consultation and referral (teamwork), non-discrimination and involvement in research and education of future midwives.[28]

The Executive Committee went through three different reviews of proposed statements that resulted in a Draft #4 of the code that was sent out to the ICM MAs for discussion and comment before the 1993 ICM Council meeting in Vancouver, Canada. This mailing included a background paper on how the draft code was developed, including:

- ✓ the need for culturally sensitive wording;
- ✓ that whenever possible the ICM code would promote a global (universal) level of morality – reflecting universal ethical principles; and
- ✓ consciously excluding reference to the law or legal entities.[29]

The draft Code was adopted unanimously by the 1993 ICM Council.[30] The *International Code of Ethics for Midwives* contained an Introduction, Preamble as well as four sections with three-seven moral statements each related to:

- Midwifery Relationships;
- Practice of Midwifery;
- The Professional Responsibilities of Midwives; and
- Advancement of Midwifery Knowledge and Practice.

As this was a relatively new area of knowledge for many midwives and MAs, the ICM Board of Management commissioned the publication of a booklet to increase understanding and use of the 1993 Code. The booklet contained the Code, the glossary of terms used in the Code, the ethical analysis of each statement in the Code, a brief history of the development of the Code and suggestions on how midwives could use the Code in their practice, education, or research activities.[31]

The Code was reviewed and revised slightly during the ICM Council meeting in Manila, Philippines, 1999, and then again per schedule in 2008, 2014 and 2020. Minor wordsmithing with few exceptions occurred with each review, a testament to the careful consideration of global understanding of concepts by the Executive Committee in 1991 that adopted universal, culturally sensitive words throughout.

The first important additions occurred in Section I with the addition of a statement related to the midwife as a person of moral worth in 1999[32] along with the statement on violations of human rights.

> I. g The Midwife has responsibilities as a person of moral worth, including duties of moral self-respect and the preservation of integrity
>
> III. d Midwives understand the adverse consequences that ethical and human rights violations have on the health of women and infants and will work to eliminate these violations.[33]

The next additions to the ICM code occurred in the Preamble and in Sections I and III. The first paragraph of the <u>Preamble</u> remained the same, but now includes a second paragraph first added in 2008.[34]

> The aim of the International Confederation of Midwives (ICM) is to improve the standard of care provided to women, babies, and families throughout the world through the development, education and appropriate utilization of the professional midwife. In keeping with this aim, the ICM sets forth the following code to guide the education, practice and research of the midwife. This code acknowledges women as persons with human rights, seeks justice for all people and equity in access to health care, and is based on mutual relationships of respect, trust, and the dignity of all members of society.
>
> The code addresses the midwife's ethical mandates in keeping with the Mission, the International definition of the Midwife, and standards of ICM to promote the health and wellbeing of women and newborns within their families and communities. Such care may encompass the reproductive life cycle of the woman from the pre- pregnancy stage right through to the menopause and to the end of life. These mandates include how midwives relate to others; how they practice midwifery; how they uphold professional responsibilities and duties; and how they are to work to assure the integrity of the profession of midwifery.[35]

One addition to Section III in 2014 offered further guidance on the responsibilities of midwives who conscientiously object to a given service requested by a woman and their role when human rights are violated. They include:

> III. d. Midwives with conscientious objection to a given service request will refer the woman to another provider where such a service can be provided.[36]

The latter followed the adoption of a revised statement of *Mission* and another Core Document in 2011, *Bill of Rights for Women and Midwives*, discussed below. All current ICM Core Documents can be found on the ICM website under Core Documents: www.internationalmidwives.org

PHILOSOPHY AND MODEL OF MIDWIFERY CARE (2005)

For centuries midwives have provided health services (care) for women, newborns and families as trusted members of their communities. Midwives expressed their deeply held beliefs about the naturalness of women's childbearing experiences for most women over the years in the way they provided midwifery care. In other words, midwives believed that why they provided care was just as important as how they provided care for others. From an organisational perspective, the ICM in its early years was guided by its constitutional Aims and Objects that led to written statements of Vision, Mission and Ethics in the 1990s. It was a natural next step for ICM to clearly define both the midwifery philosophy and model of care based on these documents so that all the world could more clearly understand who a midwife was/is and what the essence of midwifery care entails. When the first ICM Glossary of Terms was adopted in 2011 following the release of the updated ICM Essential Competencies for Basic Midwifery Practice and the adoption of the new standards for education and regulation (Chapter 12), the term Midwifery Philosophy was included. It read, *'A statement of beliefs and values about the nature of midwifery – whether in practice, education, regulation, management or research.'*[37] However, what midwives believed about the nature of midwifery was yet to be defined.

In the early 2000s the ICM Board began to discuss the need to put on paper what midwives believed about childbearing care and how that care should be given, knowing that it was their beliefs about childbearing and women's roles in it that often set them apart from others providing these services. This discussion led to a beginning statement of philosophy, followed by the distinguishing characteristics of midwifery care labelled the 'midwifery model of care.' Nester Moyo, ICM Project Director at the time, drafted two documents that were presented for discussion during the 2002 ICM Council meeting in Vienna, Austria.

The initial draft of two documents (philosophy and model of care) were discussed at length during the 2002 Council meeting resulting in the several recommendations that were sent on to the 2004 Executive Committee meeting in Trinidad for discussion and finalisation. The suggestions from the Council working group were that the two documents be merged into one and edited into a shorter version with simple, positive language and reference to the ICM *Definition of the Midwife*. In addition, it was suggested that the philosophy come first in the document followed by the model of care, and that the document include a statement of purpose and how it would be used.[38]

The Executive Committee worked on the integration of the two documents and their wording, adopting the revised statement as in the interim document sent on to the 2005 ICM Council in Brisbane, Australia, for final review and approval.[39] The 2005 draft was based on the ICM Definition of the Midwife updated in 2005, the 1999 *Vision statements for Women and for Midwives*, the 2002 update of the International *Code of Ethics for Midwives* and the newly adopted 2002 *Essential Competencies for Basic Midwifery Practice*.

The revised document, *Philosophy and Model of Midwifery Care*, that was presented to the 2005 ICM Council included the first page on Background highlighting the reasons for having the statement, beginning with the ICM Definition of the Midwife and research indicating that midwife-led continuity models of care are associated with benefits for mother and newborns. It also noted that the standard of midwives being the professional of choice for childbearing women was based on the ICM's requirement for competency-based education and respect for human dignity, compassion and the promotion of human rights for all persons.[40]

When the one-and-a-half page statement of philosophy and model of midwifery care was presented to the ICM Council in 2005, it was adopted with agreed word changes from the 2004 Executive Committee. Wording from the *Definition of the Midwife* was used for inclusion of the concepts of 'reproductive health'.[41] This Core Document was a culmination of work begun in 1972 and throughout the 1990s[42] to clarify to the global audience who a 21st-century midwife was/is and what constitutes midwifery care.

A key element of the philosophy is the belief in the *normal physiologic processes of pregnancy and childbearing* for most women that carry *significant meaning to the woman, her family and the community*. Key elements of the midwifery model of care include promoting, protecting and supporting women's human, reproductive and sexual health and rights with respect for ethnic and cultural diversity and advocating for non-intervention in normal childbirth. Empowerment of women through information and support is one basis for the partnership model of care.

In addition, midwives agree the need to maintain their own competence and practice in collaboration with other health professionals when needed. The 2014[43] version of the *Philosophy and Model of Midwifery Care* that remains in effect in 2022 can be found on the ICM website: www.internationalmidwives.org

BILL OF RIGHTS FOR WOMEN AND MIDWIVES (2011)

The proposed *Bill of Rights for Women and Midwives* came from the Asia-Pacific region in 2011. It was thoroughly discussed during the ICM Council meeting with the decision to delay voting on the document while directing the Asia-Pacific regional delegates, specifically Karen Gilliland, to continue editing the document based on key discussion points during Council.[44] They were asked to submit the final document to the ICM Council within three months. Though that deadline was not met, the attribution at the bottom of the current document states that the statement was adopted in Durban 2011 (though actually during 2012 yearly Council meeting) and reviewed and adopted in Toronto in 2017.[45] Chapter 14 has some details on this statement as well.

The background of this ICM Position Statement [now Core Document] called 'for governments globally to recognise and support accessible and effective midwifery care as a basic human right of all women, babies and midwives'[46]. The justification related, in part, to the growing global concern for ongoing violence against women, lack of gender equity and the fact that midwifery is a predominantly female profession serving women. The document states:

> 'The *Bill of Rights for Women and Midwives* addresses those basic human rights of women and midwives that have been systematically denied and adds another framework to approach governments when demanding change to improve midwifery and maternity services.'[47]

The background page goes on to acknowledge the ICM's role in meeting the United Nations' Sustainable Development Goal 3 (3.1 reduction of maternal mortality ratio; 3.7 ensuring universal access to sexual and reproductive health care services) and Goal 5 (Achieve gender equality and empower all women and girls).

The Bill of Rights statement for women and for midwives reflects the earlier vision statements and code of ethics adopted by the ICM Council in 1993 and the position statement, 'Midwives, Women and Human Rights' adopted in 2002.[48] An additional section on 'Women's and Midwives' Rights' bring in the ICM Council's 21st-century focus on a 'system of regulation that will ensure a safe, competent and autonomous midwifery workforce for women and their babies' in addition to workforce planning so that governments have sufficient midwives to meet the needs of women and babies.

Of interest historically is Statement 4: 'The midwifery profession has the right to be recognised as a separate and distinct profession.'[49] This statement continues the centuries-old debate about whether midwifery is a distinct profession in its own right that arose initially in Europe (Chapter 3) and continues to be a problem for midwives in some areas of the world. This statement highlights the deliberate efforts of the ICM during the last 50 years to develop the documents needed to settle this debate once and for all, including the code of ethics, essential competencies that define the unique scientific bases of midwifery practice and standards for education and regulation that demonstrate the profession's commitment to be responsible for setting the standards for midwives' education and practice.

The 2017 update[50] of the position statement was based on agreed concepts contained in the updated ICM core documents and key updated position statements that addressed ICM's beliefs about midwifery care.

DEFINITION OF MIDWIFERY (2017)

The ICM Council agreed the definition of the term 'Midwifery' following a 2-year process of updating the 2011 ICM Glossary of Terms and mandate by the 2014 Council for a task force to draft such a definition.[51] Therefore, the newest Position Statement [now Core Document] adopted by the ICM Council in 2017 was the *Definition of Midwifery*.[52] This definition was not included in the ICM Glossary of Terms when first adopted by the ICM Board in 2011.[53] The final definition adopted by the 2017 ICM Council was a 'Position Statement', not a core document, and was added to the ICM Glossary of Terms 2017.[54]

The definition of 'Midwifery' acknowledges midwifery as a profession with a 'unique body of knowledge, skills and professional behaviours drawn from disciplines shared by other health professions such as science and sociology but practised by midwives within a professional framework of autonomy, partnership, ethics and accountability'[55]. The rest of the document explains the midwifery approach to care, the autonomy and competencies of the midwife, and education based on the ICM global standards. The document also includes such statements as 'only midwives practise midwifery' and that other health professionals (nurses and doctors) providing care to women and newborns 'do not possess the competencies of a midwife and do not provide midwifery skills, but rather aspects of maternal and newborn care.'[56] Not every MA agreed with these statements of exclusiveness, but they were outnumbered in the final vote. Though these statements seemed self-serving and necessary at the time, it may be too early to tell what their effect will have on long-standing partnerships with other health professionals providing sexual, reproductive, maternal and newborn care in many areas of the world.

SUMMARY

The ICM Council delegates over the years have agreed several Core Documents considered essential to the autonomy, growth and strengthening of the midwifery profession and their MAs. ICM has accepted the responsibility as a global health professional organisation representing professional midwives throughout the world to make known what it believes about the midwifery profession including how it defines midwives, midwifery, ethics and the philosophy and model of midwifery care. These documents are essential advocacy tools to inform governments, policymakers, partners, midwifery associations and individual midwives on who and why midwives are important to the world's health. During the 21st century, ICM Council delegates agreed to convert the position statement on human rights to a core document and moved the essential competencies and global standards on education and regulation to a separate category of 'standards' as described in Chapter 12, without changing the importance of any of these documents. Together these ICM documents and standards provide a solid foundation for the work of the ICM during the next 100 years.

100 Years of the International Confederation of Midwives

1 'Profession.' Merriam Webster Free Dictionary, downloaded from web on 1 November 2013.
2 HO Thompson, JE Thompson. 'Toward a professional ethic.' Journal of Nurse-Midwifery 32: 2, March/April 1987, pp 105–110. The section on 'Background on professions' pp 106–107 details various characteristics of professions.
3 ICM. ICM Glossary of Terms 2011, updated June 2017. The Hague: ICM, 2017, p 2.
4 ICM. ICM Glossary of Terms 2011, updated June 2017. The Hague: ICM, 2017, p 1.
5 The early definition and code of ethics were titled 'Position statements' and then changed to distinguish between Position Statements and those documents that were 'core' to all the activities of the ICM. The original 'core' documents included the definition of the midwife and the code of ethics, expanding in the 2000s to include the Essential Competencies for Basic Midwifery Practice, the Philosophy and Model of Midwifery Care, and the global standards for education and regulation. As of 2020 the ICM website added the human rights statement and definition of midwifery to Core documents and excluded the competencies and standards as 'Core', but important to the work of midwives and ICM throughout the world.
6 WHO. The Midwife in Maternity Care: Report of a WHO Expert Committee. Geneva: WHO Technical Report Series No 331, 1966, p 8.
7 WHO. Maternity Care in the World. Report of a Joint Study Group of the International Federation of Gynaecology and Obstetrics and the International Confederation of Midwives. England: CM Printing Services, 1976, p ix.
8 WHO. Maternity Care in the World. Report of a Joint Study Group of the International Federation of Gynaecology and Obstetrics and the International Confederation of Midwives. England: CM Printing Services, 1976, p ix.
9 WHO. Maternity Care in the World. Report of a Joint Study Group of the International Federation of Gynaecology and Obstetrics and the International Confederation of Midwives. England: CM Printing Services, 1976, p x–xi.
10 WHO. Maternity Care in the World. Report of a Joint Study Group of the International Federation of Gynaecology and Obstetrics and the International Confederation of Midwives. England: CM Printing Services, 1976, p xxii.
11 ICM. Council Minutes Washington, DC, 1972. MIN … The date of adoption by the ICM Council was 1972 as printed on the bottom of the official document, 'Definition of the Midwife' and referred to in several sources.
12 Betty Cowell & David Wainwright. Behind the Blue Door: The History of the Royal College of Midwives 1881–1981. London: Bailliere Tindall, p 3 notes, 'The College by 1977 represented 70 percent of midwives in the country and thus in a strong position to make a submission to the Royal Commission on the National Health Service As a preliminary, the College stated its endorsement of the definition of "midwife" accepted by the Council of the International Confederation of Midwives five years earlier [1972].'
13 ICM. Executive Manual. Chiswick, London: ICM, 1996. Document explaining the structure and key activities of the ICM with the 'Definition of the Midwife' included on the final page. The historical note at the bottom that reads, 'Jointly developed by the International Confederation of Midwives and the International Federation of Gynaecology and Obstetrics; Adopted by the International Confederation of Midwives Council 1972; Adopted by the International Federation of Gynaecology and Obstetrics 1973; Later adopted by the World Health Organization. Amended by the International Confederation of Midwives Council, Kobe, October 1990; Amendment ratified by the International Federation of Gynaecology and Obstetrics 1991 and the World Health Organisation 1992.
14 ICM. Position statement: Definition of the Midwife. London: ICM, 1972, 1990.
15 ICM. ICM Council Meeting Minutes, Kobe, Japan, 1990. The definition was reviewed with minor changes, with the amendment ratified by the International Federation of Gynaecology and Obstetrics in 1991 and the World Health Organization 1992 as noted on the bottom of the ICM Position Statement in 1990. ICM. ICM Council Minutes, Vancouver, Canada, May 4–6,11, 1993. Min 93.20.8 Definition of the Midwife revision defeated at this meeting.
16 ICM. ICM Council Minutes, Brisbane, Australia, 18–21 July 2005. Agenda 05.21.3 Definition of the midwife: agreed to delete all 'she' and use the term 'midwife' throughout the definition to include 'male or female' and change 'family planning' to 'sexual and reproductive health', p 17.
17 ICM. ICM Definition of the Midwife. The Hague: ICM, Adopted by the International Confederation of Midwives Council meeting, 19 July 2005. Supersedes the ICM Definition of the Midwife 1972 and its amendments of 1990. No further mention of WHO or FIGO endorsement.
18 ICM. ICM Council Minutes, Brisbane, Australia, 18–21 July 2005. Agenda 05.21.3 Definition of the Midwife: agreed to change 'family planning' to 'sexual and reproductive health', p 17.
19 ICM. ICM Council Meeting Minutes 14–17 June 2011. Min. 10.1, Adoption of updated Definition of the Midwives, p 18. 'Dr Sally Pairman, Taskforce Chair, pointed out that the intention was to create an ICM definition that was consistent with standards, revised competencies and underpins the education a midwife has.'
20 The definition in 2021 remains the same as downloaded from www.internationalmidwives.org, 29 January 2021.
21 ICM. ICM Council Meeting Minutes, Kobe, Japan, July 2005. Agenda Item: Definition of the Midwife, adopted 19 July 2005. ICM. Definition of the Midwife. The Hague: ICM, July 2005.
22 ICM. Core Document: ICM International Definition of the Midwife. The Hague: ICM, Revised and adopted by ICM council 15 June 2011.
23 ICM. ICM Council Minutes Brisbane, Australia, 18–21 July 2005. Min 05.21.3, p 18 references acceptance of 'women's health, sexual health or reproductive health and childcare.'
24 ICM. Core Document: International Definition of the Midwife. Revised and adopted at Toronto Council Meeting, 2017. Due for next review 2023. Downloaded from www.internationalmidwives.org 29 January 2021.

25 ICM. ICM Council Minutes, Vancouver, Canada, May 4–6, 11, 1993. Min 93.22 International Code of Ethics for Midwives, 'carried unanimously' p 19.
26 The Thompsons were instrumental in the development of the first Code of Ethics for the American College of Nurse-Midwives in the early 1990s and had been teaching health care ethics since the early 1980s. Hank was an Old Testament Scholar and ordained clergy and Joyce was a nurse-midwife. Together they provided a philosophical, theological and practical approach to ethics and bioethical decision making. JE Thompson and HO Thompson. Bioethical Decision-Making for Nurses. Norwalk, CT: Appleton-Century-Crofts, 1985.
27 J Thompson. Summary of ICM Ethics Workshop in The Hague, August 1987. Prepared April 1991. Personal papers of JET.
28 Background on the International Confederation of Midwives Code of Ethics: The Process of Development. 15 December 1991, Madrid, Spain, p 1. [Personal papers of Joyce Thompson]
29 ICM. Background on the International Confederation of Midwives Code of Ethics: The Process of Development. 15 December 1991, Madrid, Spain, p 2. [Personal papers of Joyce Thompson]
30 ICM. ICM Council Minutes, Vancouver, Canada, 4–6, 11 May 1993. Min. 93.22 International Code of Ethics for Midwives, pp 19-20.
31 ICM. International Code of Ethics for Midwives, with Explanatory Notes and Glossary. Barley Mow, London: ICM, 1993, Booklet.
32 ICM. ICM Council Meeting Minutes, Manila, Philippines, May 1999. Agenda item 37.1 revised.
33 ICM. ICM Council Meeting Minutes Manila, Philippines, May 1999. Agenda item 37.1, International Code of Ethics for Midwives, addition of I g, 'The Midwife has responsibilities as a person of moral worth, including duties of moral self-respect and the preservation of integrity,' and III D, 'Midwives understand the adverse consequences that ethical and human rights violations have on the health of women and infants and will work to eliminate these violations.'
34 ICM. ICM Council Minutes, Glasgow, Scotland 28–31 May 2008. Min. 6.1.0: Code of Ethics, 'revisions adopted as presented,' p 30.
35 ICM. Core Document: International Code of Ethics for Midwives. The Hague: ICM, 2017. Preamble, p 1. This paragraph was added initially in 2008, refined in 2014. ICM. ICM Council Minutes, Glasgow, Scotland 2008. Agenda item 21.1: Position statements, pp 27–30.
36 ICM. ICM Council Minutes, Prague, Czech Republic, 2014. Agenda item 9.1.: International Code of Ethics, p 20.
37 ICM. Glossary of Terms 2011. The Hague: ICM. "midwifery philosophy", p 7.
38 ICM. ICM Council Minutes Vienna, Austria April 2002. Min. 02/23.1. D. Model of Midwifery Care (C-012) and Philosophy of Midwifery Care (C-013), pp. 22-23: 'Group acknowledged work completed by Nester Moyo in preparing the documents, particularly in bringing together ideas from sources across the world. There was a suggestion that the documents are returned to the Executive Committee for further development and review.
39 ICM. ICM Council Minutes, Brisbane, Australia, 2005. Agenda item 25.2.1: Midwifery Philosophy and Model of Care, p 27.
40 ICM. Core Document: Philosophy and Model of Midwifery Care. The Hague: ICM, 2011; revised 2017, p 1.
41 ICM. ICM Council Minutes, Brisbane, Australia, 2005 Agenda item 05.25.2.1. Philosophy and model of midwifery care, p 27. Agreed amendments suggested by 2004 Executive that included: delete 'pregnancy and childbirth are profound experiences' and insert 'childbearing is a profound experience' and Point 3 will read, 'Midwives are the most appropriate care providers to attend women during pregnancy, labour, birth and the post-partum period'.
42 Refer to Chapter 8 for ICM's Vision, Mission and Strategic Directions and earlier discussion of the Definition of the Midwife and Code of Ethics in this chapter.
43 ICM. ICM Council Minutes, Prague, Czech Republic, June 2014. Agenda Item 9.2, p 4.
44 ICM. ICM Council Minutes, Durban, South Africa, 14–17 June 2011. Agenda 17, p 26.
45 ICM. Core Document: Bill of Rights for Women and Midwives. The Hague: ICM, 2011; 2017.
46 ICM. Core Document: Bill of Rights for Women and Midwives. The Hague: ICM, 2011; reviewed and adopted at Toronto Council meeting, 2017.
47 ICM. Core Document: Bill of Rights for Women and Midwives. The Hague: ICM, 2011; 2017, p. 1.
48 ICM. ICM Council Minutes Manila, Philippines, 1999. Agenda item 53.21 referred document to Executive Committee in 2001. Final adoption 2002. ICM. ICM Council Meeting Minutes Vienna, April 2002. Agenda item 02.22.3.4. Midwives, Women and Human Rights, adopted in principle, p 14.
49 ICM. Core Document: Bill of Rights for Women and Midwives. The Hague: ICM, 2011; 2017, p 3.
50 ICM. ICM Council Minutes, Toronto, Canada, 2017. Agenda item 8.2 Bill of right for women and midwives, p 42.
51 ICM. ICM Council Meeting Minutes Prague, Czech Republic 24-30 May 2014. Agenda 11, pp 6–7.
52 ICM. Core Document: Definition of Midwifery. The Hague: ICM, 2017.
53 ICM. Glossary of Terms. The Hague: ICM, 2011.
54 ICM. ICM Council Minutes, Toronto, Canada, 2017. Agenda item 11.1 Definition of Midwifery, p. 44.
55 ICM. Core Document: Definition of Midwifery. The Hague: ICM, 2017, paragraph 1.
56 ICM. Core Document: Definition of Midwifery. The Hague: ICM, 2017, paragraphs 1 and 4.

Chapter 12: *ICM's Global Competencies and Standards*[1]

'I was engaged with the ICM over a 12-year period from 1999 to 2011 as a Board and Executive member, and finally as President. This was a challenging and ultimately very successful decade for the organization. During this time midwifery emerged from relative obscurity in most health care systems, to being recognized as the essential professional cadre for achieving high quality maternal and newborn care in low-resource countries. At the same time, midwives 'came of age' in terms of achieving leadership status in academia, clinical practice, and regulation in many countries globally, and taking leadership positions at policy tables. During this time, the MDGs and Safe Motherhood Initiatives ultimately highlighted the role of midwives to save lives. The ICM demonstrated leadership by developing global standards to build a qualified and competent midwifery workforce for all countries.'

Bridget Lynch (Canada)

INTRODUCTION

The decade of the 1990s heralded new elected leadership within the ICM from Australia (Margaret Peters), the United States (Joyce Thompson), as well as the Treasurer position remaining in the United Kingdom (Sr Anne Thompson, Ruth Bennett, Julia Allison and Ruth Ashton) where the ICM Headquarters was located. One outcome of the election of midwifery leaders from outside Europe was increasing the international scope of thoughts and ideas that would strengthen midwifery and the services they provided to women in their reproductive years. These thoughts and ideas were based on the personal experiences of the elected midwives who had many years of international midwifery work in English- and French-speaking countries in sub-Sahara Africa and South Asia, as well as memberships on various global health organisations such a UNICEF and the WHO.

One consequence of the ICM being the first Non-Governmental Organisation to sign on to the global Safe Motherhood Initiative (SMI) in 1987 was the adoption of exciting and new ideas. Pre-Congress workshops, based on the four pillars of the SMI, in collaboration with the WHO and UNICEF, being a prime example (Chapter 9). It was ICM's ongoing commitment to the SMI together with midwife leaders and supporters at the WHO (Barbara Kwast, Paul Van Look) that led to the renewed discussion of what midwives needed to know and to do in their countries to save lives.

The brief history of the development of the ICM's competencies for practice, the midwifery education standards that included these competencies, and the regulation standards that would allow midwives to practice full-scope midwifery as defined by the essential competencies are discussed in this chapter. These documents were global in nature and were welcomed by the ICM Member Associations (MAs) to advocate and inform governments, policymakers and major donors and other stakeholders on what was needed for midwives to carry out their vital role in SMI and sexual and reproductive health services. The updated versions continue in global use and can be found on the ICM website: www.internationalmidwives.org.

ESSENTIAL COMPETENCIES FOR BASIC MIDWIFERY PRACTICE[1]

Background

In January 1996, the ICM Board of Management initiated a formal process through which a global statement of essential competencies for midwifery practice was developed and reviewed for relevance to the political, educational and practice environments of the ICM MAs. The ICM established a global task force representing its member associations to define the essential content of any basic midwifery education programme rather than letting other health professions define midwifery practice. The intended purpose of such a document was that midwives, their employers and regulatory authorities would have a clear understanding of the scope of work that can be expected of the competent/fully qualified midwife. Thus, the document clearly defined the midwifery knowledge, skills and professional behaviours that can be fully and appropriately utilised and makes sure that the midwifery scope of practice is neither exploited nor constrained. The concept of midwifery competence in the context of midwifery education and practice is defined as *'the combination of knowledge, psychomotor, communication and decision-making skills that enable an individual to perform a specific task to a defined level of proficiency'*[2].

ICM Council Adopts *Provisional ICM Essential Competencies for Basic Midwifery Practice* – 1999

The first version of the essential competencies was developed in a two-phase project, led by the ICM Deputy Director (Joyce Thompson, USA). The initial global competency list of knowledge, skills and professional behaviours (KSBs) was generated with use of a Delphi survey conducted with key informants, ICM Executive Committee members and international experts from 1996 to 1999. The ICM Council approved the Board of Management's recommendation to adopt the *Provisional ICM Essential Competencies for Basic Midwifery Practice* in 1999 along with the proviso that they be field-tested during the coming triennium with results reported back to Council in 2002.[3]

The task analysis field survey[4], directed by an ICM evaluation consultant (Dr Judith Fullerton, USA) and Project Research Assistant (Kelly Brogan, USA), was conducted in 22 countries with ICM MAs from 2000 to 2002, funded by a grant from USAID. The field survey generated evidence in support of the content validity of the core competency list. The survey data were supplemented by an extensive literature review to provide evidence supporting the items included in the final essential competencies document.[5] The competencies document included items designated as 'basic' or 'core', i.e. those that should be an expected outcome (the mandatory content) of midwifery pre-service education, and other items designated as 'additional' knowledge or skills.[6] Additional items were defined as those that could be learned or performed by midwives under either of two circumstances: (a) midwives who elect to engage in a broader scope of practice, consistent with the globally emerging concept of 'advanced practice nursing/ midwifery' and/ or (b) midwives who have to implement certain skills to make a difference in maternal or neonatal outcome when circumstances compel such action.

ICM Council Adopts ICM Essential Competencies for Basic Midwifery Practice – 2002

The first set of midwifery competencies were adopted by the ICM Council in 2002.[7] A total of 254 distinct statements of KSBs were organised under six domains of midwifery practice:

<u>Domain #1:</u> Competency in social, epidemiological and cultural context of maternal and newborn care.

Domain #2: Competency in pre-pregnancy care and family planning.
Domain #3: Competency in the provision of care during pregnancy.
Domain #4: Competency in the provision of care during labour and birth.
Domain #5: Competency in the provision of care for women during the postpartum period.
Domain #6: Competency in postnatal care of the newborn.[8]

The statement of midwifery competencies has undergone periodic updates in order to keep pace with emerging evidence of best or safe practice.[9] The various subsequent versions of the document were developed using Delphi study methods, modified to accommodate paper-based, and later, as technology advanced and became widely available, to the global community of midwives, through computer-mediated survey strategies. The aim of each of these studies was to generate consensus (or agreement on a position) among a representative sample of midwifery experts and stakeholders internationally about the essential competencies required of a midwife globally, incorporating emerging evidence of best practice. Adoption of these competencies reflected the ICM's support for the scope of midwifery practise.

Updated ICM Essential Competencies – 2010/2011

The updated version of the competency document was agreed by the ICM Board in 2010 and endorsed by the ICM Council in 2011[10], following a two-phase, five-step study, conducted from January 2009 through to December 2010, via a postal survey process. A total of 111 individual surveys representing 178 respondents were returned by respondents from 37 ICM member and five non-member countries with ICM MAs. The 2011 version was amended in 2013, in response to feedback received from global partner organisations, to reflect even further emergence of evidence supporting best practices in reproductive, obstetric and neonatal health care.[11]

The 2002 version of the essential competencies served as the foundation for the revision of the competency statements (Phase 1). The bibliographic (peer-reviewed) and global (e.g. organisational) literature was reviewed in the interest of gleaning new information in the broad domains of reproductive and newborn/young child (up to 2 months) health care that may have emerged in the decade since the initial list of KSB statements was affirmed by and for the ICM. The literature review focused on new studies that provided evidence supporting retention of current competency statements and that provided evidence of changes in recommended policy or practice that would support deletion of a current competency statement. It also focused on policy, position and clinical practice statements that were promulgated since 2000 by the ICM, WHO and other reproductive and child health policy-focused organisations that would lead to the inclusion of new/additional competencies, and/or amendment (change) from the current content.

A new competency domain related to 'Competency in facilitation of abortion-related care',[12] was developed at the direction of the ICM Council and Board in response to requests from ICM regional MAs, primarily in countries where unsafe abortions were the major cause of maternal deaths. The knowledge and skills statements related to this competency domain were newly generated after an exhaustive review of the literature and consultation with subject content experts.

2017 Update of the ICM Essential Competencies

The next update research process was initiated in 2017 by the ICM Education Standing Committee Chair (Michele Butler, UK) and midwives from each ICM Region who crafted the third version of the statement of competencies. This three-round survey was conducted completely online and enabled the most robust response of all competency studies to date. A total of 90 of the ICM's then 105 member associations participated in at least one of the survey rounds, with equitable distribution across all the ICM regions, three language groups, and higher- and lower-resource countries. The organising framework for report of the findings used four (rather than the original seven) domains of midwifery care. The fourth domain incorporated the sub-domains of antenatal care, care during labour and birth, postnatal care and sexual and reproductive health (including abortion-related care). The overall findings from this study indicated that the basic scope of midwifery practice remained unchanged from the 2013 task list; however, several skills were re-designated as advanced practice or optional skills, and several new advanced/optional skills were introduced.

The evidence-based results of the 2017 study were never published by ICM.[13] The ICM Board of Directors authorised an independently crafted document that was published in 2018. That document reflected only basic midwifery skills omitting reference to any advanced or optional skills and citing a list of skills that were not linked to the opinions expressed by the membership in the research process. An addendum to the 2018 document was published by the ICM in October 2019 to emphasise the role of a midwife in preventing, detecting and stabilising complications, i.e. critical content that had been omitted in the 2018 document, but was essential to the support of midwifery practice in these challenging situations.

The 2017 ICM version did not have the same level of details of KSBs as earlier versions and therefore became potentially less useful to international midwifery consultants in countries where midwifery education was just beginning or was being upgraded, requiring clearly defined KSBs. The ICM Board began working with a donor to develop an updated competency assessment tool in 2021 that can be used in tandem with the new Midwifery Education Accreditation Programme (MEAP) tool.

MIDWIFERY EDUCATION STANDARDS AND GUIDELINES (2010)

> 'Midwives are taking action to make sure they are well prepared for their professional role, including ongoing education and updates. But how do/can midwives deal with some of the other devastating injustices forced upon women simply because they are born female?'[14]

Background

There appeared to be agreement among many European midwifery associations in the 1930s that the basic education of the midwife should be three years where the person did not already hold a nursing qualification.[15] Though the topic of how a midwife should be educated and for how long, this three-year time frame did not reappear in writing until 2010. The formal adoption of the programme lengths for direct entry and post-registration education in midwifery occurred with the ICM Board's adoption of the ICM Global Standards for Midwifery Education in 2010 that were endorsed by the ICM Council in 2011, as discussed below.

The discussion of whether ICM needed to create and publish midwifery education standards was carried out over several decades and took on increasing importance once the Essential Competencies were published in 2002 defining the core content of any midwifery education programme. The need for such standards centred around the fact that many individuals and governments throughout the world were using the title, 'midwife' but not all midwives had the same preparation. These individuals had varying levels and quality of formal and informal education, different scopes of practise and varying levels of competence. In addition, many countries needing midwives did not have a midwifery education programme and were asking the ICM for guidance on how to establish such a programme.

Another impetus for defining standards for basic midwifery education programmes came from ICM's representatives on the WHO Global Advisory Group on Nursing and Midwifery (GAGNM) to the Director General of the WHO.[16] This group was in the process of developing standards for basic education of nurses and midwives[17] using consultants from Sigma Theta Tau International (SSTI). SSTI is an honorary nursing organisation that recognises professional nursing education beginning at the baccalaureate level. This fact meant that any midwifery education programmes at the certificate or associate degree level (2-year college) would not be able to meet the WHO standards. The ICM was not willing to agree to those standards.

Finally, the core reasons why the ICM needed to develop midwifery education standards included the fact the ICM represents the world's midwives, it has a long-time goal to strengthen midwifery worldwide, and thus needed global consensus on how one educates a competent midwife as defined by the International Definition of the Midwife.[18]

Development of the Standards and Guidelines

Following the 2008 ICM Council directive to the ICM Education Standing Committee (ESC) to establish global standards of midwifery education in keeping with core ICM documents,[19] the ICM President, Bridget Lynch, appointed Joyce Thompson (USA) and Angela Kamara (Liberia) co-chairs of the Education Standards Task Force (TF) in January 2009. Eleven additional members were confirmed in April 2009 representing all ICM regions, the three official language groups, a member of the ICM Board and ESC, along with a representative from the WHO. The Task Force reviewed existing literature on standards and accreditation of health professional education programmes in several countries along with education/accreditation standards available from MAs and other sources.[20] Based on these documents, the TF drafted a Preface, Standards and Glossary of terms in May 2009.

The Institutional Research Board (IRB)[21] approval for an international modified Delphi study was received in August 2009 from Western Michigan University (USA) to obtain feedback from ICM MAs and midwifery educators.[22] The research question was:

> 'What are the elements of quality that should be reflected in any type of midwifery education programme that prepares a person to meet the ICM Definition of the midwife and the ICM Essential competencies for basic midwifery practice?'

The quality indicators in the proposed standards included: 1) midwifery leadership of the programme; 2) minimum length of midwifery programmes (direct-entry or post-registration); 3) minimum entry level of students and other qualifications; 4) qualifications of midwifery teachers and clinical preceptors/teachers; 5) use of competency-based teaching and learning strategies and minimum content of curriculum beginning with essential competencies; 5) criteria for learning resources/practice facilities and 6) ongoing processes of evaluation of students, teachers, curriculum and programme using valid tools.[23]

ICM Adopts Global Standards for Midwifery Education with Guidelines – 2011

The outcome of three rounds of the Delphi process resulted in two documents. The first was titled ICM *Global Standards for Midwifery Education*, and the second was titled, *Companion Guidelines*. The Standards document included an Introduction and Preface explaining the purpose of the standards noting they were minimal standards that could 'be expanded to include higher expectations and to reflect country specific needs for curriculum content and cultural appropriateness.'[24] In addition, the Preface included the founding values of trust, continuous quality improvement, integrity, lifelong learning and autonomy of the profession upon which the standards were based. The ICM Education Standing Committee became the responsible arm of the ICM for questions relating to the Standards and for monitoring their use and needs for updates. Both documents were adopted by the ICM Board in 2010 and endorsed by the ICM Council in 2011.[25]

The final approved education standards were organised into six categories:
  I.   Organisation and Administration
  II. Midwifery Faculty
  III. Student Body
  IV. Curriculum

100 Years of the International Confederation of Midwives

  V. Resources, Facilities and Services
  VI. Assessment Strategies.

Each category had from five to eight specific standards with sub-standards where needed. For example, <u>Category I has six standards</u> that address institutional support and the budget needed to run the programme, stating; 'The head of the midwifery programme is a qualified midwife teacher with experience in management/administration'[26]. <u>Category II has eight standards</u> defining the qualifications of a midwife teacher and clinical preceptor/clinical teacher, including the need to fit the ICM Definition of the Midwife. <u>Category III has seven standards</u> that address admission policies, non-discriminatory practices and the need for clearly written student policies along with mechanisms for students' active participation in programme governance and committees.

  Of interest to many midwife teachers is Standard III.6 that reads: 'Students have sufficient midwifery practical experience in a variety of settings to attain, at a minimum, the current ICM Essential Competencies For Basic Midwifery Practice'[27]. Both this standard and Standard I.5 (head of programme is a qualified midwife) have been used successfully as advocacy tools for obtaining the needed support to establish a midwifery education programme run by midwives and with sufficient clinical sites to allow each student to attain all the essential competencies. This advocacy is a work in progress in many countries starting new midwifery programmes or attempting to strengthen existing programmes.[28]

  <u>Category IV has six standards</u> relating to Midwifery Curriculum, with four sub-standards under Standard IV.2 relating to the purpose of the programme in meeting ICM competencies, etc., and two sub-standards relating to length of programmes under Standard IV.4. Standard IV.5 has resulted in several additional education documents produced and shared by ICM relating to the promotion of adult learning and use of competency-based teaching, learning and evaluation strategies[29]. <u>Category V has five standards</u> relating to the need to keep students and teachers in a safe environment for learning, needed equipment and other teaching and learning resources[30], and having sufficient teachers and practical learning sites available for the number of students admitted into the programme. <u>Category VI has five standards</u> relating to the use of valid and reliable formative and summative evaluation methods for student progress, curricular review and evaluation of clinical sites.

100 Years of the International Confederation of Midwives

The Companion Guidelines offered a two-column approach. The first column offers suggestions on how to meet the Standard including examples to illustrate what was meant. The second column highlights the type of evidence, with some examples, that a programme might use to determine when and whether they have met the standard.[31]

The development of the education standards in 2010–2011 resulted in other education resources produced by ICM consultants for use by MAs (Chapter 9). Many midwifery teachers, especially in resource limited countries where midwifery was/is relatively new, used one or more of these documents and found them very useful. They were also used by the ICM and other midwifery education consultants to strengthen midwifery education in areas of the world where needed. *The ICM Glossary of Terms*[32] was the only education resource on the ICM website in 2021, though contact information for the Education Standing Committee is available. The parallel development of the core documents on competencies, education standards and regulation highlighted the critical need for congruence in terminology across these three (and essentially all) of ICMs documents.[33]

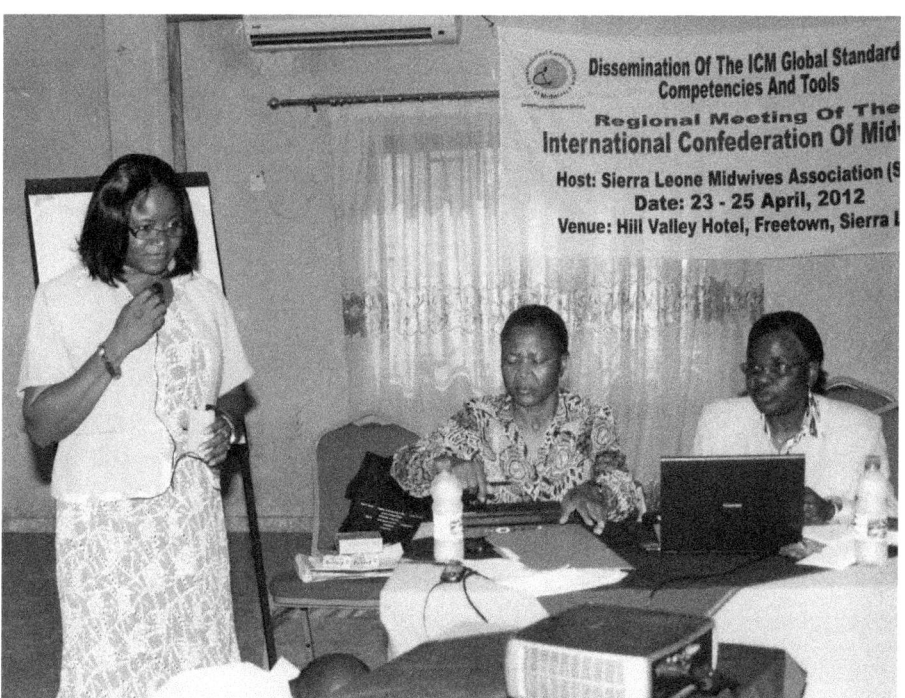

Midwives disseminating ICM global standards for midwifery – ICM Archives at Wellcome Collection

Similar to the ICM competencies, *the Global Standards for Midwifery Education with Companion Guidelines* are considered 'living' documents. That is, they require review and updating periodically to reflect changing evidence in competency-based teaching, curriculum design and content needed (competencies) in midwifery. The first revision was completed in 2013, with a few major changes. First, the statement about minimum education prior to entry (secondary school) and the consensus-based minimum length of direct entry (3 years) and post-nursing (18 months) education programmes were moved from the Preface to an actual standard (IV.a, IV.b). These agreed standards were often 'lost' in the Preface. The new placement of these standards statements under Standard IV provided the opportunity to explain why and how these could be achieved in the *Companion Guidelines* in response to queries from countries in South Asia, Latin America, the Caribbean and Europe. Based on common queries related to the Education standards, the Guidelines were expanded to offer suggestions for new programmes which may not have a prepared midwife head of programme or qualified midwifery teachers, suggesting use of international midwifery education consultants until the country cadre of midwifery teachers could be prepared.[34]

As noted earlier, the ICM Education Standing Committee is responsible for monitoring and updating the Education Standards. The co-Chairs of this committee (Melissa Avery, Mary Barger, Ans Luyben) carried out further studies to determine the use and effectiveness of these standards since 2012.[35] These efforts have led to the ICM creating the Midwifery Education Accreditation Programme (MEAP) that was being field-tested in 2021–2022.

MIDWIFERY REGULATION STANDARDS AND TOOLKIT

The third essential ICM document that was developed during the first decade of the 21st century at the same time as the Education Standards was *Global Standards for Midwifery Regulation (2011)*[36], addressing the question of how a midwife and midwifery practice should be regulated at the country level. These standards were developed in response to requests from midwives, midwifery associations, governments, UN agencies and other stakeholders. The goal of setting midwifery regulatory standards was to promote the development and adoption of legal and/or regulatory mechanisms that would protect the public (namely, the baby, women and families) by making sure that the midwives providing health services were prepared according to competency standards and provided high quality care for 'mothers and babies'[37].

It is important to note that the midwifery regulation standards were based on ICM Core documents, including the *Definition of the Midwife*, the *International Code of Ethics*, the *Philosophy and Model of Midwifery Care*, the *Essential Competencies for Basic Midwifery Practice*, the *Global Standards for Midwifery Education* and selected Position Statements. Without these core documents and agreed Position Statements, midwifery regulation standards most likely would have been further delayed.

Background

Midwifery regulation was a topic of discussion among MAs, ICM leaders and individual midwives since the beginning of the Confederation in 1922. Questions of how to prepare a qualified midwife and how to regulate midwifery practise for the benefit of childbearing women pervaded the early IMU congresses (Chapter 3). The first *Definition of the Midwife* in 1972 left the description of midwifery regulation to the legal authority in a given country as noted by, 'has acquired the requisite qualifications to be registered and/or legally licensed to practise midwifery.'[38] The ICM Council agreed to certain aspects of regulation that would fit all MAs and in 1990 adopted its first Position Statement on regulation titled, *Appropriate Legislation for Midwives*.

The ICM Council in 1999[39] was asked to adopt a framework based on an earlier position statement, *Legislation to Govern Midwifery Practice*. Due to lack of time at the Council meeting, the Executive Committee in 2001 took up the discussion and drafted a proposed statement, *Framework for midwifery legislation and regulation*, that was presented and adopted at the 2002 ICM Council.[40] The adoption of this Framework included 'the need to establish guidelines for the development of regulatory standards to further enable member associations to achieve regulatory processes appropriate for the practice of midwifery in their country.'[41] In 2005, the ICM Council adopted an updated position statement that listed a set of statements about what midwifery regulatory legislation should provide, and these statements were used by the Regulation Standing Committee (RegSC) to develop the Standards discussed below.

Development of Regulation Standards

The need to establish a Regulation Standing Committee was agreed by the ICM Council in 2008. The Asia-Pacific region took a strong interest in the drafting and gathering feedback from ICM MAs on the proposed global standards for midwifery regulation. Bridget Lynch, ICM President (2008–2011), appointed Sally Pairman (New Zealand) and Louise Silverton (UK) as co-chairs of the Regulation Standing Committee and Task Force to establish global midwifery regulation standards in 2009. The co-chairs then added other members of the Task Force from all ICM regions who worked together to draft the initial standards document during a meeting in Hong Kong in April 2010.[42] The initial draft of regulation standards was based on information obtained from an extensive literature review on midwifery regulation and during regulation workshops, such as the ICM Asia-Pacific Regional meeting in India in November 2009 and the ICM/UNFPA South Asia midwifery meeting in Bangladesh in March 2010.

The draft standards were endorsed by the full Task Force, translated into English, French and Spanish, and disseminated to the ICM MAs for feedback. The consultation process included both written feedback and focus group discussions initially, before a formal questionnaire was sent to all MAs with a request to send on to the appropriate regulatory body in their country for feedback. Responses to two rounds of the questionnaire were received from 33 countries (33 per cent total membership) representing all ICM regions. Additional focus group discussions were held with regulators in Europe, Canada, South-East Asia and the South Pacific. The Task Force amended the initial draft standards and sent to the ICM Board for approval in February 2011. The ICM Council approved the regulation standards in June 2011 in Durban, South Africa.[43]

ICM *Global Standards for Midwifery Regulation* (2011)

The final approved *Global Standards for Midwifery Regulation* included statements of purpose, founding values and principles, principles of good regulation, a glossary of terms[44], the intended use of the standards and the actual global standards for midwifery regulation with an accompanying explanation for each standard. The full document was 24-pages long.

<u>Purpose of Regulation</u>
The approved document stated that: 'regulatory mechanisms, whether through legislation, employment or other regulation, aim to ensure the safety of the public'. This is achieved through the following six main functions:
1. Setting the scope of midwifery practice
2. Setting/approving standards for pre-registration midwifery education

3. Registering midwives
4. Re-licensing midwives who remain competent after registration
5. Disciplining midwives found to breach standards
6. Setting a code of conduct and ethics.[45]

The standards are deliberately generic and take a principled approach to midwifery regulation to provide a benchmark for global standardisation of midwifery regulation. They cover Model of Regulation, Protection of Title, Governance and Functions. Co-Chair Sally Pairman stated that the Task Force saw the process of re-licensing as an annual or triennial exercise. The principled approach used as a framework for midwifery regulation was meant to enable governments to set regulations appropriate to each country, and therefore were not prescriptive for a particular country.[46]

Midwifery Regulation Toolkit (2016)

At the time that the ICM Council members adopted the Global Standards for Midwifery Regulation in 2011, MAs requested some type of document (guidelines, toolkit) to help them work with regulatory bodies in their own country to implement and/or strengthen the legal recognition of midwives practising full-scope midwifery according to their competencies. The co-chairs of the ICM Regulation Standing Committee began working on a toolkit in December 2013, with a draft presented to ICM Council in 2014.

The draft toolkit was based on five principles: positive engagement, transparency, accountability, sustainability and partnership. It was further divided into the following sections: Introduction and purpose of regulation; gap analysis; achieving change; barriers to change; skills and tools. Two workshops were scheduled during the 2014 Triennial Congress and delegates were urged to provide feedback regarding the toolkit. Upon receipt of the feedback the team reviewed and revised the document before sending a revised version to the Board for circulation to the 2016 ICM Council.[47]

The 2016 Annual Council approved the Regulation Toolkit.[48] The purpose of the Toolkit is to support MAs by providing a very practical guide to work with regulatory bodies who are at different stages of a midwifery regulatory process to implement the global standards, tools and competencies. It has been disseminated and made available on the ICM website.[49]

SUMMARY

This chapter highlights the incredible expansion of the influence of the ICM on global midwifery and women's health during the first two decades of the 21st century and the autonomy of the profession by setting these standards. The ICM's role in defining the midwife's essential competencies, the minimum standards for the education of midwives and a principled approach to the regulation of midwives and midwifery practice have nearly eliminated any doubt about who is a competent midwife and what that midwife can do to contribute to the health of women, their newborns and their families throughout the world. Midwives' contributions to the Millennium Development Goals and the more recent Sustainable Development Goals are fully accepted based on these ICM global competencies and standards. The reader can contact the ICM for access to current documents in addition to using the ICM website: www.internationalmidwives.org

100 Years of the International Confederation of Midwives

1. The core of the essential competences section was written by Dr Judith Fullerton, ICM Consultant who carried out the multi-country study of the draft Essential Competencies for Basic Midwifery Practice developed by a team of international midwifery experts and the ICM Regional Representatives during 1996-1999, led by Dr Joyce Thompson, ICM Deputy Director. Dr Fullerton was also the leader of the 2011 update study, and consultant to the 2017 update.
2. ICM. *Glossary of Terms* 2011. The Hague: ICM. 2011, updated 2017, p 3. J Fullerton, A Ghérissi, P Johnson, J Thompson. Competence and competency: Core concepts for international midwifery practice. *International Journal of Childbirth*. 2011; 1:1, pp 4–12.
3. ICM. *ICM Council Meeting Minutes, May 1999, Manila, Philippines*. Chiswick, London: ICM. Agenda item 99.38: Provisional Essential Midwifery Competencies, carried unanimously, p 36.
4. Nester Moyo. The ICM's provisional midwifery competencies: field-testing. *International Midwifery* 14:4 (July/August 2001), p 4.
5. J Fullerton, R Severino, K Brogan, J Thompson. The International Confederation of Midwives' study of essential competencies of midwifery practice. Midwifery 2003; 19, pp 174–190.
6. J Fullerton, J Thompson. Examining the evidence for the international confederation of midwives' essential competencies for midwifery practice. Midwifery 2005; 21:1, pp 2–13.
7. ICM. *ICM Council Minutes April 9–11, 2002, Vienna, Austria*. The Hague: ICM, 2002, Agenda item 02/21.2, p 21. Council agreed all the specific KSBs that raised some concern during the final Delphi round.
8. ICM. *Essential Competencies for Basic Midwifery Practice*. The Hague: ICM, 2010.
9. J Fullerton, J Thompson, R Severino. The International Confederation of Midwives essential competencies for basic midwifery practice: An update study, 2009–2010. Midwifery 2011, 27:4, pp 399–408. http://doi:10.1016/j.midw.2011.03.005
10. ICM. *ICM Council Minutes, 14–17 June 2011, Durban, South Africa*. The Hague: ICM, 2011, 'Vote: Essential competencies for basic midwifery practice, p 22.
11. J Fullerton, J Thompson. 2013 Amendments to International Confederation of Midwives *Essential Competencies and Education Standards* Core Documents: Clarification and Rationale. International Journal of Childbirth 2013. 3:4, pp 184–194.
12. ICM. Essential competencies for basic midwifery practice. The Hague: ICM, 2010; revised 2013, pp 18–19.
13. M Butler, J Fullerton, C Aman. Competence for basic midwifery practice: updating the ICM Essential Competencies *Midwifery* 2018; 66, pp 168–175. http://doi:10.1016/j.midw.2018.08.011
14. JE Thompson. Midwives and human rights: Dream or reality? Midwifery 18:4, 188–192, 2002.
15. ICM. *A Birthday for Midwives: Seventy-Five Years of International Collaboration*, pp 2–3. 'At Prague in 1925 and in Vienna in 1928, the member associations were clearly united behind the call for a minimum of three years education for the profession …'
16. J Thompson. The WHO Global Advisory Group on Nursing and Midwifery. *Journal of Nursing Scholarship*, 34:2, 111–113, (Second Quarter) 2002.
17. ICM representatives on the GAGNM argued that the WHO should not be developing standards of midwifery education since the ICM represented all midwives. In addition, the fact that the WHO standards would require a baccalaureate degree as an entry requirement would go against the ICM policy that such education needed to be based on competencies and not the 'recognition' of completion of a programme of study. The WHO Standards were published in 2009.
18. ICM. *International Definition of the Midwife*. The Hague: ICM. 2005. The updated definition included reference to the 2002 IC*M Essential Competencies for Basic Midwifery Practice* as a requirement, and these competencies were viewed as the core content of any basic midwifery education programme.
19. ICM. ICM Council Minutes 28-31 May 2008, Glasgow, Scotland. The Hague: ICM, 2008. Agenda item 5.4/2 Education Standing Committee, p 12. Joyce Thompson asked the ESC to consider developing education standards and Andrea Steifel agreed to consider this.
20. Key documents reviewed include ICM Core documents and position statements related to midwifery education and educators, WHO *Midwifery Modules & Midwifery Toolkit* (draft), WHO *Global standards for the initial education of professional nurses and midwives* (2009), USA Accreditation Commission for Midwifery education (2008), ESCSACN's *Professional nursing and midwifery standards*, European Union and United Kingdom midwifery standards, as well as Task Force members' regional and/or national standards in use at the time.
21. Most research projects (national and international) involving humans or animals are required to go through review for permission to carry out the study and publish any findings. Research universities have some form of Institutional Review Board (IRB) to protect study subjects from harm or abuse.
22. JE Thompson, JF Fullerton, A Sawyer. The International Confederation of Midwives' Global standards for midwifery education (2010) with companion guidelines: The process. *Midwifery* 27:4, 2011, 409–416. Doi:10.1016/j.midw.2011.04.001.

23 JE Thompson, JF Fullerton, A Sawyer. The International Confederation of Midwives' *Global standards for midwifery education* (2010) with companion guidelines: The process. *Midwifery* 27:4, 2011, 409–416. Doi:10.1016/j.midw.2011.04.001.
24 ICM. *Global Standards for Midwifery Education*. The Hague: ICM, 2010. Preface, p 1
25 ICM Board of Management, 2010. ICM. *ICM Council Minutes, 14–17 June 2011, Durban, South Africa*. The Hague: ICM, 2011, pp 22.
26 ICM. *Global Standards for Midwifery Education*. The Hague: ICM, 2010/2-17. Standard I.5, p 4.
27 ICM. *Global Standards for Midwifery Education*. The Hague: ICM, 2010; 2017. Standard III.6, p 6.
28 Use of the ICM global competencies and standards throughout the Latin America and Caribbean region, with the support of UNFPA-LAC Regional Office, has resulted in improved midwifery education in many countries of the region. [Personal experience of JET.]
29 ICM. *Global Standards for Midwifery Education*. The Hague: ICM, 2010; 2017. Standard IV.5. p 7. J Fullerton, J Thompson, P Johnson. Competency-based education: The essential basis of pre-service education for the professional midwifery workforce. *Midwifery* 2013. http://dx.doi.org/10.1016/j.midw.2013.07.006. JB Thompson, JT Fullerton, C Carr, P Elgueta, E Hebert, A Luyben. Global Workshops in Midwifery Competency-Based Educational Methodologies: Lessons Learned. *International Journal of Childbirth* 7 (1), pp 4–17, 2017. http://dx.doi.org/10.1891/2156-5287.7.1.4.
30 None of these education tools appear on the ICM website in 2021.
31 ICM. *Global Standards for Midwifery Education 2010*: Companion Guidelines. The Hague: ICM, 2010, p 1 footnote.
32 ICM. *Glossary of Terms*. The Hague: ICM, 2011; updated 2017.
33 The formulation of the ICM Glossary of Terms was initiated during the ICM Conference in Durban SA, by discussion among the leaders of these various Task Forces and with additional input from the ICM Board.
34 JT Fullerton, JE Thompson. 2013 Amendments to International Confederation of Midwives' *Essential Competencies and Education Standards* core documents: Clarification and rationale. *International Journal of Childbirth* 3 (4), pp 184–194, 2013.
35 Mary K Barger, Melissa Avery, Ans Luyben. A Needs Assessment for Recognizing Midwifery Education Programs that Meet the International Confederation of Midwives Global Education Standards. *International Journal of Childbirth* 7(2), 2017.
36 ICM. *Global Standards for Midwifery Regulation*. The Hague: ICM, 2011.
37 ICM. *Global Standards for Midwifery Regulation*. The Hague: ICM, 2011, p 1. Note that the reference to 'mothers' is inconsistent with Constitutional aims and mission statement of the time that addressed midwifery care for women during their reproductive cycle.
38 FIGO/ICM Joint Study Project. *Definition of the Midwife*, 1972.
39 ICM. *ICM Council Meeting Minutes, May 1999, Manila, Philippines*. London: ICM, 1999. Agenda item 53.12, p 40 notes that the position paper was not considered due to lack of time and was referred to the Executive Committee meeting in 2001.
40 ICM. *ICM Council Meeting Minutes, April 2002, Vienna, Austria*. The Hague: ICM. Agenda item 22.3.1, p 14.
41 ICM. *Framework for midwifery legislation and regulation*. The Hague: ICM, Position statement, 2002.
42 ICM. *Global Standards for Midwifery Regulation (2011)*. The Hague: ICM, p 3: Process of development.
43 ICM. *ICM Council Meeting Minutes, 14–17 June 2011, Durban, South Africa*. The Hague: ICM, 2011, pp 20–21.
44 Joyce Thompson remembers the co-chairs of the Competencies, Education and Regulation standards task forces sitting together in a hotel lobby in Durban, South Africa, sharing a list of definitions in English that were deemed essential to understanding the education and competencies documents, and asking the Regulation task force members to add their needed definitions. There was much discussion of which terms to include, and then the fun began of agreeing draft definitions so they could be sent out to member associations for comments/edits. This was done twice (2011 and prior to the 2017 Council meeting) to make sure the terms were appropriate and understood in all three languages of the Confederation.
45 ICM. *Global Standards for Midwifery Regulation (2011)*. The Hague: ICM, p 4.
46 ICM. *ICM Council Meeting Minutes, 14–17 June 2011, Durban, South Africa*. The Hague: ICM, 2011, pp 20–21.
47 ICM. *ICM Council Meeting Minutes, 27–30 May 2014, Prague, Czech Republic*. The Hague: ICM, 2014, p 29.
48 ICM. *ICM Council Meeting Minutes 2016*.
49 ICM. *ICM Council Meeting Minutes, 13–16 June 2017, Toronto, Canada*. The Hague: ICM, 2017, p 16.

Chapter 13: *Regional Member Associations' Perspectives on the ICM*

'ICM helped Spanish midwives during the dark period of 9 years (1986-1994) without any midwifery training running in Spain. During this time, ICM Board members have been of support in all the actions and negotiations between the Spanish Midwifery Associations and the Ministry of Health and Ministry of Education. At the end in 1992, we got a new law and we could reopen the midwifery training curriculum in 1994.'
Gloria Seguranyes Guillot (Regional Representative 1990–1996)

INTRODUCTION

The global nature of the ICM and the goal of representing midwifery associations and midwives in all areas of the world led to a decision early on to have official appointed/elected representatives in a given geographic region. This decision also reflected the reality that most of the work of the ICM is carried out by its Member Associations (MAs) organised into regions. The European Region's MAs have the longest history, followed by the Americas, with the Eastern Mediterranean Region being the newest (Refer to Annex G for ICM Member Charts). As noted in the vignette at the beginning of this chapter, the ICM Board occasionally supported individual MAs in their struggle to move midwifery forward.

Number of Regions

The number of ICM Regions remained stable at four (Africa, Americas, Asia-Pacific and Europe) from 1981 until 2017, when some of the MAs in Europe, Africa and Asia-Pacific Regions joined together to create the Eastern Mediterranean Region (Chapter 5). Efforts to represent midwives and their associations throughout the world, to listen to their concerns, were important to the ICM and decisions on its policies and work. Such two-way sharing was challenging at times due, in part, to limited communication vehicles until the mid-1990s and lack of MA financial support for their named representative to stay in contact with all the MAs in their region. In addition, each of the ICM Regions had a large geographic area with a variety of cultures and language groups to cover – an enormous task for even the most eager representative!

Regional Survey Questions

In order to gain a regional perspective on the impact/value of the ICM for this history book, a survey questionnaire was sent to each regional team in 2019 with responses from the Americas, Anglophone Africa, Asia-Pacific and the Eastern Mediterranean Regions. Unfortunately, after several requests, no one from the European Region responded, hence no specific European information could be included here. Responses to five of these questions are the foci of this chapter beginning with when the midwifery association was accepted into membership of the ICM[1] followed by a brief history of midwifery development in that country. The MA dates are as of 2019 when the surveys were completed. The authors extend the disclaimer that the membership charts in this chapter reflect only those MAs who responded to the survey. Likewise, some of the dates given by the MAs in 2019 were not those recorded by ICM Headquarters, so both dates are listed where appropriate with ICM dates in parentheses. See Annex G for complete 2021 charts of the ICM MAs by Region.

Each Region's introduction and chart of membership begins the chapter, followed by a summary of responses focusing on:
1. the value/impact that ICM membership had on the Member Association,
2. the value/impact that the Member Association had on the ICM and
3. the MAs expectations of the ICM for the future.

ANGLOPHONE AFRICA [Jemima Dennis-Antwi and MAs]
Historical Background

The ICM's association with Africa began in the early 1950s when the Gold Coast Midwives Association (GCMA)[2] joined the ICM in 1954 to champion the cause of midwives and midwifery on the African continent. Over the years, midwifery evolved in many African countries, especially within the areas of education, regulation and association strengthening, leading to growth of a competent midwifery workforce within the 18 countries that form the membership so far in the Anglophone Africa Region. This growth was epic in that it occurred within associations whose midwives were often undervalued, underpaid and financially unable to travel beyond their own country without assistance. In more recent years, the ICM's drive towards strong leadership for equitable, gender-sensitive and quality midwife-led care[3] has informed policy decisions and advocacy in further strengthening and repositioning midwives and midwifery services for improved reproductive, maternal, newborn, child and adolescent health (RMNCAH) in the Africa Region.

Member Associations

The section below summarises the responses of 12 of the 18 Anglophone African countries in membership of the ICM who responded to the questionnaire sent to countries between 26 November 2019 and 30 June 2020.[4] Table 13.1 describes the country, name of the midwifery association and year that it became a member of the ICM.[5]

1. **Table 13.1 Anglophone Africa**

Country, Name and Year Midwifery Associations Accepted for ICM Membership

Country	Name of Association	Year
Ghana	Gold Coast Midwives Association (GCMA)[6]	1954
	Ghana Registered Midwives Association (GRMA)	1982*
Nigeria	National Association of Nigerian Nurses & Midwives (NANNM)	1957; 2014*
Sierra Leone	Sierra Leone Midwives Association	1969; 1982*
Liberia	Liberian Midwives Association	1982* (1985)
Ethiopia	Ethiopian Midwives Association	1990* (1993)
South Africa	The Society of Midwives of Southern Africa	1994*
Zimbabwe	Zimbabwe Confederation of Midwives	1997* (1999)
Malawi	The Association of Malawian Midwives (AMAMI)	1998* (1997)
Zambia	Midwives Association of Zambia	2011* (2012)
Rwanda	Rwanda Association of Midwives (RAM)	2014* (2013)
Namibia	Independent Midwives Association of Namibia	2015*
Kenya	Midwives Association of Kenya (MAK)	2016*

*=ICM current members in 2019; where two dates listed denotes lapse in

membership often due to lack of ability to pay fees. Dates in parentheses are those held by ICM HQs.

Value/Impact of ICM Membership on Anglophone Africa MAs

ICM MAs in Anglophone Africa reported several common themes in response to the impact that joining the ICM had/continues to have on the MAs and the midwives. First and foremost was the enhanced visibility and/or recognition of midwives and midwifery in their countries, supported by strong associations.

<u>Visibility & Association Strengthening</u>: Membership in ICM enhanced the visibility and strengthened the voices of midwives in Ghana, Liberia, Namibia, Rwanda and Zambia with their governments, NGOs and UN agencies as well as with regional and international partners. For example, Zambia reported a three- to four-fold increase in members because of their visibility and ICM-led projects they participated in. Deserving midwives and stakeholders are often recognised for their hard work and commitment to saving mothers and their newborns. Many strategies have been adopted to create awareness about the work of the MAs and the ICM. These have included seminars, stakeholder engagements, community outreach programmes (South Africa). One example of association development occurred after Hagar Mapondera attended the 1984 ICM Congress in Sydney, Australia and then participated in the 1987 Pre-Congress workshop in The Hague, the Netherlands. She was motivated to start the Zimbabwe Confederation of Midwives, though it took several years to become a reality.

The ICM Young Midwifery Leaders (YML) programmes have afforded MAs (e.g. Malawi, South Africa and Zimbabwe) the ability to develop their leadership skills in youth mentoring, association strengthening and the opportunity to apply the myriad ICM policies and standards for midwifery education, practice and regulation (Namibia). Zambia and Zimbabwe consider that their association with the ICM has been the backbone to their recognition as very strong stand-alone associations. Their associations are now confident in representing midwifery in any meetings or platforms where midwifery issues are discussed.

<u>Recognition for Midwifery and Midwives:</u> African midwives' attendance at ICM Triennial Congresses provided opportunities to present scholarly papers and time for building networks for collaboration. Hosting the 29th ICM Congress in

Durban, South Africa in 2011, was an important milestone in global recognition for African midwives as it was the first Congress to be held in Africa.

These events placed midwives and MAs at the centre of maternal health care and the ICM became recognised as the provider of international guidelines in midwifery at country and regional levels. This link created a level of authenticity to MAs' assertions and policy engagements with governments and stakeholders, including representation at National Committees of the Ministries of Health (e.g. Zambia, Ethiopia, Ghana, South Africa, Rwanda, Sierra Leone). This recognition also facilitated efforts to separate midwives' associations from nurses' associations, leading to midwifery independence and self-recognition and an increase in local membership (e.g. Nigeria, Zambia and Zimbabwe). As a result, the Zimbabwe Confederation of Midwives (ZICOM) has been a strong advocate for the recognition of midwifery as a separate profession from that of nursing which hitherto was non-existent.

Since 2009, the annual celebration of the International Day of the Midwife (IDM) in most African countries whose midwives were dually qualified meant that they no longer needed to participate in celebrations during the International Day of the Nurse in order to be acknowledged. MAs in Ghana and Uganda, however, had been participating in IDM celebrations since 1991. These IDM celebrations provided a visible platform for midwives to speak about their work, concerns and need to advocate for better reproductive, maternal newborn, child and adolescent health (RMNCAH) for quality health outcomes.

<u>Use of ICM resource materials, policy initiatives and guidelines:</u> ICM resources have enhanced not only the visibility and status of midwives and their associations at country and regional levels but serve as invaluable resources during advocacy/lobbying efforts. For example, the development of the ICM Midwifery Services Framework (MSF) resulted in a number of African countries piloting it. A notable introduction was that of Ghana led by Jemima Dennis-Antwi, funded by Jhpiego-Ghana and facilitated by ICM international consultants. The product of the MSF was used to inform the development of a 5-year Strategic Plan for midwifery (2019–2023) developed by Jemima Dennis-Antwi for the Ghana Ministry of Health. In addition, the ICM global standards on regulation have been instrumental in helping countries such as Rwanda, Uganda, Ethiopia, Ghana, Sierra Leone and Liberia in setting new regulatory policies or revising obsolete Acts of Parliament on midwifery practice.

All 12 responding Anglophone MAs in Africa, informed by the ICM global standards and competencies, have advocated for and ensured reviews of midwifery curricula to meet the ICM educational standards for producing competent midwives. Most countries have also upgraded and expanded the recognition of new midwifery graduates, ranging from professional certification, diploma and bachelor to masters level midwifery programmes in countries. In some countries (e.g. Ghana, Ethiopia, Nigeria, Rwanda, South Africa, Zambia, Zimbabwe), the Millennium Development Goals (MDGs) gave impetus to the development of direct-entry education, with qualified applicants entering midwifery programmes without first qualifying as nurses.

The ICM *Newsletter* which covers various topics and midwifery activities globally keeps midwives well informed. ICM's toolkits have helped the midwives to be strong advocates for women and midwifery issues, along with ICM's Policy and Position Statements pertinent to the health issues found throughout Africa.

Capacity Development with Involvement in ICM Projects with Donors: MAs throughout Africa have benefited from ICM activities and projects supported by global donors related to the Safe Motherhood Initiative, MDG #4 (newborn/child) and #5 (maternal), and, more recently, Sustainable Development Goals #3 (health for all) and #5 (gender equity). Each of these projects has focused on the improvement of the sexual and reproductive health of women and their families, especially in high burden countries in Africa. Examples of African midwives' involvement in ICM projects include Helping Mothers Survive and Helping Babies Breathe (HMS and HBB) workshops that strengthened the capacity of midwives to provide evidence-based, quality midwifery care. In Zambia, the successful implementation of the 10,000 Happy Birthdays Project led to the follow on one-year project supported by the Rotary Club of Norway and hosted by the Rotary Club in Lusaka Central. The ICM and partners supported Ethiopia and Rwanda MAs in implementing a 50,000 Happy Birthdays Project in 2018–2019. The Project increased their capacity in managing huge grants, thus increasing the MA's visibility at national and international levels. In Rwanda over 6,000 health care providers were trained in HMS/HBB.

More African midwives are involved in capacity-building in response to ICM's global advocacy campaigns such as 'The world needs more midwives more than ever'. Education, deployment and retention of midwives have remained high on Governments' priority lists. Capacity building for continual competency of midwives in practice included training workshops and seminars in Respectful Maternity Care (RMC), management, adolescent sexual and reproductive health (ASRH), HBB, management of obstetric complications such as Post-Partum Haemorrhage (PPH) and eclampsia, Competency-Based Education (CBE). These have made a great impact by contributing towards reduction of maternal and neonatal mortality and the provision of respectful midwifery care. These efforts also helped midwives access information and realise opportunities for conducting research. Opportunities were opened up for a number of the midwives to present scientific papers at local, regional and international conferences.

A large project that gave impetus to the growth of midwifery in Africa was the ICM/UNFPA *Investing in Midwives Program* of 2009–2013. As part of the programme, Dr Jemima Dennis-Antwi, then the ICM Regional Technical Adviser for Anglophone Africa, was requested to support the Sierra Leone MA to conduct the first Gap Analysis for Midwifery Strengthening in Sierra Leone with focus on midwifery education, regulation and association. The information generated contributed to further deliberations around midwifery strengthening in Sierra Leone and informed subsequent initiatives.

Global Leadership Building: The Ghana MA has a long history of being involved at the global midwifery level. As noted in Chapter 3, Madam Fredrica Kwarley Aba Addo visited the United Kingdom (UK) in 1933 and contacted the Royal College of Midwives, briefed them about the GCMA and sought information about how to join the International Midwives' Union (IMU), forerunner of the ICM, which until that time had admitted only European based midwives' associations. More recently, ICM membership exposure gave impetus for African midwives to apply for ICM global positions. Such persons who have served as ICM staff include: Nester Moyo (Zimbabwe), Abigail Kyei (Ghana), Jemima Dennis-Antwi (Ghana), Rachel Ibinga Koula (Gabon), Martha Bokosi (Malawi) and Liliane Ingabire (Rwanda). At the ICM Board level, Address Malata was elected Vice-President, and the following have served as ICM regional representatives for Anglophone Africa: Priscilla Owusu-Asiedo (Ghana), Gloria Betts (Sierra Leone), Christine Achurobwe (Uganda), Kathlyn Ababio (Ghana), Deliwe Nyathikazi (South Africa), Jemima Dennis-Antwi (Ghana) and Hilma Shikwambi (Anglophone Africa).

Partnerships and Affiliations: The ICM membership has resulted in different donors and partners working with African MAs to improve the competencies of midwives and the quality of maternal and newborn health services. For instance, the ICM has helped link the Midwives' Association of Zambia (MAZ) to funders such as Laerdal Global Health, American Academy for Paediatrics, IPAS, ZAGO, SIDA, UNFPA, WHO, UNICEF, Rotary Club of Norway, White Ribbon Alliance (WRA), Lugina Midwifery Research Network (LAMRN), Sanofi Espoir Foundation and Johnson and Johnson. Work with other ICM MAs and their in-country organisations such as Nursing and Midwifery Councils, Associations of Gynaecologists and Obstetricians, Medical Associations and Nurses Union were also enhanced.

Impact of Anglophone African MAs on the Growth and Development of ICM as an Organisation

Strategic Documents and Position Statements: African ICM MAs have contributed to the development of global midwifery strategic documents and position papers which are used for advocacy and putting midwifery on the global map. They have broadened the strategic planning base of the ICM and supported the inclusion of the perspectives and experiences drawn from African realities to better advocate for the midwife, mother and baby wherever they find themselves in the world.

Dissemination of ICM's Policies: The ICM's visibility in different African countries increased and its advocacy tool as the global representative of midwives was enhanced as the number of MAs increased. MAs have regularly advocated for and disseminated the ICM policies and guidelines. The number of associations that have joined and continue to join have increased the ICM representation of midwives (i.e. database) in the world thereby giving the ICM access to a larger number of women, adolescents and children who will benefit from the richness of the ICM and its MAs. Collaboration with UN agencies has been on the basis of the African membership in the ICM, thereby giving the ICM a voice for the voiceless members in Africa.

Networking with Development Partners: Enhanced communication and networking with African Ministries of Health (MOHs) and in-country development partners through and with MAs are a positive force for the ICM. In the 21st century it is much easier for the ICM to network and communicate with African MAs across the continent and to unite and address the regional issues affecting midwifery in the 21st century.

AMERICAS REGION: NORTH AMERICA /CARIBBEAN (Dr Pandora Hartman & MAs)
Historical Background

The history of midwifery development in the North America/Caribbean Region dates back to the colonial period which laid the foundations for both the successes and challenges that shape the region today. The ICM MAs in this region provided a brief history of the development of midwifery in the Caribbean, USA and Canada as background for understanding the importance of their subsequent membership in the ICM.

Caribbean Islands: Midwifery was an important factor in the economy of the islands as the slaves were expensive commodities. After the transatlantic slave trade was stopped, women's bodies became a reproductive commodity. An example of this can be seen in the mention of midwifery and the need for training of midwives which appears in the records of Trinidad as early as 1826 during British rule when property owners appealed for help from the Governor of the Colony over the loss of their slaves in childbirth. They advocated for better training of the birth attendants/ midwives who attended the birth of slaves. The then Governor of Trinidad and Tobago, Sir Ralph James Woodford, appealed to the Medical Board, started by Don Chacon, for assistance. The Medical Board then commenced the registration of women who could read and write. They were required to pass an oral exam and upon success they were given a ticket to practice midwifery.

USA: Before and after the turn of the century (1900) in the USA there were many attempts to systematically and deliberately dismantle midwifery systems by the medical societies and public health departments. This spurred the need for organisation and support that could only be found through local and international professional associations, such as the ICM.[7] The marginalisation of the traditional apprentice model midwifery was possible because of the unequal system. The importation of European midwifery models changed the context of the Americas in the 1920s. This split midwifery into distinctive 'camps' that adversely affects advancement of the profession even today. Generally, midwives were recruited from or initially trained within the UK to scale up midwifery services in the Americas. With the exception of Canada, much of formalised midwifery education was undertaken only after completion of a minimum of 3 years of nursing education.

Early midwifery services were grounded in volunteerism and service to others outside of and within employment as midwives. By the 1950s, all but 12 of the 250 midwives of the American College of Nurse-Midwifery at the time worked overseas in missions which influenced early leaders in the decision-making process around pursuing ICM membership. This spirit of service holds true today, as many of the region's ICM MAs maintain active global health sections which have provided countless volunteer hours and technical assistance to midwives in other countries over the decades. 'Our membership with the ICM and its philosophies bonds us in service as global citizens; we must give back where we can.'[8]

Canada: Indigenous midwives in Canada have held a distinct role within the Indigenous, First Nations, Inuit and Métis communities, which included all aspects of the health of women and their families throughout the life cycle. Over the last 100 years, the colonial system took away the practice of indigenous midwifery. It is only due to the resilience and commitment of indigenous midwives that their practice has continued. Today indigenous midwives are represented by the National Aboriginal Council of Midwives (NACM), officially formed in 2008.

Settlers in Canada had a different experience from the indigenous people. The French settlers imported midwives under order of the King of France. Later, in the 20th century, nurse-midwives were recruited, often from the UK, to work in remote communities where physicians were not available. In Newfoundland, British midwives were recruited to work in the Grenfell Mission. Some nursing schools offered postgraduate certificates in midwifery to support the outpost settings. However, similar to its US counterparts, midwifery was marginalised. There was also an active campaign to discredit the midwife with roots in medicine in the late 19th century that endured late into the 20th century. A grassroots movement, born out of social activism and the struggle for women's rights, resulted in the development of a parallel midwifery practice in Canada. These early midwives' desire for learning and sharing of experiences led them to chart new territory in a region unlike Europe.

Member Associations

The first ICM MAs from this Region were the American College of Nurse-Midwifery (ACNM) and the American Association of Nurse-Midwives (AANM) who were accepted into ICM membership in 1956, then joining together as the American College of Nurse-Midwives in 1969 resulting in the name change in the ICM records. The same thing happened in Canada when the International Section of the Ontario Midwives Association, the Midwives Association of British Colombia, the Alberta Association of Midwives and the Quebec Association of Midwives joined together to form the Canadian Association of Midwives in 2002. In 2021 there were ten full MAs in North America and the Caribbean as listed in Table 13.2. Numbers of the ICM MAs do not adequately reflect the impact of the ICM in the region as many of the smaller Caribbean Community Market (CARICOM) island midwives' groups exist under the umbrella of the Caribbean Regional Midwifery Association (CRMA), an associate member of the ICM that derives many of its executive board members from official ICM MAs.

Table 13.2 North America & Caribbean Country, Name and Year Midwifery Associations Accepted for ICM Membership

Country	Name of Association	Year
United States of America	American College of Nurse-Midwifery (ACNM)	1956
	American Association of Nurse-Midwives (AANM)	1956
	American College of Nurse-Midwives (ACNM)[9]	1969*
	Midwives Alliance of North America (MANA): International Section	1981*
	National Association of Certified Professional Midwives (NACPM)	2014*
Jamaica	Jamaica Midwives' Association (JMA)	1966; 1981*

Trinidad & Tobago	Trinidad & Tobago Association of Midwives (TTAM)	1990; 1999*
Canada	Midwifery Association of British Colombia (MABC) Association of Ontario Midwives (AOM) Alberta Association of Midwives (AAM) Regroupment Les Sages-Femmes du Quebec (RSFQ) Canadian Association of Midwives (CAM)[10]	1982 1984 1991 1999 2002*
Barbados	Barbados Nurses Association: Midwives Group	1998*
Guyana	Midwives Association of Guyana (MAG)	2012*
Haiti	Association des Infirmieres Sages-Femmes d'Haïti (AISFH)	2006*
Suriname	Suriname Organization of Midwives (SOM)	2006

*= ICM current members in 2019; where two dates are given, there was a lapse in membership.

Value/Impact of ICM Membership on North American and Caribbean Midwifery Associations

Recognition for Midwifery and Midwives: Membership in the ICM has contributed all over the region to increased recognition of the professional profile of midwives and midwifery. It is universally reported amongst all that baseline tools and continuing professional development sessions developed under the auspices of the ICM have helped the MAs in the Americas become more vocal and politically involved. Another key factor in this political involvement has been the technical support provided by the Regional Representatives to empower the early ICM executives to utilise research to improve the ICM. A case example can be seen in the extensive use of the ICM *Global Standards for Midwifery Education with Guidelines (2010; 2013)* to strengthen direct-entry midwifery in the USA resulting in increased access to midwives through multi-state recognition of midwifery credentials that are not dependent upon prior licensure as a nurse. This in turn has raised the professional profile of midwives in the United States.

Impact on Midwifery Education, Regulation and Practice: Utilising the ICM's core documents has significantly enhanced the regulatory and educational standards within countries in the Americas, which has led to better prepared midwives and greater access to care for childbearing women. The services that midwives have provided over the centuries in the region have varied and, since the early 21st century, have been supported by the ICM core documents and global standards.[11] Membership in the ICM allowed local associations to strengthen the local midwifery profession by improving the capacity of its members to provide quality care for clients and their families during pregnancy, childbirth, the post-natal period and for family planning services through expansion of education programmes based on ICM documents. Dissemination and use of the ICM's global standards landmark documents have shifted midwifery educational pathways with refinement of the definition of a midwife influencing adaptations from Ministries of Health to recognition from the US Department of State. For example, the Trinidad and Tobago Association of Midwives (TTAM) has been able to redefine the role of the midwife as an independent practitioner and to enhance the professional status and image of its members because of the information from the ICM's website that was easy to access.

An early example of the ICM's value to its MAs comes from Jamaica during the Black Sash campaign whereby all the nurses and midwives in the country wore black sashes. This visible campaign in 1966, the same year that the association joined the ICM, generated such a movement that the government was compelled to undertake a formal inquiry into the condition of midwives and nurses as service workers. This memorable campaign resulted in changes to pension status, formalisation of duty hours and allowed for supervisory level advancement within the public service system that governs the health workforce. The ICM's *Global Standards for Midwifery Regulation (2011)* have helped to generate significant momentum once again for the legal recognition and regulation of the varying pathways to midwifery practice that are found in the region. Though there is still work to be done, the regulation standards have supported midwives' efforts to lobby for change within countries.

Another example of the value of using ICM's competencies and standards comes from Ontario, Canada, where midwifery regulation was first enacted in 1991. Since that time 11/13 provinces and territories have regulated and funded midwifery and at the time of writing (end 2020) the mountainous sparsely populated Yukon Territory was drafting regulations to govern midwifery practice in this remote area. The work based upon the foundations of regulatory standards continues in Canada with advocacy for Federal Occupational Classification of Midwifery to allow midwives to work in federal jurisdictions, the inclusion of midwifery in the student loan forgiveness programme (loan forgiven if graduate works in federal facility) and the call for the return of birth to indigenous communities and midwives.

<u>Triennial Congresses & Regional Conferences Bring Global Exposure</u>: The Americas hold a history of ongoing participation by ICM MAs since the 1954 Triennial Congress in London, UK. The experience of MAs participating during Council meetings also helps to develop MAs and is counted as one of the highlights of ICM membership. These ICM congresses and regional conferences have served dual networking and global exposure purposes that have broadened the perspective and awareness of participants far beyond the value of any continuing professional development courses. For example, with its history of segregation of African American and Caribbean diaspora midwives, the hosting of the ICM Congress by ACNM in 1972 in Washington, DC, provided an important opportunity for American midwives of colour to meet other midwives of colour from around the globe. The 'seeing of others like me' established vital reconnections to the African continent which contributed to the election of the first African American vice president (Betty Carrington) of the ACNM in 1973.

The early and ongoing ICM Congresses have also served to combat misinformation about the practice of midwifery. Remembrances from Hattie Hemschemeyer's address, 'Maternity Care Within the Framework of the Public Health Service' follow:

> 'Were we prejudiced? In reviewing the findings, we think not. The audience had been informed by an earlier speaker that there were no midwives in the United States. This created a rather awkward situation for any representative from the United States who was obliged to rise as a visible contradiction to what was being presented. We know that at least one person went away from the Congress better informed about midwifery in this country. We wonder how many more had their ears, minds, and hearts alerted to Nurse-Midwifery U.S.A.'[12]

The historical accounts of the Canadian Association of Midwives (CAM) paint a similar story of immediate professional uplifting directly related to ICM

Congress involvement. CAM reports that siting the 1993 Congress in Vancouver, British Colombia, represented a major pivotal point in the national midwifery movement in Canada adding to the increased use of midwives during the 70s and 80s as consumers pushed for childbirth choices. The MABC had 27 members at the time, and when they won the bid to host the Congress 6 years prior, there was no regulated midwifery in Canada. The British Columbia (BC) Government selected the ICM Congress to announce plans for regulation of midwifery in BC on the opening day of that Congress. The 2017 ICM Triennial Congress brought 2,000 midwives from around the world to Toronto, Canada. This was unsurpassed in raising the national profile of midwives as the Canadian Federal Minister of Health chose this Congress as the venue for announcing the first ever $6-million investment for indigenous midwifery. During this and other congresses, Canadian midwives have valued the relationships built and support provided by midwives from around the world. Strong international midwifery alliances and partnerships have positively impacted midwifery growth in Canada with every Congress exposure.

Partnerships and Affiliations: The ICM works as an important liaison between midwifery associations and brings midwives to the larger international stage such as with the UN and the WHO. Reports such as *The State of the World's Midwifery*, universal standards and advocacy toolkits are used around the region to improve the lives of the families that midwives serve. Any midwife, no matter how remote, can know that they are connected with other midwives across the world through the ICM with coordinated activities such as the International Day of the Midwife which is a celebrated and highly anticipated event for most of the region.

Impact of the North Americas/Caribbean MAs on the Growth and Development of ICM as an Organisation

The impact of the Americas' regional MAs on the growth and development of the ICM as an organisation is not hugely appreciated outside of possible contributions from dues payment to the overall operations of the organisation and, thus, its ability to stand as a voice for midwives. There is, however, a huge recognition of the impact of the region's production of global midwifery leaders and ICM's core documents and standards that have helped to guide the direction of the ICM as an organisation.

Global Leadership Building for the ICM: The Americas have developed several association members who were successful in being elected or hired into the headquarters of the ICM. The Americas can count two Secretary Generals/Chief Executives (Frances Cowper-Smith, Canada, and Frances Ganges, USA) emerging out the of ACNM and CAM. Notable midwifery leaders from the Americas include elected midwives Joyce Thompson (ACNM), Deputy Director (1993–1999) and Director (1999–2005); Bridget Lynch (CAM), Deputy Director (2005–2008) and President (2008–2011) and Debrah Lewis (TTAM), Vice President (2014–2017). Appointed officers included 1969–1972 Congress Host President Lucille Woodville (ACNM), 1990–1993 Congress Host President Carol Hird (MABC) and 2014–2017 Congress Host President Bridget Lynch along with Dorothea Lang (ACNM), long-time ICM representative to the United Nations in New York City. North America and the Caribbean MAs have been ICM Regional Representatives each triennium, including Dorothea Lang, Margaret (Peg) Marshall serving as the representative for Latin America (1993–1999), Lee Saxell (CMA) and Diane Holzer (MANA). Frances Ganges (ACNM) was hired as the ICM Chief Executive, managing the ICM Secretariat for five years (2013–2017).

The strength of the ACNM, its international expertise and its forward-looking leaders contributed to the development of several of the ICM Core Documents over the years. These included the first iteration of the ICM *Code of Ethics* (1993), the ICM Vision and Mission Statements in 1996, the *Essential Competencies for Basic Midwifery Practise* in 2002 and the *Global Standards for Midwifery Education with Guidelines* (2010; rev. 2013). These ICM documents were based in large measure on ACNM documents of similar names that were shared with the ICM. Each was amended for international acceptance by the global community of midwives during ICM workshops.

The twinning of CAM and Tanzania (initiated and seed funded by the ICM) has grown into a long-term partnership that has blossomed between the two associations. This twinning approach has influenced relationships with other midwifery associations and partners and has become a successful model for CAM's global programmes. This twinning is grounded in the ICM's three pillars: education, regulation and association, with funding from the Canadian Government (Global Affairs Canada), and in partnership with UNFPA, Jhpiego and other NGOs. The Americas have now partnered with midwifery associations in Benin, Ethiopia, Democratic Republic of Congo, Haiti, Tanzania, Somalia and

South Sudan. These successes further serve to raise the global profile of the ICM with national governments.

AMERICAS REGION: LATIN AMERICA AND MEXICO [Alicia Cillo, Anita Román, Sandra Oyarzo and MAs][13]
Member Associations

Latin American ICM MAs were very active at regional level following the 1969 ICM Triennial Congress that was held in Santiago, Chile. Regional meetings without support of ICM throughout the past 40 years and the lack of full Spanish translation of educational sessions during ICM Congresses led to multiple discussions of breaking away from the ICM, though that did not happen. Latin America and Mexico currently have nine active full ICM members (Table 13.3). This section is based on reports from four of them (Argentina, Chile, Mexico, Paraguay).

Table 13.3 Latin America and Mexico
Country, Name and Year Midwifery Associations Accepted for ICM Membership

Country	Name of Association	Year
Chile	Colegio de Matronas de Chile AG [College of Midwives of Chile]	1969; 1982*
Paraguay	Associacion de Obstetras Paraguayas (AOP) [Midwives Association of Paraguay]	1981*
Brazil	Associacao Brasileira de Obstetrizes i Infermeiros (ABENFO) [Association of Nurses & Midwives of Brazil]	1982; 2010*
Ecuador	Federación Nacional de Obstetrices y Obstetras del Ecuador (FENOE) [National Federation of Midwives of Ecuador]	1996; 2005*
Argentina	Colegio de Obstetrices de la Provincia de Buenos Aires (COPBA) [College of Midwives of the Province of Buenos Aires]	1999*
Peru	Colegio de Obstetras de Peru (COP) [College of Midwives of Peru]	2003; 2005*

Uruguay	Asociación de Obstetras de Uruguay (AOP) [Midwives Association of Uruguay]	2010*
Costa Rica	Asociación de Profesionales de Enfermería Obstetricia de Costa Rica (APEOCR) [Association of Professional Nurse Midwives of Costa Rica]	2019*
Mexico	Asociación de Parteras Profesionales (APP) [Association of Professional Midwives]	2019*

*= ICM current members in 2019; where two dates listed, there was a lapse in membership.

Value/Impact of ICM Membership on Latin American and Mexican Midwifery Associations

The ICM MAs in Latin America and Mexico reported several common themes in response to the impact that achieving full membership in the ICM had or continues to have on their midwifery association and midwives. These themes were similar to those expressed in other ICM Regions, beginning with increased visibility and recognition for the profession and practise of midwifery.

Recognition for Midwifery and Midwives: Chile and Argentina are among the oldest ICM MAs in Latin America; Mexico and Costa Rica are the newest. The Mexican Association for Professional Midwives (APP) was the first group of midwives in Mexico to receive full membership in the ICM, giving the association national and international status. Both the College of Midwives in Chile and the Province of Buenos Aires' Midwifery Association in Argentina agreed that ICM membership has meant greater recognition of the profession and the important work of midwives in their countries. ICM involvement also provided national, regional and international status for the MAs. Paraguay mentioned that joining the ICM in 1981 was vital as it was necessary to have a guild that could represent midwives nationally and internationally in view of the multiple situations in the county trying to undermine midwifery.

Association Strengthening: The use of the ICM's core documents and standards supported the three pillars of education, regulation and association, especially for newer MAs struggling to build strong associations. These ICM documents empowered leadership and advocacy efforts of individual associations, such as in Paraguay where the midwifery association was strengthened, empowered with strong voices and used good practices in partnerships for the achievement of midwifery legislation. The development of the ICM/UNFPA Young Midwifery Leaders (YML) Programme in the region in 2013 was an important step in association strengthening in preparation for succession planning. In fact, one of the YML participants from Paraguay became President of the MA in that country and another YML is currently the Vice President of the MA in Argentina, demonstrating that young midwives can strengthen the midwifery associations.

Use of ICM's Resources, Policies and Guidelines: It was noted by all the respondents that having the ICM tools to assume leadership and face the challenges that arise periodically is important. Argentina in particular praised the availability of the ICM documents that allowed midwives to position themselves with evidence before the authorities responsible for midwifery practice, education and regulation (Ministries of Health and Education, local and national Legislators). Advocacy documents are used to promote the profession, empower midwives with voices and improve access to quality sexual reproductive health and rights-based services.

Global Leadership Building: ICM membership has led to the selection of Board members from Latin America, including the roles of Regional Representative and the recent election of the first ICM Vice President (Sandra Oyarzo) in 2020. Exposure to ICM also supported Chile's appointment of the First Director of Midwifery in the Ministry of Health, Giorgia Cartes.

ICM Triennial Congresses and Regional Conferences: Participation of MA presidents and their members in regional and international meetings with other midwives has led to increased support and sharing of experiences with midwives all over the world. In addition to establishing networks with midwives around the world, knowing their realities and learning from achievements has been extremely enriching! As the Mexican MA noted, exchange of experiences with colleagues from other countries and having advice and support from the ICM Regional Representative and colleagues with a lot of experience was very helpful in establishing a strong association. In addition, ICM provided training workshops that strengthened the midwives and MAs along with regional meetings and

Congresses where individual midwives could present papers and listen to the voices of other midwives, especially once ICM Triennial Congresses provided education sessions in Spanish.

Value/Impact of Latin American and Mexico MAs on the Growth and Development of ICM

Broadening the ICM's Remit/Perspective with Latin Influence: The growth and development of ICM's MAs in Spanish-speaking Latin America and Mexico have contributed to the expansion of ICM's remit to truly represent all the midwives of the world. In addition, Latin influence in the development of ICM policies and position statements is vital to aggressively strengthen and unite the voices of midwives within the ICM to achieve its strategic goals and activities more fully. Latin American midwives have also served in leadership roles within the ICM, including Americas Regional Representatives (Alicia Cillo, Mirian Solis, Sandra Oyarzo).

Increasing Number of ICM MAs: The commitment of the strong Spanish-speaking MAs (Argentina, Chile, Uruguay) to twin with newer and/or developing midwifery associations led to increasing the number of ICM MAs in the 21st century; notably the return of Brazil (ABENFO) and newest ICM MAs in Costa Rica (APNM) and Mexico (APP). For example, Costa Rica was advised to form an independent midwifery association separate from the nursing college, which they did. The ICM MA's efforts in this region to promote, disseminate and use the ICM global competencies and standards, with support of UNFPA-LACRO, has strengthened the influence of the ICM overall and led to increasing the interest of midwifery groups in the Region to join the ICM and participate in activities.

Conclusion (Sandra Oyarzo)

The work in the region is greatly strengthened by the active and interactive work between all the Presidents of the ICM MAs and the team of UNFPA consultants in the Latin America and Caribbean Regional Office (LACRO), and the partners of PAHO/WHO, the Regional Group to Reduce Maternal Mortality, and midwifery networks in Latin America and the Caribbean sub-Regions, the Implementing Partner at the University of Chile which is also a PAHO/WHO Collaborating Centre in Midwifery. The use of open access platforms and applications such as WhatsApp have allowed for increased participation and equity of access for midwives in the region, strengthening teamwork. The active participation of the ICM Regional Representative is very necessary to continue to maintain close and effective networking.

ASIA-PACIFIC/WESTERN PACIFIC REGION [Karen Guilliland, Ann Kinnear] Introduction

At the 1984 ICM Congress in Sydney, Australia, a decision was made to host Regional meetings at each Council meeting. It also decided that each of its four Regions would host a meeting in their regions in between Council meetings. The aim of the Regional meeting was to initiate policies that reflected the Regional needs and implement policies developed at the previous Council meetings (Chapter 5). The ICM leadership also hoped to establish a better co-operative network between each regional MA that could give assistance to each other and enlarge the ICM membership within the region.[14] The name of this region was changed several times, including more recently being divided into two regions: South-East Asia and Western Pacific Regions.[15]

The Region covers a huge geographical area crossing from one hemisphere to another. The geographical boundaries are extreme in their differences with a mix of resource rich and resource poor countries. This combined Region demonstrates the best and worst of maternal and newborn outcomes. In addition, ICM's MAs are very diverse in terms of culture, language, geography and their association with the ICM. Communication was difficult in the 1980s. The Region called on the ICM to increase the Region's representation on Council over many years, though it remained at two.

Historical Background

The history of midwifery development across the Asia-Pacific/Western Pacific Region is varied and arises from the old to the new.

Japan: In Japan, historical books dating from around the 8th century describe how women observed childbirth. The Traditional Birth Attendant became a specific role in the 17th century and, in the latter half of the 19th century, midwifery education leading to a Midwife License commenced and became established in the early 20th century. The system changed drastically after World War II when midwifery education was based on nursing registration and became part of the nursing profession as it remains today.

China: In the 19th century, the births in China including Hong Kong were conducted by women named 'Wen Po' who acquired knowledge and skills from an experienced 'Wen Po'. In 1910, the Hong Kong government established the Hong Kong Midwives Board (now the Midwives Council of Hong Kong). It is separate from the Nursing Council and is a unique, independent regulator of midwives under the Midwives Registration Ordinance of Hong Kong. The Hong Kong Midwives Association has three representatives on the Midwives Council of Hong Kong.

Others: Other countries have a younger history of midwifery development. The Philippine Midwifery Act was passed in 1992, but there has been a Philippine association of midwives in membership of the ICM since 1981. In the early 1990s, New Zealand established midwives with equal pay and equal rights as the medical profession through their role as Lead Maternity Carers. In Australia, midwives were regulated by the different Australian Territorial governments in differing ways. The Australian Capital Territory was the first to recognise midwifery as a separate profession from nursing. In 2010, Australia established the Health Practitioner Regulation National Law which provided national registration and a separate register for midwives and nurses. It was not until some eight years later that midwifery was recognised as a distinct profession in the National Law.

Member Associations

This report is a combination of Asia-Pacific, Western Pacific and South-East Asia regions from those MAs who responded. In 1984 there were 11 Associations in the Western Pacific Region: Japan (with two Associations and all others one); Korea, Hong Kong, Philippines, Indonesia; New Zealand, Australia and Sarawak, Malaysia, Taiwan, Mauritius. In 2020 there were 23 ICM MAs in the combined Western Pacific, Asia-Pacific and South-East Asia regions (Table 13.4).

Table 13.4 Asia–Pacific Country, Name and Year Midwifery Associations Accepted for ICM Membership

Country	Name of Association	Year
Australia	Australian College of Midwives, Inc. (ACMI)	1972*
Indonesia	Indonesian Midwives Association	1979*
Sarawak	Sarawak Midwives Association (SMA)	1980*
Hong Kong	Hong Kong Midwives Association (HKMA)	1981*
Japan	Japanese Midwives Association (JMA) Japanese Nursing Association, Midwives Section (JNA)	1981* 1981*
New Zealand	New Zealand College of Midwives (NZCOM)	1981*
Philippines	Integrated Midwives Association of the Philippines, Inc. (IMAP)	1981*
Taiwan	Midwives Association of the Republic of China (MARC)	1982*
Japan	Japan Academy of Midwives (JAM)	1989*
Sri Lanka	Sri Lanka Nurse Midwives Association (SLNMA)	1992*
Cambodia	Cambodia Midwives Association (CMA)	1995*
Philippines	National Capital Region Midwives Association, Inc. (NCRMA)	1996*
Vietnam	Vietnam Association of Midwives (VAM)	1996*
India	Society of Midwives of India (SMI)	2003*
Papua New Guinea	Papua New Guinea Midwifery Society (PNGMS)	2006*
Mongolia	Mongolian Midwives Association (MMA)	2010*
Philippines	Philippine League of Government & Private Midwives, Inc. (PLGPMI)	2011*

Kyrgyzstan Republic	Kyrgys Alliance of Midwives (KAM)	2014*
Tajikistan	Tajikistan National Association (TNA)	2014*
Timor Leste	Associação das Parteiras de Timor-Leste	2015*
Nepal	Midwifery Society of Nepal	2016*
Myanmar	Myanmar Nurse & Midwives Association (MNMA)	2019*

*=ICM current members as of 2019.

Value/Impact of ICM Membership on Asia-Pacific/Western Pacific Midwifery Associations

All MAs in this region spoke of their desire to be part of a global midwifery movement, a midwifery community with important common interests and rights, as their key motivation for joining the ICM. This meant that their midwife members had opportunities to attend ICM Triennial Congresses, improving learning, networking and understanding of global midwifery.

Visibility and Association Strengthening: Membership in the ICM assisted MAs in their growth and development as well as positioning midwifery within individual countries. For some, it influenced the development of midwifery education and practice (Japan) ensuring midwifery education and practice met global standards and competencies (Hong Kong, Japan). For Australia, this meant obtaining a clear idea of the value of being a MA and gaining recognition as midwives. The Japan Midwives Association stated that the existence of the ICM as an entity distinct from the International Council of Nursing supported the status of midwives as independent professionals.

ICM's Core Documents and Advocacy: The ICM has had significant influence on MAs and midwifery in member countries in several areas. ICM's standards and publications have provided benchmarks for MAs in raising local standards and their use in advocacy. In Hong Kong, membership in the ICM built credibility and quality assurance to such an extent that they have witnessed increased trust from obstetricians. This trust also includes improvement in public acceptance of services provided by midwives. The provision of excellent platforms to broaden midwifery knowledge supports women for normal birth. ICM's constant dissemination of new global trends in maternal and child health is shared with midwives. The midwives of Hong Kong have acted as a bridge between midwives in mainland China and the ICM through professional ties and sharing new knowledge from the ICM. The organisational structure of the ICM, including the vision and mission, has influenced the strengthening of the organisation and governance of the Philippine League of Government and Private Midwives.

Participation in ICM meetings: The local celebrations of the International Day of the Midwife, participation in local conferences sponsored by the ICM, and ICM Regional meetings have led to local policy development. The development of regulatory standards under an ICM banner using ICM material promoted respect and understanding of ICM at national and regional levels.

Value/Impact of Asia-Pacific/Western Pacific MAs on the Growth and Development of the ICM

ICM Leadership: All MAs reported that the ICM has benefited from their active engagement across several areas. Many midwives from MAs have stood for election and served as elected Director of ICM (Margaret Peters), Deputy Director (Judi Brown) and representatives of the former Asia-Pacific Region and the current Western Pacific Region (Japan, New Zealand, Australia, Hong Kong). These individuals provided significant leadership and connectivity among midwifery groups of the region and expanded ICM's global remit. Participation in ICM Councils provided the ICM with contributions to planning, critical analysis of midwifery issues worldwide and decision making in terms of governance.

Contributions to ICM's Financial and Management Successes: MAs in this region have hosted ICM Triennial Congresses (1984 Sydney, Australia; 1990 Kobe, Japan; 1999 Manila, Philippines; 2005 Brisbane, Australia) and Regional meetings, thus contributing to ICM's dissemination of knowledge, research and standards, governance and finances. The financial success of the Sydney Congress in 1984 enabled a substantial contribution to the then challenging financial position of ICM. Similar positive financial outcomes of the Kobe Congress in 1990 helped move Safe Motherhood efforts forward in low resource countries (LRC).

100 Years of the International Confederation of Midwives

<u>Support for Regional Meetings:</u> The Australian MA (ACMI) established a bank account for the region and deposited $7,000 from the 1992 Regional conference profit that year. This enabled the next three regional meetings to have a seeding fund of about $2,000 towards the planning and organisation of the next association hosting meetings. Australia and Japan were the main MAs that provided/fundraised for start-up funding for regional meetings up until 2000 when New Zealand took over the account and also began signing sponsors and contributing funds. Kimberly-Clark and Johnson and Johnson were two of the first commercial companies supporting Regional meetings. This Region was the most active in holding Regional meetings, leading the way in demonstrating the true value of such meetings and its ICM Regional Representatives.

<u>Increasing ICM Membership</u>: In 1998 the 5th Regional meeting, 'Asia Pacific Midwives: Sharing Responsibility for Tomorrow, History for Safe Motherhood', was held in New Delhi, India. It was hosted by the ACMI and created in conjunction with the ICM/WHO Safe Motherhood workshops. This was a historic meeting as it was held in a country <u>without</u> an ICM MA with the objective to encourage midwife identity and ICM membership in India and South Asia, which was accomplished. The high resource countries (HRC) in this Region demonstrated their ability to raise funds in their own countries for regional ICM activities, an important model for all the other Regions. For example, ACMI gained funding from Australian AID to sponsor ten midwives from Pacific countries and the Midwives Division of the JNA also sponsored ten midwives. NZCOM sponsored a delegation of five Maori midwives from the Maori Midwives organisation 'Nga Maia'. They were the first indigenous midwives to present at an ICM conference.

Regional MAs have been active participants in the ICM twinning programme (Vietnam with Japan, Papua New Guinea with Australia). Some MAs expanded twinning efforts and built relationships with newer midwifery groups who were later accepted into ICM Membership; for example, the Japanese Midwives Association working with the Mongolian Midwives Association.

<u>Development of ICM's *Global Standards for Midwifery Regulation*</u>: The Asia-Pacific Region took a strong interest in the drafting and gathering feedback from ICM MAs on the proposed global standards for midwifery regulation. Sally Pairman (New Zealand) was appointed co-Chair of the ICM Regulation Standing Committee and

Judy Ng Wai Ying was appointed as the other Asia-Pacific member. Board member for Asia-Pacific, Karen Guilliland, was appointed as the Regulatory Liaison to the Committee. Mary Kirk (Australia) followed in this Board role from 2011. The standards were adopted in 2011 by the ICM Council (Chapter 12).

EASTERN MEDITERRANEAN REGION [Dr Roa Altaweli & MAs]
Historical Background

The Eastern Mediterranean Region (EMR) was formed in June 2017 during the ICM council meeting. The creation of an Eastern Mediterranean ICM region overcame the issue of ethnically defined regions and increased representation of MAs in this region. Some MAs from other regions were moved to the EMR region. These included Afghanistan and Pakistan from Asia-Pacific; Morocco from Africa West and South Sudan and Yemen from Africa East; and Lebanon, Tunisia, Palestine and United Arab Emirates (UAE) from Southern Europe.

ICM's association with the EMR began in 1982 when the midwifery association of Lebanon was the first one accepted into ICM membership and further strengthened when Morocco was admitted into ICM in 1991 to champion the cause of midwives and midwifery in the region. Over the years, midwifery has evolved in many Eastern Mediterranean countries, especially within the areas of education, regulation and association strengthening, leading to growth of a competent midwifery workforce within the 15 countries that form the membership so far in the Eastern Mediterranean Region.

Member Associations

The section below describes the perceptions of 11 of 15 countries of the Eastern Mediterranean Region with ICM MAs who responded to the questionnaire between 19 November 2019 until 30 December 2020. The 2021 number of EMR ICM MAs is 18 in 15 countries.[16]

Table 13.5 Eastern Mediterranean Country, Name and Year Midwifery Associations Accepted for ICM Membership

Country	Name of Association	Year
Lebanon	Association des Sages-Femmes de la Faculté de Médecine [Lebanese Order of Midwives]	1982; 2019*
Morocco	Association Marocaine de Sages-Femmes (AMFSF)[Moroccan Association of Midwives]	1990 (91)*
Afghanistan	Afghan Midwives Association	2005*
Pakistan	Midwifery Association of Pakistan	2006 (7)*
Yemen	National Yemeni Midwives Association (NYMA)	2010 (11)*
Somaliland	Somaliland Nursing & Midwifery Association	2014*
Tunisia	Association Tunisienne des Sages-Femmes [Tunisian Association of Midwives]	2014*
Somali	Somali Midwives Association (SOMA)	2016*
Saudi Arabia	Saudi Midwifery Group (SMG)	2018 (16)*
Iran	Iran Scientific Association of Midwifery (ISAM)	2018 (19)*
Iraq	Iraqi Midwives Association	2019*

*=ICM member in 2019. Dates in parentheses are dates held in ICM records vs the dates submitted by the MA.

Value/Impact of ICM Membership on Eastern Mediterranean Midwifery Associations

All listed MAs described the significant impact they have had locally and internationally since their membership in the ICM. It was an achievement for most of the countries to be accepted into membership, and especially prestigious for the midwifery association in Yemen.

Recognition/Visibility: All countries considered that their membership in the ICM has been the backbone to their recognition as very strong stand-alone midwifery associations. This recognition from global midwives and other key stakeholders including governments and donor agencies provided the most impact for many MAs in the region. MAs are now confident in representing midwifery in any meetings or platforms where midwifery issues are discussed. Being an ICM MA in some countries not only enhanced their visibility but also strengthened the voices of their midwives with the government, NGOs, UN agencies as well as regional and international partners. For example, midwives in Somalia became confident members of their association because of its membership with the ICM. Lebanon confirmed that ICM membership also added value to their members who now realised they had joined a global network of midwives. ICM membership for the Moroccan midwives' association resulted in being recognised as representative of the midwifery profession in that country based on their capacity to meet the ICM principles and global standards of practice.

Midwives and midwifery are becoming recognised as essential to maternal health care. Such recognition also facilitated the separation of midwives' associations from nurses' associations, thereby setting the pace for independence and self-recognition and an increase in local membership. Being an ICM MA made other national and international organisations respect and appreciate the role of the association and midwives in Yemen.

Association Strengthening and Advocacy: ICM's activities and tools to strengthen MAs have been essential for relatively young MAs. ICM membership helped many countries, such as Lebanon and Saudi Arabia, to develop midwifery associations nationally. Many strategies have been adopted to create awareness about the work of the MAs and the ICM. These have included seminars, stakeholder engagements, community outreach programmes and sharing ICM's global standards for midwifery education and regulation. ICM advocacy materials such as policy and position statements and the *State of the World's Midwifery* reports, have facilitated strong advocacy efforts with governments. They have helped midwives become strong advocates for women and midwifery issues while advocating for the midwifery profession and for evidence-based practice. The ICM *Newsletter* which covers various topics and midwifery activities globally keep the midwives of Pakistan and Lebanon well informed and connected.

ICM's Resource Materials, Policy Initiatives and Guidelines: the ICM's basic pillars and guidance through standards and sharing of evidence-based practices became the road map for midwives and midwifery in many MAs in this region. ICM's leadership role in the development of the definition of the midwife and the delineation of the midwifery scope of practice based on the essential competencies were vital to MAs in the Region. For example, Somaliland adapted the ICM competencies, ethics code, *Midwifery Scope of Practice* and the midwifery philosophy in their curricula. In addition, the ICM's global standards for midwifery education and regulation provided a professional framework that is being used by midwifery associations, midwifery regulators, midwifery educators and governments to strengthen the midwifery profession, raise the standard of midwifery practice, and strengthen MAs' credibility within their country and the Region.

Capital Investment in Midwives: The ICM helped midwives access information and opportunities to conduct research. A number of the midwives have had opportunities to present scientific papers at local, regional and international levels.

Conferences and Global Exposure: The first combined regional ICM conference for Eastern Mediterranean, South-East Asia and Western Pacific regions was held in Dubai, UAE, in 2018. Attendance at regional and global ICM congresses by Eastern Mediterranean midwives has given academic exposure and the chance to build networks for collaboration. For example, Somaliland benefited and learned a lot from the ICM Triennial Congress and Council meetings, and other ICM sponsored conferences and meetings. Exchange of experiences between countries such as the twinning between Morocco and KNOV (Netherlands) and building the network of Arab countries' MAs were very beneficial. Afghanistan introduced the name of the ICM at the national level and mentioned the ICM's cooperation in all countries in meetings and programmes.

Global Leadership Building: Exposure to the ICM also gave motivation for Eastern Mediterranean midwives to apply for ICM global positions. The midwives who have served on the ICM Board or standing committees, among others, include ICM regional representatives for Eastern Mediterranean: Rafat Jan (2017–2020) and Roa Altaweli (2020–2023).

Impact of EMR MAs on the Growth and Development of ICM as an Organisation

a. MAs have been committed to paying ICM membership fees to help support the running of ICM.
b. MAs have contributed to the development of global midwifery core documents, strategic planning and position papers which are used for advocacy and putting midwifery on the global map.
c. MAs have expanded the planning base of the ICM and supported the ICM to include perspectives and experiences drawn from the Eastern Mediterranean Region to better advocate for the midwife, mother and baby worldwide.
d. As ICM's visibility in different Eastern Mediterranean countries increased, the number of MAs from the Region increased, thus increasing the ICM's representation of midwives globally. The increased number of MAs from the EMR region has given the ICM access to a larger number of women, adolescents and children who will benefit from the richness of the ICM. MAs have regularly disseminated ICM's policies and guidelines and advocated for their use. Some collaborations with the UN agencies have been on the basis of the Eastern Mediterranean membership, thereby giving the ICM the voice for the voiceless members in the Eastern Mediterranean region.
e. Enhanced communication and networking with Eastern Mediterranean Ministries of Health and Development partners through MAs such as in Iraq. It is much easier for the ICM to network and communicate with Eastern Mediterranean MAs across the continent and to unite and address the regional issues affecting midwifery.
f. Iran Scientific Association of Midwifery (ISAM) is new in the ICM and has well-educated members (BS, MS and PhD) with very excellent potential to improve ICM's aims, vision and mission. ISAM could also help the ICM with needed exchange programmes.
g. MAs participated in ICM studies, research, awareness campaigns, several trainings in different countries, events and ICM elections.

REGIONAL EXPECTATIONS FOR THE FUTURE OF ICM[17]

Following is a brief summary of future expectations of ICM from four Regions. Many address the challenges listed in Chapter 17. Of importance to future leaders of the ICM are the differences in expectations depending on the region of the world surveyed.

Future Expectations of the ICM from Anglophone Africa MAs[18]

a. <u>Relationship building and capacity strengthening</u>: the ICM needs to keep the good relationships with its MAs and work closely with members in strengthening MAs in Africa to improve the quality of midwifery education and quality of services. In addition, the MAs will expect to work in partnership with ICM in grant management. ICM will champion unified associations in countries and avoid splintering and divisions.

b. <u>Midwifery research</u>. Provide more support for the Africa region to build a database of publications to tell the story of midwifery in Africa. There is need for a guiding document for research competencies for midwifery educators.

c. <u>Increase partnerships and collaborations</u>: Based on the current contribution of 50,000 Happy Birthdays Project in capacity building of midwives, continue working in partnership at country level.

Future Expectations of the ICM from North America and Caribbean MAs[19]

1. Continue to <u>grow as an organisation</u> that connects midwives globally
2. <u>More fully recognise the differing needs of MAs</u>
3. Focused <u>intent on development of marginalised communities:</u> grow and achieve a more representative and diverse midwifery workforce
4. <u>Support student needs and availability of clinical sites</u> for learning
5. Advocate for sustainable health systems that allow midwives to thrive in an increasingly globalised world.

Future Expectations of the ICM from Spanish-speaking Latin America and Mexico MAs[20]

1. Support <u>local and national projects</u>
2. Continue to <u>promote research</u> through national congresses with support from the international scientific committee

Future Expectations of the ICM from Asia-Pacific/ Western Pacific Region MAs[21]

1. Continue in a <u>strategic role</u> around midwifery practice, education and research to improve maternal and child health within and across nations

2. Maintain contemporary publications and advice
3. <u>Diversify the ICM official languages</u> to include Japanese to increase the number of Japanese midwives who can participate in ICM activities

Future Expectations of the ICM from Eastern Mediterranean Region MAs[22]

1. Provide <u>internships in the ICM office</u>
2. <u>Professional development</u>: MAs expect more support for and opportunities for professional development through training (in person or online).
3. <u>Midwifery research</u>: the ICM needs to provide more support for the Eastern Mediterranean region to build a database on publications to tell the midwifery story of the Eastern Mediterranean region.
4. <u>Leadership/increased midwife recognition/profiling</u>: MAs expect more support in recognition of their role in improving maternal and child health and their contribution in reduction of maternal and infant mortality rates. There is a need to support MAs to identify the midwifery profession as a unified profession around the world and to be recognised by the governments of their respective countries, increase the midwifery workforce and maintain an optimum level of the quality of midwifery education and practice.
5. <u>More partnerships and collaborations</u>: the ICM needs to be a champion in advocating for women's health rights, advocating for women's empowerment for their health and eliminating Female Genital Mutilation (FGM) (FGM practice in Somalia is 99 per cent) and strengthening communication and coordination among the midwives and the ICM along with more twinning programmes between member associations.

Common Expectations from All Regions Include:

1. <u>Promote use of the ICM standards</u>: Continually promote the ICM global standards for harmonisation of education, regulation, association strengthening in countries
2. <u>Leadership/raise profile of midwives</u>: Continue raising the profile of midwives with representation at regional and international levels and sustain leadership at all levels globally

3. <u>Capacity building</u>: for young midwife leaders, how to influence health policies, get involved in national decision-making and advocate for improved health
4. <u>Continue to be a strong global voice for</u> midwifery and for the reproductive <u>health and</u> <u>rights of women and families</u>: Continue reciprocal partnerships with women, other health professionals and international organisations such as the WHO, UNFPA and FIGO
5. <u>Promote and advocate for midwives</u> and the <u>value of midwifery care</u> to governments and other policymakers to improve midwives' autonomy and to promote reproductive health
6. <u>Achieve midwifery regulation</u> around the world
7. Continue <u>proactive response of the ICM in any future crisis</u>, such as the COVID-19 pandemic
8. <u>Strengthen ties</u> within and between ICM regions
9. <u>Support Global and regional networking</u>

SUMMARY

Many similarities across regions describing the value of the ICM and its activities and documents and the impact of MAs on the ICM are described in this chapter. Differences, though few, are primarily related to the low status of women/midwives in a given region, limited educational opportunities and slow economic development of countries, leading to an increased need for financial support and twinning of associations. Though MAs and their midwives face many challenges across the globe, it has been important for MAs to listen to the expectations of the ICM and conversely for the ICM to hear its MAs' concerns. With this mutual working together, the future can be brighter for all. As noted earlier, any midwife, no matter how remote, can know that they are connected with other midwives across the world. They are empowered with strong voices and associations through the ICM, its activities and documents to carry out the Aims of the ICM. The overwhelming agreement was that membership in the ICM was mutually beneficial to the ICM and to the Member Associations charged with improving the health of women, newborns and families with well-qualified and supported midwives.

100 Years of the International Confederation of Midwives

1. The responses to MA status included some responses that did not match the 2021 ICM database or archival records. Where differences were noted, they are included in the respective tables of membership as the first date followed by the reported date following a '/'. The possible explanation of this variance is that the MA may have reported when their application was sent to the ICM, while staff at the ICM recorded dates of official action by the ICM Council. In addition, the MAs listed on regional charts were those who responded to the survey resulting in some newer members in the region not included. Annex G has the complete MA list through 2021.
2. GCMA was the predecessor of the Ghana Registered Midwives' Association that came into existence with independence in 1957 and the country's name was changed from Gold Coast to Ghana. As noted in Chapter 3, the GCMA was in existence in the 1930s when a representative tried to join the IMU and was told the IMU was for European associations at the time.
3. ICM 2017–2020 Strategic Plan found on the website.
4. The dates on the Table of membership in parentheses represent what the country reported if different from ICM records.
5. The original report from Anglophone Africa contained a list of individuals who had led the association, and did not include information from those MAs who did not respond. Annex G has list of former and current ICM members by Region as of 2019.
6. GCMA was a member of the ICM in 1954 until there was a name change to GRMA in 1957 when the country changed its name from Gold Coast to Ghana at independence. There was no lapse in membership.
7. Helen Varney & Joyce Beebe Thompson. A History of Midwifery in the United States: The Midwife Said 'Fear Not'. New York: Springer Publishing Company, 2016. Chapters 3 and 4.
8. Suzanne Wertman, ACNM member. Interview by Pandora Hardtman.
9. The two nurse-midwifery associations that became members of ICM in 1956 merged to become the American College of Nurse-Midwives in 1969, continuing as an ICM Member Association without a break in membership.
10. The four Provincial midwifery associations in Canada with ICM membership since the 1980s merged into one in 2002, becoming the Canadian Association of Midwives without a lapse in ICM membership.
11. The sharing of ACNM documents during the late 1990s and early 2000s formed the basis for establishment of the ICM Essential Competencies for Basic Midwifery Practice (2002) and the ICM Global Standards for Midwifery Education (2010).
12. Hattie Hemschemeyer. Quoted in Ruth Coates & Marion Strachan. Bulletin of the America College of Nurse-Midwifery. 2:3 (September 1957).
13. The Latin American report was translated from Spanish into English by Joyce Thompson.
14. Carol Hosking, 1985 (New Zealand Delegate).
15. ICM. ICM Council Meeting Minutes (virtual), June 2020. Agenda item 4.2.
16. The original report from EMR contained a list of individuals who had led the association.
17. Anglophone Africa, the Americas, Asia-Pacific and Eastern Mediterranean regions were the only ones to respond to the 2020–2021 survey.
18. Anglophone Africa report written by Jemima Dennis-Antwi, Ghanaian midwife.
19. North America and Caribbean report written by Pandora Hardtman, US midwife.
20. Latin America and Mexico report written by Alicia Cillo, Argentine midwife and Anita Roman, Chilean midwife.
21. Asia-Pacific report compiled by Ann Kinnear (Australia) and Karen Guilliland (New Zealand) midwives.
22. Eastern Mediterranean report compiled by Roa Altaweli, Saudi Arabian midwife.

Chapter 14: *Women, Midwives and the ICM*[1]

'... Joining forces with women succeeds in making the reestablishment of the Midwifery Model synonymous with reclaiming women's control over childbirth. Extending the Midwifery partnership to the professional organisation, development and maintenance of Midwifery gives us a unique identity, social recognition and protects women's choices and self-determination.'

New Zealand College of Midwives' Statement 1993

INTRODUCTION

For centuries midwives have worked 'in partnership' with women, families and communities to achieve good outcomes for pregnancy and birth but the definition of 'partnership' was wide and varied. The ICM relies on the day-to-day practice of every midwife working with women in a way that makes a positive difference to the woman's well-being. Women and midwives as partners are therefore an obvious and natural bond to build that gives strength to both. Individual and collective midwifery partnerships with women are an ethical, philosophical and practice stance that the ICM members have been continually developing and building on over many years.

Since the early days of the 100-year-old Confederation emphasis has been placed on protecting motherhood as well as improving the status of the midwife, a profession dominated by women. The value accorded to women as persons from an ICM perspective dealt with both midwives' struggle for autonomy and midwifery services directed at protecting childbearing women, preventing needless maternal and newborn deaths and ensuring basic human rights. The reader may view this approach as 'speaking for' rather than encouraging the 'voices' of women that occurred later in ICM's history, though not a negative approach for those women and their newborns who were dying at high rates for lack of care, food and low social status. However, concern for the status of midwives was at the core of valuing women who were both the majority of midwives globally and those receiving midwifery services.

The ICM has been increasingly aware since the early 1990s that partnering and working with women's organisations and other organisations committed to the reproductive health of girls and women at an international and organisational level is essential to ensure that midwifery policy and health services place women and newborns in the centre of care. But this organisational activity can only be successful and transformational if its foundational and professional objectives are firm and credible. The content in this chapter explores the ongoing efforts of midwives working with women directly and the ICM's representatives working with other organisations who share a common vision for healthy women and families. The ICM's story is truly the story of women.

WOMEN'S WORK

> 'I have always believed that the midwife is to be a Korowai – a cloak. Her role is to surround the woman with warmth, wisdom, comfort, and protection so that the woman, in turn, can birth well. The Korowai is woven with great skills and the technique of its making has its own whakapapa wahine (women's story). From generation to generation the knowledge of such making is passed down. So too with midwives. We are taught the art and skill of midwifery from the woman who wove and the women who wore the korowai. Our patterns and feathers are individually unique but they share the same purpose - nurture of the woman and her baby.'
>
> Jackie Pearse, New Zealand Midwife, Lawyer, 2004

A common feature of women's work is that it is often invisible, stereotyped, subject to prejudice and assigned a lower value than men's work,[2] despite the fact the WHO reported that 70 per cent of the world's health workforce are women.[3] Women's health services are equally lacking priority in most countries when compared to other health services. Midwifery is a predominantly female profession providing care almost exclusively to women and their newborns and, as such, midwives and midwifery services are also often further undervalued. This inequitable environment ultimately adversely impacts or compromises the care that midwives are able to provide to women.

The ICM, as the only international organisation representing midwives, has had to look for innovative and effective ways to counter the invisibility of women's work and women's voices. These efforts were driven forward when the Australian College of Midwives, Inc. (ACMI) became a member of the ICM in 1972 and the New Zealand College of Midwives became a member of the ICM in 1981, adding these strong feminist midwifery voices to ICM's quest to represent all the midwives in the world.

Purposefully encouraging and building partnerships with women both as clients and in organisations with mutual goals so that women and midwives make a louder voice together is now an established ICM strategy. It has taken the vision, persistence and commitment from all the midwives leading the ICM over the decades to demand improvements to the status of midwives and to women's childbearing experiences and other aspects of reproductive health.

WOMEN AS MEMBERS OF ICM MEMBER ASSOCIATIONS

The ICM has always endeavoured to carry out its dual aims of promoting the health of women and childbearing families and strengthening its Member Associations (MAs) (Chapter 10). Since the early 1950s, the ICM has carried out much of this work with global organisational partners, such as the WHO and the FIGO. However, the concept of midwifery as an individual and collective partnership between women and midwives took on new meaning during the 1990 ICM Council meeting in Kobe, Japan, when delegates from the New Zealand College of Midwives (NZCOM) challenged the ICM Council to recognise New Zealand's consumer/woman membership as part of their ICM MA.[4] The ICM Executive attempted to disallow the NZCOM from ICM membership[5] on the grounds that their women members (7 per cent of their membership) were not midwives and therefore the College was not eligible to be a member based on the criteria for membership written in the ICM Constitution of the day.[6] New Zealand argued that its partnership with women in all aspects of midwives' professional lives was a philosophical and political necessity and therefore under its constitution the ICM could not discriminate against a member 'foundered upon reasons of philosophical, religious or political nature'.[7] After much debate Council accepted New Zealand's membership. NZCOM gave notice of its intention to bring the topic of partnership with consumers back to the 1993 ICM Congress.[8]

In March 1992 NZCOM attended an ICM Asia-Pacific conference in Melbourne to gauge the region's support for consumer representation and partnership. NZCOM took Judi Strid from the women's consumer activist group, the Auckland Women's Health Council, to speak. Some of the obstacles identified were apprehension about working with non-professionals; fear that consumers may take over; cultural issues where health professionals are expected to speak on behalf of consumers.[9] The Region agreed for two remits to go forward to the 1993 ICM Council in Vancouver calling for the endorsement of the right of NZCOM to operate in partnership with consumers and further endorsement for this partnership on a global basis.

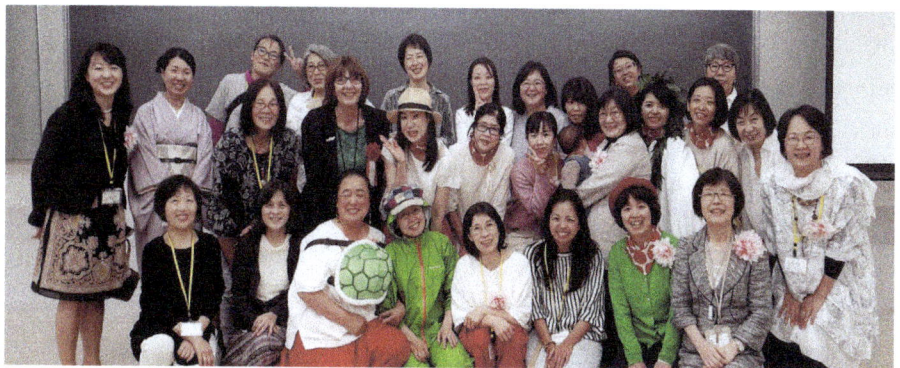

Japanese midwives and the Japanese consumer group "Appletree" working together for change in Japan – Courtesy of Karen Guilliland

The NZCOM delegates proposed changes to the ICM constitution in 1993 (seconded by the Alberta Association of Midwives, Canada) that would enable any member association to have a specific consumer membership category, but this proposal lost.[10] The rationale for this lack of support centred on Council's view of 'the importance of retaining an exclusively midwifery professional voice for negotiation with bodies such as the WHO and the need to find other ways of expressing partnership with women.'[11] The ICM Constitution remains silent on consumer membership to the present time but the 1996 Constitutional amendment added the word 'primarily' to Clause 6; *Qualification for Membership. An Association applying to become a member shall ... 1) consist <u>primarily</u> of midwives ii) have duties and objectives that are in harmony with those of the Confederation.* This single word has enabled consumer members in MAs in those countries who work in partnership with women this way.[12]

THE ICM'S VISION FOR WOMEN AND FOR MIDWIVES

In 1993 the NZCOM delegates proposed a revision to the 1990 position statement *The Midwifery Partnership* with a name change. This motion was seconded by Midwives Alliance of North America (MANA) with a title change to *The Midwifery Partnership with Women*, and was adopted unanimously.[13] It began with: 'Midwifery is a profession based upon a partnership between women and midwives.'[14] These words are now overt in many ICM documents since 1993 though they caused a polarising debate at the time. Extracts from the NZCOM proposal introduced this chapter.[15] Debate focused on the need to respect cultural differences and demonstrate flexibility in developing different models of partnership. This position statement was revised and re-ratified in 2005 by the vast majority of MAs as *Partnership between Women and Midwives* with more emphasis on women's informed consent,[16] a key element in the ICM's *International Code of Ethics for Midwives* that was first adopted in 1993 (Chapter 11).

Listening to Women

One of the major challenges of consumer–midwife partnerships was to listen to the voices of women and childbearing families and then work with women and families to act on those needs, including empowerment and woman-friendly policy changes. Many midwives and midwifery associations carried out this partnership very well throughout history, but others needed help in understanding how best to be a partner with the women one is serving.

New Zealand had a strong partnership between midwives and women which, with information from the ICM Headquarters, enabled a change to their national health legislation that recognised midwifery as an autonomous profession separate from nursing and medicine in 1990. It also legitimised every woman's right to choose a midwife as her lead maternity carer and embedded partnership/continuity of care into the national maternity service.[17] It was the first country to do so. Midwives Karen Guilliland, Sally Pairman and Sue Bree led the midwifery changes with consumers in New Zealand while they were the NZCOM delegates to the ICM in the 1990s. They all went on to become ICM Regional Representatives, Standing Committee Chairs and Board members over two decades, and Sally as its CEO from 2014 onwards. As such, these women had a major influence on ICM's international and regional policy and commitment to partnership and continuity of care, especially in the Asia-Pacific Region. MA countries with huge birthing populations such as the Philippines, Indonesia, Japan and Canada modified New Zealand's Midwifery partnership model for practice[18] and standards of practice as components of their midwifery education curricula. Other ICM MA countries that followed suit in the 1990s and early 2000s were Australia, Bangladesh, Italy, Sami Peoples of Lapland Finland, Ethiopia, Turkey and Portugal highlighting how the midwifery partnership with woman resonated with a wide range of cultures. Many others learnt about partnership from the ICM's regional and international congresses.

ICM's Statement at the 4th World Conference on Women – 1995

The opportunity to share the ICM's support for women and their health with the world came in Beijing, China. The ICM's Deputy Director (Joyce Thompson) presented the official ICM statement to the 4th World Conference on Women in September 1995. This statement began with sharing the January 1995 ICM Executive Committee endorsement of the following statement, *'In looking forward to the 21st century, midwives and women share many of the same concerns and will work together toward achieving the vision that empowers both women and midwives to be fully respected as persons who are also productive members of all societies'*.[19] The statement went on to pledge the ICM's support to all national and international activities that promoted women as persons, reproductive health targeting the reduction of maternal mortality and lifelong women's health as an essential component of every country's development. It ended with: *'In recognition of the crucial roles that women play in the health of families and in the development of nations, the Confederation supports the inclusion of women in national debates and decisions about health policies, such policies having been developed by women themselves.'*[20] Though the statement was important, it continued to be a challenge for MAs to implement these concepts in many areas of the world where women continued to be treated as the property of men without any rights.

ICM's Vision: Empowering Women, Empowering Midwives – 1993

The concept of midwives being in partnership with women was more clearly stated and demonstrably more accepted when the ICM Council adopted its first formal statement of Vision in 1996 (Chapter 8). It was stated simply as: 'Empowering Women … Empowering Midwives'[21]. Based on the overall vision of empowerment, the 1996 ICM Council delegates recognised that midwives and women share many of the same concerns. The ICM Vision was developed, in part, based on information received from the 'Listen to Women' campaigns carried out by the American College of Nurse-Midwives (ACNM).[22] What was evident in the midwifery movement of the 1980s–1990s in the USA was the tendency for many midwives to focus internally, on solely what they needed, often to the detriment of what the women who sought their services wanted/needed – especially women who sought hospital births.[23] The 'Listen to Women' campaign in the United States resulted in a better understanding of how midwives could listen and then act on women's needs such as what was being done in New Zealand, rather than imposing the midwife's idea of what women who sought midwifery care needed.

ICM'S COMMITMENT TO WORKING WITH WOMEN AS PARTNERS

An additional ICM commitment to the partnership between women and midwives was captured during the ICM Council Meeting, May 1999, in Manila, The Philippines. The ICM Council agreed to update the Midwifery Partnership with Women from 1993[24] and to add the following to the statement Legislation to Govern Midwifery Practice that had been agreed provisionally by the ICM Executive in New Delhi, India, in February 1998: 'The consumer representation should come from within women's organisations concerned to advance the quality of care provided to women in their countries.'[25] During the discussion, Council delegates emphasised the importance of including women in the regulation of midwifery. One member noted that:

> 'It is appropriate that women who are reliant on the quality of their caregivers be included in the organisation that develops and oversees any midwifery regulation.'[26]

The ICM urged midwives to 'work with the bodies that regulate midwifery in their country and advocate for consultation with women in developing, reviewing and implementing regulation.'[27] This position was ratified again in 2017.[28]

The ICM Africa Regional Conference in 2001 followed the Safe Motherhood workshops with a theme of, 'Achieving Midwifery Partnerships with Women for Safe Motherhood.' Joyce Thompson, ICM Director, gave the keynote address titled, 'Safe Motherhood: A Call to Action for Women, Men, and Especially

Midwives'.[29] The value to the ICM of the Africa Conference in Zimbabwe in 2001 was affirmation of its Vision[30] that midwifery partnerships with women implies consultation with women, advocacy for women and empowerment of women with both voices and choices, including the midwives who offer high quality, woman-centred care. The value to the midwives and women of Africa was immense, given the low status of women in those countries who now had the support of the ICM to improve their status and strengthen their voices within their countries.

ICM's *Midwives, Women and Human Rights* – 2002

This statement adopted in 2002 was the forerunner of the Core Document, *Bill of Rights for Women and Midwives* adopted in 2011 (Chapter 11). The adoption of the ICM 2002 Position Statement focusing on the basic human rights of midwives and women followed the 1999 update of the ICM Code of Ethics. The basis of this statement came from Section 3d of the Code of Ethics that read:

> 'Midwives understand the adverse consequences that ethical and human rights violations have on the health of women and infants and will work to eliminate these violations.'

The 2002 statement was based on the belief that all efforts to empower women and to empower midwives to demand their basic human rights and understand the responsibilities that accrue to those persons exercising such rights were needed. In addition, the statement called on midwives working with women to aim for empowerment of themselves and others, including voices as well as choices for women. Support for the basic rights of women to participate in decisions about their care was further evidence of the ICM's strong support of partnerships with women and childbearing families. The influence of feminism with an emphasis on global women's rights movement was obvious in these statements and in the *International Code of Ethics* as midwives were urged to 'speak out' and foster partnerships with women's groups.

During the early 2000s, the ICM worked with many different partners in an effort to improve the status of midwives and women's health with significant results. Examples included the 2000 *Munich Declaration-Nurses and Midwives: A Force for Health* to strengthen midwifery and nursing workforces with Ministers of Health across Member States of the European Region of the WHO;[31] the 2002

Aachen Declaration on Midwifery for All[32] demanding maternity care policies form an integral part of all public health policies in Europe that was drafted with the ICM in partnership with MA conference delegates from Germany, Spain, Brazil, Czech Republic and the Netherlands; and the ongoing Alliance for Women's Health where the ICM, FIGO, WHO, UNFPA, UNICEF, the World Bank and IPPF joined together to advance women's health.[33]

ICM's Philosophy and Model of Midwifery Care – 2005

The 2005 ICM Council delegates in Brisbane, Australia, moved forward the partnership between women and midwives with greater clarity by describing how midwives were to provide women-centred services, reflecting earlier statements of the ICM *International Code of Ethics for Midwives*. The ICM *Philosophy and Model of Midwifery Care* was revised, further reinforcing this partnership with women. It stated:

> 'Midwifery care takes place in partnership with women, recognising the right to self- determination, and is respectful, personalised, continuous and non-authoritarian.'[34]

Another significant step forward during the 2005 Council meeting was the adoption of the Position Statement, *Midwifery: An Autonomous Profession*, where professional autonomy was linked with partnership: 'Midwifery … maintains its contract with society in partnership with women and communities.'[35] The active participation of the ICM at the consumer organised 'Women Deliver' (WD) global conferences starting in 2007 reflected the ICM's ongoing commitment to work with women and consumers to improve health for all. The midwifery conference that precedes each WD conference demonstrates that the ICM platform at this important event continues to grow.[36]

ICM's *Bill of Rights for Women and Midwives* – 2011

Another important core document created in 2011 reinforced the vision for women and for midwives as partners for healthy nations. The proposed *Bill of Rights for Women and Midwives* was drafted by the NZCOM, debated, approved by the Asia-Pacific Region at its conference in Hyderabad, India in 2009[37], and ratified by the ICM Council globally in 2011. The 2011 rights' statements for women and for midwives reflected the earlier code of ethics adopted by the

ICM Council in 1993, vision statements first adopted in 1996 and the position statement, 'Midwives, Women and Human Rights' adopted in 2002.[38] The current document states, 'The Bill of Rights for Women and Midwives addresses those basic human rights of women and midwives that have been systematically denied and adds another framework to approach governments when demanding change to improve midwifery and maternity services'[39] (Chapter 11). The background page goes on to acknowledge the ICM's role in meeting the United Nations' Sustainable Development Goal 3 (3.1 reduction of maternal mortality ratio; 3.7 ensuring universal access to sexual and reproductive health care services) and Goal 5 (Achieve gender equality and empower all women and girls).

ICM's *International Definition of Midwife* rev. 2011

The midwifery partnership with women was specifically referred to for the first time in the 2005 revised International Definition of the Midwife and Scope of Practice.[40] One of the important updates reflecting ICM's partnership with women occurred in 2011 with the addition of the underlined words below in the Scope of Practice statement:

> 'The midwife is recognised as a responsible and accountable professional <u>who works in partnership with women</u> to give the necessary support, care and advice during pregnancy, labour and the postpartum period…'[41]

ORGANISATIONS SHARING A COMMON VISION OF WOMEN AND MIDWIVES AS PARTNERS

A proposed position statement, Partnership and the International Confederation of Midwives, at the 1999 Council meeting in Manila, The Philippines, demonstrated a move to operationalise partnerships and asked ICM MAs to inform headquarters of organisations worthy of partnership. 'The establishment of relationships/partnerships is beneficial to the ICM, making it more effective by extending its influence beyond the midwifery profession and in the achievements of its aims and objectives.'[42] This proposal was returned to the 2002 ICM Council in Vienna, Austria, and adopted.[43] The White Ribbon Alliance is one important partner example.

The White Ribbon Alliance

In 2003 Judith Brown, Deputy Director of ICM, was elected to the Decision-Making Committee of the White Ribbon Alliance (WRA), 'a grassroots movement for safe motherhood that builds alliances, influences policies and inspires action to save women's lives …'[44]. The ICM established an enduring partnership with WRA in 2003 built on the launch of the WRA during the 1999 ICM Congress in the Philippines by its founder, Theresa Shaver, an American nurse-midwife. The ICM signed a Memorandum of Understanding (MOU) with the White Ribbon Alliance in 2009 which 'formalised ICM's engagement with the coalition and contributed to the coalition campaigns'[45]. In 2010, the WRA facilitated a global petition from the ICM, the International Pediatric Association (IPA), the International Council of Nurses (ICN) and the International Federation of Gynecology and Obstetrics (FIGO) on behalf of their combined 14.3 million members. This petition was presented at the G8 Summit held in Huntsville, Ontario, Canada, with a call to commit an extra $10 billion to help women birth safely. What power this partnership demonstrated!

Other ICM Partnership Efforts

In 2003 the ICM introduced the new programme, 'Strengthening Midwives Associations', as visible public support for positive relationship-building with the community.[46] The influence of the global women's rights movement was obvious as midwives were urged to 'speak out' and foster partnerships with women's groups.

In 2004 the ICM noted that: 'Effective partnerships continue to hold the key to the ICM's Achievements'[47]. The global reach of ICM's partnerships concerned with women and midwives, their health and their voices continue to expand. One example was the *Islamabad Declaration on Strengthening Nursing and Midwifery* that was agreed between ICM/WHO/FIGO/ICN in Pakistan in 2007.[48]

In June 2006 the Board's strategic planning efforts gave priority to reviewing their partnership philosophy and representation in the global arenas, increasing links with aligned organisations.[49] This was the same year that the ICM instigated formal 'Twinning' Projects between MAs with one country association 'twinned' with another to mentor and support them. There had been small examples of informal twinning in preceding years. In 2007 ICM's partners and collaborative work were discussed as core business with Criteria for Core Partners and Criteria for Partner projects and funding developed.[50]

Criteria for Core partners (e.g. WHO, PMNCH, FIGO) required:
- An essential relationship for impact and influence
- Represents women's reproductive health/newborn health
- International and professional
- Relationship mutually beneficial and interdependent
- Common purpose
- Aligned core business.

Coalition partners; (e.g. WRA, UNFPA) required:
- Mutual benefits for public information
- Projects that are mutually beneficial
- Projects related to core business
- Relationship is time limited
- Work is international[51]

The review of the ICM's partners and representation efforts leading up to the 2008 ICM Council meeting in Glasgow, Scotland, resulted in the Council's revision of the organisation's Vision and Mission statements to be more woman centred. MAs from Canada and New Zealand led the discussion on indigenous midwifery as part of the efforts of the ICM to be more inclusive and woman centred, recognising cultural differences. Brazil spoke on their consumer-led humanisation of birth movement working together with midwives, and Slovenia proposed that the midwives' journey to professionalism is to work through partnership and consultation.[52] Another equity step forward was the term midwife 'expert' was removed from definitions and replaced with midwives as 'specialists'. This was in line with the belief that women worked as partners with midwives and brought their own expertise in their care.[53]

Partnerships with Global Health Groups/Agencies

A new position statement titled *Collaboration and Partnerships for Healthy Women and Infants* proposed by the ACNM and the Midwives Alliance of North America was passed during the 2008 ICM Council meeting in Glasgow, Scotland.[54] The statement called for more collaboration and partnership-type working with like-minded groups and agencies. It also recognised that: 'It is appropriate that midwives lead the way to expand the traditional partnerships for care, to include other health professional groups, policymakers and global agencies that share a common vision of healthy women and newborns throughout the world.'[55] The understanding of the power of partnerships was articulated clearly throughout the statement. For example: 'The power of partnerships goes beyond what each individual, group or agency can do alone, thereby maximising the effectiveness of strategies to promote the health of women and newborns.' It goes on to say:

> 'Collaboration between midwives, other health professionals and consumer groups, and between ICM and other international partner organizations, should be constructive and focused on women's and newborns' needs at every level.'[56]

There are an increasing number of projects that the ICM began undertaking to strengthen its partnership with women and for women's health. They include being a key contributor to the 'What Women Want' Campaign launched in 2017, a global advocacy campaign to improve quality maternal and reproductive health care for women and girls and strengthen health systems.[57] MAs participated in the 2017 International Day of the Midwife advocacy activity titled, 'I Believe in Partnership.' Midwives were invited and encouraged to share their views, stories, photos and videos to showcase their partnership with women and their families. These videos, photos, views and stories were shared for two months resulting in approximately 100,000 Twitter impressions and over 70,000 people reached through the ICM's Facebook.

In 2018 the ICM, in partnership with UNFPA, began developing a series of workshops on Respectful Maternity Care (RMC). These addressed the education and support needed to change the behaviour of health workers caring for women during pregnancy and birth and counter the disrespect and abuse of women in many countries.[58]

The ICM Advocacy Toolkit developed in 2020 shows how far the concept of working with women had come. It highlighted the need to get the support of women:

> 'We can't do any of this without the support of women. It makes no sense to fight for midwifery if women don't want it. Women need to know that midwifery exists, and to demand it. Midwives need to build their grassroots base.'[59]

THE ICM's ORGANISATIONAL STRUCTURE SUPPORTING WOMEN AS PARTNERS AND LEADERS

The early history of the IMU was formed within the social context of women's work and its value (Chapter 2). The structure of the IMU was confusing at times, held together primarily by Frans Daels, a Belgian Obstetrician (Chapter 3). As ICM evolved since 1954, many MAs considered the Constitution too complex and unwieldy with little in it to reflect and enable women's ways of working. The NZCOM, supported by the Royal College of Midwives (UK) and the Midwives Association of British Columbia (Canada), put forward a Resolution to the 1996 ICM Council Meeting in Oslo, Norway, 'that the organisational structure of ICM and the constitution be reviewed to enable implementation of the Global Strategy and a working group developed to develop a plan.' They submitted that 'this woman centred vision of empowerment for women and midwives needs to be reflected in the structure, function and processes of the ICM.' Members called for 'a more flexible and empowering organisation than the present structure and constitution allow.' The process (Rules of Order) used for decision-making during Council meetings, dictated by the Constitution of the day, was perceived by some MAs to obstruct free thinking and limit debate on key issues. Some MA delegates also noted that 'ICM relies heavily on unpaid women's work and as it moves towards the 21st Century and the challenges of its Global Strategy, this voluntary approach is no longer appropriate.'[60] This resolution was adopted. A Constitution Review working group was set up and MAs were asked to indicate any amendments they had, keeping in mind the *Global Vision* and strategy of empowerment.

All leadership of the ICM during its 100-year history struggled under the global discrimination directed at female-dominated professions and female-led organisations in its efforts to make the organisation stronger and midwives more visible. This tenacious and long-standing work by many midwives and their supporters underpins today's successes as noted throughout ICM's history. Some suggest that perhaps it is not surprising that the last two decades within the context of global recognition of gender inequalities gave midwifery leaders more confidence in reclaiming midwifery as a partnership between midwives and women.

The Strategic Plan 2021–2023 shows the increasing maturity and inclusiveness position that the ICM holds. It states: 'The strategic plan positions ICM as a partner, advocate, technical adviser, and knowledge base for midwives' associations and midwives around the world, allowing the organisation to grow and expand in tailored ways that will make the largest impact on the profession of midwifery, with broader impacts on gender equality, human rights, diversity, and universal health coverage.'[61]

SUMMARY

When researching the minutes of ICM Board and Council meetings over the last 50 years, it is clear that the MA countries who have contributed significantly to the notion of the empowerment of women and midwives through partnership were consistent over several decades. Unsurprisingly, they are countries which themselves are egalitarian with strong women leadership and influence or have strong women's movements supporting midwives seeking change. Countries such as Canada, the Netherlands, New Zealand, the United Kingdom and the United States of America have historically led innovation and change in many areas of women's rights. Midwifery is no exception and these country gains gave the ICM's leadership more confidence to claim partnership with women as essential to midwifery and the story of the ICM.

The ICM has come a long way in the gender empowerment role. It has defined Midwifery as a partnership relationship between midwives and women with continuity of care an essential part of this model (Chapter 11). Its core documents, standards, guidelines, position statements and projects promote this relationship model of care. Despite many years of seemingly slow progress on specific gender empowerment activities while the ICM worked tirelessly to identify and promote the status and role of the professional midwife globally, the ICM has moved forward rapidly in the early 21st century to reinforce that the lives of women and midwives are intrinsically intertwined.

Many believe that midwifery is essential to gender equality throughout the world and that the ICM needs to reflect modern feminist thinking. The ICM recognises it must always keep women at the centre of everything it does if the status of both women and midwives are to be strengthened. At the close of the first century of ICM's story, the ICM has embedded working in partnership with women into its organisational culture. This partnership has sped up the ICM's progress and has given, and will continue to give, the ICM the strength of vision and voice to achieve the goal of 'a world where every childbearing woman has access to a midwife's care for herself and her newborn'[62] and that midwifery care is evidence-based and collaborative with the women themselves.

100 Years of the International Confederation of Midwives

1. This chapter was contributed by Karen Guilliland, New Zealand midwife and long-time member of ICM leadership. It was derived, in part, from: Karen Guilliland and Sally Pairman. The Midwifery Partnership-A model for Practice. First edition; Monograph Series 95/1 Department of Nursing and Midwifery Victoria University, 1995. Second edition; New Zealand College of Midwives, 2010. Additional content was added in the editing process in keeping with the format of the book.
2. World Health Organization, International Confederation of Midwives, The White Ribbon Alliance. *Midwives Voices, Midwives' Realities: Findings from a global consultation on providing quality midwifery care.* Geneva: World Health Organisation; 2016.
3. World Health Organization. *Delivered by Women, Led by Men: A Gender and Equity Analysis of the Global Health and Social Workforce.* Human Resources for Health Observer 24 (English, French): March 2019 ISBN: 978-92-4-151546-7.
4. ICM. *ICM Council Meeting Minutes, Kobe, Japan, 2–4, 9 October 1990*. Minute 90/6: Matters Arising, 'The New Zealand delegate raised the question of consumer membership. It was pointed out that ICM was a federation of associations of midwives, p 3.
5. The New Zealand College of Midwives was awarded full membership by the ICM Council in 1981.
6. ICM. *ICM Constitution*, 1987. Qualifications for membership, para 6: association shall '(i) consist of midwives recognized by their government or professional organisations as being competent to practice midwifery; (ii) maintain its complete unity, independence and method of working; (iii) undertake to pay financial dues in such form and within such time limits as many be decided by the council,' p 4.
7. Karen Guilliland and Sally Pairman. International Confederation of Midwives: 23rd Triennial Congress, Vancouver, Canada. *New Zealand College of Midwives Journal*, 9 October 1993.
8. ICM. *ICM Council Meeting Minutes, Kobe, Japan, 2–4, 9 October 1990*. Minute 90/25.2, p 14.
9. Judy Strid. 'Women and Midwives': The International Conference of Midwives Asia Pacific Region. *NZCOM Journal*, June 1992.
10. ICM. *ICM Council Meeting Minutes, Vancouver, Canada, 4–11 May 1993*. Item 93.28.5, p 25. The suggested change in wording of membership was proposed again in 1996 and defeated. ICM. *ICM Council Meeting Minutes, Oslo, Norway, 21–23 May 1996*. Agenda Item 44.5 p 22.
11. ICM. *ICM Council Meeting Minutes, Vancouver, Canada, 4–11 May 1993*. Item 93.28.5, p 25.
12. https://www.internationalmidwives.org/assets/files/general-files/2020/07/_icm-articles-of-association-constitution_june-2020.pdf Qualification for membership is now under Article 4 of the 2020 Constitution.
13. ICM. *ICM Council Meeting Minutes, Manila, May 1999*. London: May 1999, Agenda 51.11, p 38.
14. ICM. *ICM Council Meeting Minutes, Vancouver, Canada, 4–11 May 1993*. Item 93.20.16, pp 18–19. The title was changed in 2005 to 'Partnership Between Women and Midwives' and can be downloaded from ICM website: http://www.internationalmidwives.org.
15. ICM. *Board papers. Resolution: Position Statement. The Midwifery Partnership with woman.* FD.Coun-Resjc 1993.
16. ICM. *ICM Council Meeting Minutes, Brisbane, Australia, 19–21 July 2005.* Item 25.1.11, p 25. https://www.internationalmidwives.org/assets/files/statement-files/2018/04/eng-partnership-between-women-and-midwives1.pdf. Accessed 12 March 2021.
17. Department of Health. *Nurses Amendment Act 1990 Information for Health Providers.* Wellington, New Zealand. October 1990.
18. Karen Guilliland and Sally Pairman. *The Midwifery Partnership-A model for Practice.* First edition; Monograph Series 95/1 Department of Nursing and Midwifery Victoria University, 1995. Second edition; New Zealand College of Midwives, 2010.
19. ICM. *Statement to the 4th World Conference on Women, Beijing, China, September 1995*. [Personal papers JET].
20. ICM. *Statement to the 4th World Conference on Women, Beijing, China, September 1995*. [Personal papers JET].
21. ICM. *ICM Council Meeting Minutes, Oslo, Norway, 21–23 May 1996.* Agenda Item 96.35.2 Vision Statement and Global Strategy, p 16.
22. Joyce E Thompson. 'The ACNM's Visionary Planning.' *Journal of Nurse-Midwifery* 38: 5 (September–October 1993), pp 283–284. Erica L Kathryn. 'Listen to Women: The ACNM's Vision.' *Journal of Nurse-Midwifery* 38:5 (September–October 1993), pp 285–287.
23. Helen Varney & Joyce Beebe Thompson. *A History of Midwifery in the United States: The Midwife Said 'Fear Not'.* New York: Springer Publishing Co, 2016. Chapter 18: Midwives with Women and Childbearing Families, pp 373–390.
24. ICM. *ICM Council Meeting Minutes, Manila, May 1999*. London: May 1999, Agenda 51.11, p 37, agreed a 4th bullet point that read, 'encouraging midwives' associations to involve women/consumers in their activities' p 38.
25. ICM. *ICM Council Meeting Minutes, Manila, May 1999*. London: May 1999, Minutes 53.1 Consumer consultation in midwifery legislation p 39.
26. ICM. *ICM Council Meeting Minutes, Manila, May 1999*. London: May 1999, Minutes 53.1 Consumer consultation in midwifery legislation, p 39.
27. ICM. Position Statement. Legislation to Govern Midwifery Practice. Ref 99/3/PP Adopted ICM Council, Manila, May 1999.
28. https://www.internationalmidwives.org/our-work/policy-and-practice/icm-position-statements/ Accessed 20 March 2021.
29. Joyce Thompson. Safe Motherhood: *A Call to Action for Women, Men, and Especially Midwives,* 2001. [Personal papers JET].
30. ICM. *Empowering Women – Empowering Midwives: The Vision for Women and their Health.* London: ICM, adopted by the ICM Council, May 1996.
31. ICM. The Munich Declaration – Nurses and Midwives: A Force for Health. *International Midwifery* 13: 6 (November/December 2000) p 12.
32. ICM. The Aachen Declaration on Midwifery for All: a European or global document? International Midwifery 15:3 (May/June 2002), pp 8–9 (page 9 in French and Spanish).

33 Franka Cadée. The Alliance for Women's Health: ICM + FIGO/WHO/IPPF/UNFPA/UNICEF/World Bank. *International Midwifery* 15:5 (September/October 2002), p 9.
34 ICM. *ICM Council Minutes, Brisbane, Australia, 2005*. Agenda item 25.2.1: Midwifery Philosophy and Model of Care, p 27.
35 ICM. Midwifery: An Autonomous Profession. *International Midwifery* 18: 6 (November/December 2005), p 68.
36 ICM *International Midwifery* 20:5 (December 2007), pp 57–60.
37 Personal papers of Karen Guilliland, Asia Pacific Regional Representative member of Executive Committee 1999–2002 and 2005–2011.
38 ICM. *ICM Council Minutes Manila, Philippines, 1999*. Agenda item 53.21 referred document to Executive Committee in 2001. Final adoption 2002. ICM. *ICM Council Meeting Minutes Vienna, April 2002*. Agenda item 02.22.3.4. Midwives, Women and Human Rights, adopted in principle p 14.
39 ICM. *Core Document: Bill of Rights for Women and Midwives*. The Hague: ICM, 2011; 2017, p 1.
40 ICM. Press Release: Midwives vote for revised 'Definition of the Midwife'. *International Midwifery* 18:4 (July/August), 2005 p 44.
41 ICM. *Scope of Practice of the Midwife*. Revised ICM Definition of the Midwife during 2011 ICM Council Meeting, Durban, South Africa.
42 ICM. *ICM Council Meeting Minutes, Manila, May 1999*. London: May 1999, Agenda 60.4 ICM Partnerships, 'was not considered due to lack of time,' and was returned to the proposer, p 42. ICM Council Meeting. Position Statement. *Collaboration and Partnerships for Healthy Women and Infants*. Vienna, 2002.
43 ICM. *ICM Council Meeting Minutes, Vienna, 2002*. Position Statement. *Collaboration and Partnerships for Healthy Women and Infants* adopted.
44 Judith Brown. The unifying symbol of the White Ribbon. *International Midwifery* 17:1 (January/February 2004), p 4.
45 ICM. *Triennial Report 2008–2011. The Hague:* ICM, p 20.
46 ICM. Communique with Member Associations. Background paper Ref Sam/mydoc/associ/strengthen.dec/3.
47 ICM. *International Midwifery* 17: 5 (September/October 2004), p 51.
48 Fadwa Affara. Strengthening nursing & midwifery: scaling up capacity to reach the Millennium Development Goals. *International Midwifery* 20:2 (June 2007), pp 20–21.
49 ICM. *Report of Final Board meeting June 2006*. The Hague: ICM [SvdC Doc SC].
50 ICM. *ICM Board meeting minutes 23– 25 June 2007*. The Hague: ICM. Paper B11.2, p 12.
51 ICM. *ICM Board meeting minutes June 2007*. Paper B11.2.
52 ICM. *International Midwifery* 21:2 (June 2008), pp 23–25.
53 ICM. *Draft Board meeting minutes*, 23–25 June 2007. The Hague: ICM, p 13.
54 ICM. *ICM Council Meeting Minutes, Glasgow, 2008*. Agenda 10.1, p 30.
55 ICM. *Collaboration and Partnerships for Healthy Women and Infants*. The Hague: ICM, 2008.
56 ICM. *Collaboration and Partnerships for Healthy Women and Infants*. The Hague: ICM, 2008.
57 White Ribbon Alliance. *What Women Want Campaign* 2017. https://www.whatwomenwant.org/about Accessed 2 April 2021.
58 https://www.internationalmidwives.org/our-work/other-resources/respect-toolkit.html Accessed 21 March 2021.
59 https://www.internationalmidwives.org/assets/files/advocacy-files/2020/12/icm_midwivesadvocacytoolkit_final.pdf Accessed 21 March 2021.
60 ICM. *ICM Council Meeting Minutes, Oslo, Norway, 21–23 May 1996*. Agenda Item 96.35.2 Vision Statement and Global Strategy, p 16.
61 ICM. *Strategic Plan 2021–2023*. The Hague: ICM, 2021. Can be downloaded from the ICM website at www.internationalmidwives.org.
62 ICM. Vision Statement. The Hague: ICM, 2008.

CHAPTER 15: *United Nations (UN) Agencies*

'I had been fortunate to attend a FIGO Congress in San Francisco at which Dr Petros-Barvasian, a Paediatrician who then headed WHO's maternal and infant sector, had given a Keynote address. She eloquently described the appalling state of the levels of maternal mortality with its associated infant mortality in the world's countries where most of the births took place. She also highlighted that most of the deaths occurred from largely preventable causes with an associated lack of access to a skilled attendant.

'Given that many of the countries with the worst outcomes were in the Asia Pacific Region, I thought she was the right person the give the keynote address in Sydney. The program committee agreed so we invited her to the 1984 ICM Sydney Congress. It is fair to say Dr Petros-Barvasian presented a depressing and challenging picture of the need for much commitment to universal access to skilled midwives wherever women gave birth if the situation was to improve worldwide. That, I believe, was the renewal of a strong relationship between ICM and the WHO with midwives viewed as essential to saving lives.'

Margaret Peters, ICM President 1984

INTRODUCTION

The ICM represented midwifery in many different arenas, was a member of various international networks, developed relationships with other players in the field of reproductive health including maternal and newborn care and initiated and/or co-led many projects for midwives over the years (Annex D lists partners). The guiding principles for this part of the ICM's work included the organisation's commitment to healthy women, healthy childbearing and healthy newborns within a human rights framework. These activities were in keeping with the ICM's mission, vision and triennial strategic goals and objectives. As noted in a 2002 Council agenda item:

> 'The partnerships and projects in which the ICM is involved are intended to benefit midwifery as a whole and to further the goals of the Safe Motherhood Initia-

tive which dictate much of the international activity in the field of maternal and child health care.'[1]

Much of the ICM's story is intertwined with other global organisations concerned with the health and rights of families, women, adolescents and children, especially following the establishment of the United Nations and the World Health Organization (WHO). ICM's formal recognition by the WHO as an accredited international non-Governmental Organisation (NGO) in 1957 continued joint activities between representatives of the ICM and WHO headquarters.[2]

Other UN agencies including the United Nations' Children's Education Fund (UNICEF) and the United Nations' Fund for Population (UNFPA) have been intricately linked with the ICM for decades. Content in this chapter focuses on the initial and ongoing impact these UN health partners had on the growth and development of the ICM as a respected international NGO representing the midwives of the world and on the ICM's efforts to ensure that midwives' voices are heard in international health policy fora. Details on the ICM's role on the Interagency Group on Safe Motherhood (IAG-SM) with WHO and other partners is found in Chapter 16. Other chapters provide details about the ongoing impact of ICM's collaboration with its UN partners.

THE WORLD HEALTH ORGANIZATION

'If there hadn't been an ICM, the tasks of UNFPA and WHO would be much harder.'

Luc de Bernis, Interview 2017

The WHO was the first and undoubtedly the most significant partner (though not without challenges) with the ICM over the years, resulting in the attention paid to details about the WHO and the ICM throughout this book. Upon its founding in 1948, the WHO began establishing volunteer Expert Committees to explore the various global health challenges throughout the world. There were four Expert Committees of importance to the work of midwives in the 1950s. They included the *Expert Committee on Maternity Care*, the *Expert Committee on Nursing* and the *Expert Committee on Maternal and Child Health*. Selected members of these committees became part of the *Expert Committee on Midwifery Training* in 1954 (Chapter 4), joining forces to define maternity care and the health workers involved in providing these services. The 'trained' midwife was just one of the categories defined in that report, with a paucity of information available on the education and practice of the 'trained midwife' in areas of greatest need such as Africa and South-East Asia.

Individual midwives and obstetricians were invited by the WHO as members of Expert Committees on issues related to maternity care and midwifery, especially in countries with high levels of maternal and child deaths. Marjorie Bayes was named Executive Secretary of the ICM during the 1954 ICM Congress in London. Her location in London at the Royal College of Midwives (RCM) afforded many opportunities to know of WHO activities and for the WHO to know of her position at the ICM. This resulted in her presence at many WHO meetings in Geneva, though the first official request for an ICM representative to be a part of a WHO Expert Committee did not come until 1965.

The WHO Expert Committee: The Midwife in Maternity Care – 1965

The WHO Expert Committee on the Midwife in Maternity Care met in Geneva from 19 to 25 October 1965. Alongside Marjorie Bayes as the ICM representative were a nurse-midwife tutor from Singapore (Lau Koi Eng) and chief midwife from the Catholic University in Chile (Lidia Celis) on the eight-member Committee.[3] The chair of this committee was Allan C Barnes, Obstetrician/Gynaecologist from Johns Hopkins University, USA. The purpose of the Committee was to review the work of the midwife, to define the midwife's contribution to maternity care in the light of developments and changes that had occurred since 1954, and to provide recommendations to countries on how to address these changes.[4] One major change in maternity care over the previous decade included the move of births in the home (village) to hospitals or maternity centres with short post-partum stays, primarily in urban areas, that made continuity of midwife care increasingly difficult.[5] In addition, physicians became very interested in normal births requiring a team-approach to maternity care, a difficult challenge for many midwives and physicians who were used to being in charge of births. In addition, family planning became an important part of reducing needless maternal and newborn deaths, expanding the role of the midwife in many countries of the world, though not always popular with the midwives.

Of particular importance to the ICM's early story was the collective view of this international group of maternity care experts on the need to have a clear definition of the 'midwife' in order to carry out their task. Though this definition was published as part of the Report of the Expert Committee, the note at the top of that report stated, *'that the collective views of experts ... does not necessarily represent the decisions or stated policy of the World Health Organization.'*[6] In spite of this disclaimer, the WHO is credited with this definition that preceded by seven years the ICM's agreement on a revised international definition of the midwife.[7] The 1965 WHO definition and functions of the midwife read:

> 'A midwife is a person who is qualified to practise midwifery. She is trained to give the necessary care and advice to women during pregnancy, labour, and the postnatal period, to conduct normal deliveries on her own responsibility, and to care for the newly born infant. At all times she must be able to recognize the warning signs of abnormal or potentially abnormal conditions which necessitate referral to a doctor, and to carry out emergency measures in the absence of medical help. She may practise in hospitals, health units or domiciliary services. In any one of these situations, she has an important task in health education within the family and community. In some countries, her work extends into the fields of gynaecology, family planning and child care.'[8]

This report went on to define the functions of the midwife in caring for the mother, the infant, the family and the community as well as, in some countries, the health of young children, especially when the midwife was the only health worker in that community. It is of importance to the ICM's later development of the Global Standards for Midwifery Education[9] in 2010 that this committee agreed that, 'in view of the high level of competence and responsibility required of the midwife, she should have completed secondary education ...'[10] The committee recognised that in some countries nursing registration was required prior to midwifery education, along with public health, though they recommended that in order to avoid duplication or overlapping curricula in midwifery and nursing, their education should be coordinated at national level. However, the committee concluded that not all midwives needed to be fully trained nurses, a position affirmed by the ICM to the present day with recognition of both single trained midwives and nurse-midwives.

The Expert Committee discussed the midwife's collaboration with other health workers as well as the role and functions of the auxiliary midwife and traditional birth attendant. They also devoted time to the midwife's role in posts of senior responsibility such as administration and supervision, teaching, research and evaluation. The Committee's recommendations included the need for physician support, improved training facilities and financial support for the midwife to attend refresher and ongoing educational offerings to keep up-to-date in knowledge and practice. Perhaps the concluding statement best reflects the WHO's ongoing commitment to midwives and the practise of midwifery:

> 'The Committee was firmly convinced that the work of the midwife is a permanent and essential part of maternity care throughout the world.'[11]

The ICM and the WHO: An Ongoing Relationship

The ICM and the WHO developed a synergistic relationship over the years that benefited both organisations committed to Health for All with an emphasis on the health of adolescents, women, childbearing families and newborns. More importantly, a review of the modern history of the ICM affirms that both the ICM and the WHO, often working together, have been pivotal in bringing onto the global stage the need for competent, confident midwives who are key to reaching the Millennium Development[12] and Sustainable Development Goals[13] related to the reproductive health of women, newborns, children and adolescents. Other examples include the WHO's *Midwifery Education Modules* based on the ICM's 1990 Collaborative Pre-Congress workshop; WHO's *Strengthening Midwifery Toolkit* with input from the ICM and midwife consultants; the WHO's *Core Competencies for Midwifery Educators* produced by consultant midwives and more recently ICM's input into the Global Strategy on Human Resources for Health. These are just a few of the examples of WHO-led initiatives that the ICM had an important role in their development.

Midwifery Technical Officers Within the WHO Assigned to the ICM

The inclusion of midwives as critical to the success of the UN's global goals, especially those related to gender, maternal and newborn health, helped to raise the profile of the ICM as the international organisation responsible for preparing, regulating and supporting midwifery development through its Member Associations (MAs) at regional, national and local levels.

The relationship and mutuality between the WHO and the ICM, whilst steadfast over many decades, included challenges. The WHO's support for midwives and midwifery can be traced as far back as 1955. The WHO's approach to strengthening midwifery in low-income countries through the first half of the

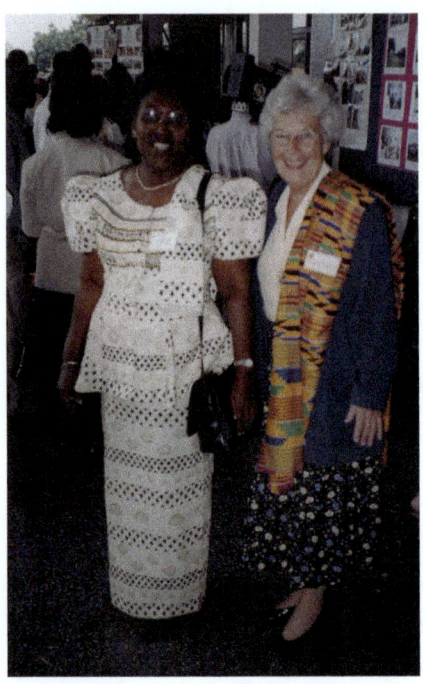

Dr Barbara Kwast with midwife Kathlyn Ababio – ICM Archives at Wellcome Collection

1960s included a reliance on midwives from European countries where strong midwifery associations had been developed, although the WHO had no senior midwife in Geneva guiding this support.[14] In addition, the WHO's reliance on medical doctors in key positions often reinforced the hierarchy with midwives at the bottom of health care professional groups. In spite of years of ICM's lobbying for a midwife at WHO headquarters, it was not until 1981 that the WHO recruited a senior midwife in the post of Public Health Nurse Midwife as a technical member of staff, who for the first time was designated as the official technical liaison with the ICM (Joan Bentley). Refer to Table 15.1 below.

Table 15.1
WHO Midwife Technical Liaison Officers for the ICM

Name	Country Origin	Title	Dates of Service
Joan Bentley	UK	WHO Technical Liaison to ICM	1981–1985
Barbara E Kwast	The Netherlands with extensive experience in Africa	WHO Designated Technical Officer to ICM	1986–1991
Sr Anne Thompson	UK with extensive experience in Africa & ICM Board member	WHO Midwifery Officer and liaison to ICM	1995–1999

Maggie Usher	UK	WHO Designated Technical Officer	1999–2001
Jelka Zupan[15]	Paediatrician at WHO	Interim WHO liaison to ICM	June 2001
Della Sherratt	UK with extensive experience in South & East Asia (SEARO)	WHO Designated Technical Officer to ICM	9/2001– 5/2005
Margaretta Larsson[16]	Sweden – seconded by SIDA	WHO Midwifery Officer and Liaison to ICM	6/2005– 6/2007
Frances McConville	UK – seconded by DFID	WHO Midwifery Advisor and Liaison to ICM	2013– present

The WHO's internal structures also created a challenge for collaboration with the ICM. The substance of the 2nd 10-year review of the WHO's work, published in 1967, indicates that the work on midwifery was split between separate departments/work programmes. The work on maternal and child health was separated from strengthening health systems and human resources, with the responsibility for both nursing and midwifery under the programme headed by the Chief Nurse.[17] This situation persisted over the years through 2020, despite repeated requests from the ICM for the WHO to appoint a Chief Midwife.[18]

The technical staff who have led most of the WHO's work around midwifery specifically, rather than general policies and strategies on midwifery and nursing as a systems issue, were recruited to the department responsible for Maternal and Child Health (MNCH) and/or Reproductive Health. The various technical officers for midwifery as the official liaison with the ICM developed a joint programme of work that was reviewed and agreed at regular intervals. The responsibility for the WHO Collaborating Centres for Nursing and Midwifery fell within the remit of the Chief Nurse Scientist, who did not always have midwifery preparation. The line management for these two departments were also very separate. Furthermore, managerial responsibility for the WHO's work at regional and country level was also separate and to some extent slightly autonomous, all of which made liaison and collaboration problematic for the ICM at times, including for its MAs at country and regional levels.

Meeting Challenges Directly for Health for All

Despite the challenges described above, the ICM continued to have a good working relationship with the WHO for decades and has had significant influence on the WHO and its policies, strategies and programmes.[19] Equally, the status of the WHO and regard given to the WHO by many of its Member States, especially those in low income countries, provided opportunities for the ICM to be recognised and respected as an NGO in official relations with the WHO and to some extent influenced ICM's own workplan.[20] This reciprocity can be seen most strongly since the launch of the global programme on Safe Motherhood in 1987 (Chapter 9). The revitalisation of the Safe Motherhood Initiatives (SMI) following the 10-year review of SMI in 1997 owes much to Sr Anne Thompson who led the WHO's work on midwifery in the later part of the 1990s and who had a significant influence on the 2000 launch of the WHO's work on the new global programme for Making Pregnancy Safer (MPS). MPS and ICM continued joint efforts with publication of the *Strengthening Midwifery Toolkit* in 2006.[21] During the 50th year celebration of WHO, its magazine devoted an entire issue to 'Midwives to the World', with the editorial by Dr Hiroshi Nakajima, Director-General of the WHO, titled, 'Midwives: Guardians of the Future.'[22] Midwives, indeed, are the guardians of the future, and the ICM and its partners are guardians of the midwives.

The midwifery WHO liaisons to the ICM all played a significant role in the joint collaboration between the ICM and the WHO on global work for strengthening midwifery over different periods of time. There were also many other midwives and nurse-midwives who supported this work as either temporary consultants/advisers and as WHO regional and country staff. ICM's observational status along with the International Council of Nurses (ICN) on the Global Advisory Group on Nursing and Midwifery (GAGNM)[23] gave the ICM a voice to the highest authority in the WHO, the Director General, and whose programme was part of the Chief Nurse's workplan. This position of the ICM was indeed useful, even critical, on separate occasions for ensuring and/or strengthening the continued technical leadership on midwifery within the WHO's technical programmes and contributing to the various World Health Assembly resolutions on nursing and midwifery.

In conclusion, this short review of ICM's collaboration and relationship with the WHO highlights that both organisations have been mutually supportive and influential at times to each other's work. Further, despite numerous challenges for the ICM with its relatively small full-time team of staff and volunteer leaders working with a large and cumbersome bureaucratic organisation, the ICM has managed to be very influential in many global health efforts. What is also clear is that on many occasions managing this process has been largely dependent on the personal relationships between ICM staff, including their broader management team, with technical staff within the WHO at various levels of the organisation. Midwives working in tandem and collaboration within both organisations have had a true impact on making pregnancy and childbirth safer across the world.

THE UNITED NATIONS CHILDREN'S FUND (UNICEF)

The United Nations General Assembly established UNICEF in 1946 to carry on the work of the United Nations Relief and Rehabilitation Agency that was providing emergency services for children and childbearing women in war-torn countries. The 1950 UN General Assembly decided that UNICEF should expand its efforts to meet the long range and continuing needs of children, especially in low resource countries. As noted by Marion Strachan, ICM's representative to the UN and UNICEF in 1970–1972, midwives were called on to meet the childbearing needs of women and their newborns at a time when one-fifth of the world's children were dying prior to their fifth birthday.[24]

Official consultative status with UNICEF was requested shortly after the World Health Organization recognised the ICM with official NGO status and was granted in 1962.[25] UNICEF shared a concern for the prevention of needless deaths and disabilities of newborns and young children with many governments. As more research was carried out, it became evident that in order for newborns and young children to survive, they needed a healthy mother. Thus, the ICM was a natural partner with UNICEF in working with childbearing women to promote safe childbirth and healthy newborns. Miss Strachan, as the ICM's representative, signed a joint statement in 1970 in which the 26 NGOs present agreed that they would encourage national affiliates in high resource countries (HRCs) to explore with their governments the possibilities of expanding bilateral and multinational programmes for children and youth. This statement also expressed the hope that more governments would use the expertise of NGOs in their health plans and work.[26]

The ICM's support and benefits from working with UNICEF was mutual. For example, the 1984 ICM Council adopted a policy on breastfeeding spelling out 'the urgent need for midwives to work much harder to increase the number of babies being breastfed' and its 'firm support for UNICEF in its work to improve survival rates of children in the world whose need is most desperate'[27]. This policy statement addressed the midwife's role in encouraging breastfeeding for at least six months following birth. It also asked midwives to 'work in cooperation and collaboration with their national governments, and with UNICEF, in order to make the work of saving infant lives more effective'[28].

There are many examples of the mutual benefits of the ICM/UNICEF partnership. One involved UNICEF's technical support and financial contribution to several of the ICM/WHO/UNICEF Collaborative Pre-Congress Workshops following the launch of the Safe Motherhood Initiatives in 1987. Another was joint efforts with UNICEF and the WHO to create the 'baby-friendly-hospital' initiative.[29] In 1997, Dr France Donnay at UNICEF New York headquarters, suggested that the ICM should have a representative from each country provide a brief update on midwifery when UNICEF health officers meet.[30]

THE UNITED NATIONS POPULATION FUND (UNFPA)

The UNFPA became a collaborating partner with the ICM in the early 1990s with both financial and technical support during ICM's collaborative pre-congress workshops addressing Safe Motherhood. UNFPA along with the WHO and UNICEF often had country and regional offices in low resource countries, thereby facilitating joint maternal and child projects with the ICM and their MAs. Of vital importance to the UNFPA leaders at the time was the meeting on 'Midwifery in the Community' held in 2006 in Hammamet, Tunisia organised by the ICM, the UNFPA and the WHO's Making Pregnancy Safer Programme (MPS). This meeting served to educate the UNFPA leaders on the potential for midwives to contribute to improved reproductive health and childbearing services.[31] This 1st International Forum on Midwifery in the Community looked at lessons learnt and considered how best to scale up access to midwifery care at the community level.[32] A Call to Action was agreed and is discussed under Joint Statements.

UNFPA-ICM Joint Initiative: Responding to a Decade of Action for Human Resources – 2008

Of note is the 2008 collaborative programme between ICM and UNFPA supported financially primarily by Sweden, the Netherlands and UNFPA. It resulted in the Swedish International Development Cooperation Agency (SIDA) and other countries placing midwives in selected UNFPA country offices. This joint project was called, 'Investing in midwives and others with midwifery skills to accelerate progress towards MDG5.'[33] This project greatly influenced UNFPA's and WHO's work and programmes along with ICM's presence in those countries described below.

From 2009 to 2013, the ICM joined with UNFPA to build national capacity in low resource countries by scaling up the capacity of midwives in order to increase skilled attendance at all births.[34] The original plan was to focus on 20 low resource countries (LRCs) in sub-Saharan Africa and Asia with the highest rates of maternal mortality and lowest rates of births attended by skilled personnel. Capacity building took the form of strengthening regulatory, education and accreditation mechanisms and promoting/strengthening midwifery associations. Country midwife advisers were placed in 30 UNFPA country offices, an international midwifery adviser located at ICM Headquarters, and four Regional midwifery Advisers were recruited and posted in the regions (Africa and South-East Asia) representing the dominant language groups of that region. The motto was to get midwives to the negotiation table for strategic planning and implementation, and to help midwives gain master's and PhD degrees to access international posts. As Vincent Fauveau (MD), UNFPA Senior Maternal Health Adviser, noted: 'Financial control was difficult, and it wasn't clear who the country Midwife Advisers (CMAs) were reporting to. The strategy followed the ICM's education-regulation-association approach and the ICM did good work at country level and with other organizations.'[35] Anneka Knutsson noted that the best outcome was having a midwife placed in 30 UNPFA country offices, with varying levels of impact to date.[36]

Mutual Respect between ICM and UNFPA

The collaborative relationship between ICM and UNFPA was and continues to be among the strongest, most respectful and least 'turf-oriented' partnership. UNFPA leaders recognised midwifery as a profession in its own right from the beginning of joint efforts, and the ICM respected the obstetricians and other health professionals for their unique roles in Safe Motherhood. In addition, Dr Luc de Bernis, UNFPA Senior Maternal Health Adviser for Africa (obstetrician), when asked if he saw a change in maternal and newborn health when ICM became an active voice in collaborative partnerships, stated:

'Many organizations contributed to the development of the Essential Interventions in reproductive, maternal, newborn, and child health (RMNCH), but we forgot the "care" elements like birth preparedness, quality of care as experienced by women, and the non-medical aspects needed to deliver those interventions. ICM has contributed to that part of the agenda.'[37]

Luc de Bernis went on to note that the international arena has grown from the strength of the ICM and vice versa, especially with regard to the global standards and competencies for midwives agreed by the ICM. UNFPA and ICM continue to collaborate on reproductive health and rights as evidenced by the UNFPA Global Midwifery Programme Strategy 2018–2030[38] published in 2018 and used as the framework for action at regional and country levels. This strategy has six strategic objectives or elements, addressing interventions and tasks for strengthening midwifery education, regulation, associations, workforce, enabling environments and midwives as integral to the national, regional and global sexual and reproductive health and rights agenda.

Strengthening Midwifery Services

A recent UNFPA collaborative project with the ICM is Strengthening Midwifery Services (SMS) that began in 2019.[39] The UNFPA project activities included workshops at ICM's regional conferences focusing on advocacy training and Respectful Maternity Care (RMC). ICM staff developed an Advocacy Toolkit that is being used by MAs and country midwife advisors. RMC workshops have been held in Africa and Latin America to assist midwives to truly understand RMC and what it means for them where they work. Other RMC workshops are in process. Another aspect of the SMS project was the establishment of the Midwifery Education Development Pathway (MEDPath) that includes a comprehensive set of evidence-based resources developed for global use and local adaptation. These education resources include updated ICM education resources developed during the early 2000s that address curriculum design; competency-based teaching, learning and assessment strategies; along with what is needed for midwifery teacher and practitioner competence and quality assurance measurement. The adoption of the ICM *Essential Competencies for Basic Midwifery Practice* and *Global Standards for Midwifery Education* provided the foundation for these resources (Chapter 12). In 2019, UNFPA worked with the WHO, UNICEF and the ICM to develop the Framework for Action: *Strengthening Quality Midwifery Education for Universal Health Coverage 2030*.

UNFPA/ICM Electronic Newsletter 2021: *A Moment for Midwives*
When the World Health Assembly (WHA) designated 2020 as the International Year of the Nurse and the Midwife, no one could have anticipated that a global pandemic would dismantle health systems the world over, placing unprecedented constraint on all health workers. The pandemic caused by COVID-19 that began in 2020 forced global changes and challenges to keep everyone healthy, especially childbearing women and newborns. The pandemic also affected many midwives directly as they practised without the essential equipment to protect themselves and the women who sought midwifery care. Many died and others were left with chronic conditions that impeded their ability to practise as a midwife. This sad situation encouraged UNFPA and ICM to develop an electronic newsletter: *A Moment for Midwives: Celebrating our Global Midwife Community Amidst the Covid-19 Pandemic*.[40]

As noted in the text below, Anneka Knutsson, Chief, Sexual and Reproductive Health Branch, UNFPA, and Franka Cadée, President of the ICM, summarised the year of the pandemic and what it has meant to midwives and the world in the Foreword to the Newsletter.

> 'We began 2020 eager to mark the International Year of the Nurse and the Midwife — a historic year when finally, midwives would receive the attention they deserve for their pivotal role in caring for women through pregnancy and childbirth, supporting their reproductive needs, and ensuring their safety, rights and dignity ... This digital magazine tells the story of 2020 from within the confines of a global pandemic. It is an ode to midwives everywhere, and UNFPA and ICM wish to extend our deepest appreciation to each and every one of you for your resilience, courage, and determination. We are honoured to stand shoulder to shoulder with you as we do our part in spearheading efforts toward increased investments in the midwifery workforce. 2021 marks the beginning of the Decade of the Midwife and real, global action towards achieving the Sustainable Development Goals. Together, we can reduce maternal and neonatal mortality and ensure respectful care for all.'

The strength of UNFPA'S ongoing support of the ICM and midwives everywhere is most evident in this response to an urgent crisis for midwives and women everywhere. Thank you, UNFPA!

THE *STATE OF WORLD'S MIDWIFERY* REPORTS (SoWMy)

Two editions of *Maternity Care in the World* were published in 1969 and 1972 from the ICM/FIGO Joint Study Group (Chapter 16). From a historical perspective one might suggest that these two global efforts to describe and support professional midwifery education and practice globally in order to improve maternity care services may have provided part of the incentive for the three *State of the World's Midwifery* (SoWMy) Reports in 2011, 2014 and 2021, led by UNFPA, WHO, UNICEF and the ICM. There were several attempts during the 1990s by Dr Eugene Declercq from Boston University and the ICM Board to seek funds to update the knowledge about midwives and their work.[41] Funds were not obtained and further efforts were halted, but not forgotten.

The SoWMy reports described the state of midwifery in the year data gathered (usually 2 years prior to publication) and any updates since the prior SoWMy report. The goal of each report was to provide an evidence-based and detailed analysis of the present and future challenges to provide effective coverage of quality midwifery services. The countries surveyed in the first two reports were those with the highest global burden of maternal, neonatal and child deaths.[42] The third report in 2021 focused more broadly on reproductive health services, including childbearing care. All countries with ICM MAs who responded to a separate ICM mapping survey related specifically to education, regulation and associations were invited to participate in addition to those countries selected with the greatest number of maternal and newborn deaths. The largest section of each SoWMy report was specific Country Briefs with instructions of how to use these to advocate for needed changes with governments and other policymakers at the country level. Each country profile included data on workforce availability, financial and geographic accessibility, vital statistics and estimates and projections to 2030. Specific data on midwives included education, regulation and associations in each country.

SoWMy 2011

In 2010–2011, the ICM worked with 26 different agencies in a UNFPA funded-project to provide a comprehensive overview of midwifery in countries with the highest rates of maternal mortality. The first *State of the World's Midwifery (SoWMy)* Report subtitled *Delivering Health, Saving Lives*, collected data from 58 countries to demonstrate the need for and value of scaling up midwifery services and strengthening midwifery associations in efforts to reduce needless maternal and newborn deaths and disabilities in keeping with the targets of Millennium Development Goal #4 (infant health) and Goal #5 (maternal health). Health Ministers at the World Health Assembly in May 2011 were given an early briefing on the results of this report highlighting the importance of the ICM's essential competencies and global standards.

The official launch of the first SoWMy report was during the ICM Congress in Durban, South Africa.[43] This launch drew significant political and press support, including having the editor of *The Lancet* present, who supported the *Lancet Series on Midwifery*, published in 2014.[44] The four papers, developed collaboratively by a multidisciplinary group of experts from around the world, put forward an evidence-based framework for action on what childbearing women and newborn infants need. The authors also advocated for new measures to identify and tackle systematic barriers to midwifery, such as inter-professional rivalries, the low status of women and poor understanding of what midwifery is and what it can achieve.[45]

SoWMy 2014

The second SoWMy report was launched during the June 2014 ICM Triennial Congress in Prague, Czech Republic. The report was subtitled *A Universal Pathway. A Woman's Right to Health*. This report was co-chaired by the ICM, UNFPA and the WHO, focusing on 75 countries that collectively represented 95 per cent of the global burden of maternal, newborn and child deaths. A separate report was prepared by UNFPA in the Latin America and Caribbean (LAC) region based on country profiles from most of the countries in the region, including those not included in the SoWMy 2014.[46] Family Care International (FCI) developed an Advocacy Toolkit funded by UNFPA and the Johns Hopkins Program for International Education in Gynaecology and Obstetrics (Jhpiego) for use in the LAC region to expand advocacy efforts to increase the midwifery workforce where needed.[47]

SoWMy 2021

The third SoWMy report was released on 5 May 2021, the 10th anniversary of the first SoWMY report. The main objectives of SoWMy 2021 were to:

a) show progress in midwifery workforce development since 2011
b) further improve the evidence base to enable stronger policy dialogue to strengthen midwifery services
c) accelerate progress on sustainable development goals (SDGs) focusing on access by women to skilled and competent midwives operating in an enabling environment
d) contribute to the monitoring of progress toward equity and 'leaving no one behind'
e) collate and share evidence on the impact of midwives and the return on investment in midwifery.[48]

The press release on 5 May 2021 began with the header: 'Fully investing in midwives by 2035 would avert roughly two-thirds of maternal, newborn deaths and stillbirths, saving 4.3 million lives per year.'[49]

As noted, this was the first time that the ICM sent out a separate survey to all MAs reflecting their efforts in education and regulation (ICM's *Global Midwives Association Map*). Likewise, the organisers and funders expanded the number of countries surveyed, using the WHO's National Health Workforce Accounts (NHWA) platform as the primary source of country data.[50] The downside of this data bank was that not all countries participated in the NHWA and/or the data were incomplete resulting in limited, inaccurate information on midwifery. A second, more troubling problem to the ICM and midwives, was the fact that all the world's nurse-midwives were classified as nurses in many countries because the NHWA does not have a separate category for nurse-midwives. Several attempts to add the nurse-midwife data element were made but it was not added prior to the 2021 SoWMy report.[51]

Another different approach was taken during the 2021 SoWMy report in that it was not exclusively related to midwives. It focused on all those health professionals providing sexual and reproductive health services, though ICM's data strengthened the unique value of midwives and midwifery services in this report.[52] From an ICM perspective, the broad definition of 'midwifery' became problematic in data collection. Integrare, a data analysis agency in Spain, was responsible for collating data and synthesising the final report, considering these limitations.

Summary UNFPA/ICM Activities

The ICM co-chaired the Steering Committee of each SoWMy report with UNFPA, the WHO and multiple other agencies. Each of these reports defined 'midwifery' as: 'the health services and health workforce needed to support and care for women and newborns, including sexual and reproductive health and especially pregnancy, labour and postnatal care.'[53] The SoWMy reports are important advocacy tools for ICM MAs, intended 'to spark an open dialogue with policy-makers about improving midwifery services and informing the post-2015 development agenda for global health.'[54] From 2021 onward, each UNFPA region will be responsible for creating their own 'state of midwifery in the region' reports.[55]

MIDWIFERY EXPERTISE SHARED WITH PARTNERS

The ICM has provided technical advice and consultation for many global partners, especially since its rebirth in 1954. ICM's leaders have served on WHO committees and influenced WHO statements about the key role that midwives play in *Health for All*. More recently, ICM representatives have provided input on several UN technical working groups, such as those to develop the Millennium Development and Sustainable Development Goals related to maternal and child health and gender equity, Every Newborn Action Plan and Every Woman Every Child advocacy campaign. ICM midwives have also provided needed consultative services during the UNFPA/SIDA/ICM Strengthening Midwifery Programme and other funded projects centred on ICM's education (WHO *Midwifery Modules, Core Competencies for Midwifery Educators*), regulation (WHO *Strengthening Midwifery* toolkit) and association (UNFPA *Strengthening Midwifery Services*) goals. ICM's input to joint statements (Chapter 16) with its partners is another example of the value of partnerships in raising the voices and visibility of ICM as well as midwives throughout the world.

SUMMARY

The partnerships with UN agencies during the last 70+ years have contributed much to the development of the ICM as a respected international health organisation concerned with the preparation of competent midwives providing quality midwifery services supported by strong midwifery associations that work together to promote the sexual and reproductive health of adolescents and women, wherever they reside. In the spirit of true partnership, the ICM has provided midwifery expertise to each of their partners as they seek improved reproductive and sexual health for all the world's people. In other words, the ICM and its partners over the century are committed to a shared vision of healthy women, healthy newborns, healthy adolescents, healthy families and healthy nations.

100 Years of the International Confederation of Midwives

1. Petra ten Hoope-Bender. 'Report on ICM Representation, Partnerships and Projects in the International Health Arena.' Vienna: ICM Council meeting, April 2002, Agenda item 24.5, p 1.
2. Candau letter to ICM Executive Secretary (Miss Bayes), 30 January 1957. Shared from WHO archives.
3. WHO. 'The Midwife in Maternity Care: Report of a WHO Expert Committee.' *World Health Organization Technical Report Series No. 331* (Geneva: WHO, 1966), p 2.
4. WHO. 'The Midwife in Maternity Care: Report of a WHO Expert Committee.' *World Health Organization Technical Report Series No. 331* (Geneva: WHO, 1966), p 3.
5. WHO. 'The Midwife in Maternity Care: Report of a WHO Expert Committee.' *World Health Organization Technical Report Series No. 331* (Geneva: WHO, 1966), p 4.
6. WHO. The Midwife in Maternity Care: Report of a WHO Expert Committee. *World Health Organization Technical Report Series No. 331*. Geneva: WHO, 1966, face page.
7. During the 1972 FIGO-ICM Joint Study Group meeting in Geneva, both organisations agreed the need to totally revise the *Definition of the Midwife* (See Chapter 11). Lucille Woodville from the USA was President of ICM at the time and Vice-Chair of the Study Group. Once the group agreed on the revision of the definition, both ICM and FIGO leaders agreed to take it to their Boards for final agreement, which was done by ICM in 1972 and FIGO in 1973.
8. *1972 FIGO-ICM Joint Study Group meeting in Geneva*, p 8.
9. ICM. *Global Standards for Midwifery Education with Companion Guidelines*. The Hague: ICM, 2010; rev. 2013.
10. WHO. The Midwife in Maternity Care: Report of a WHO Expert Committee. *World Health Organization Technical Report Series No. 331*. Geneva: WHO, 1966, p 12.
11. WHO. The Midwife in Maternity Care: Report of a WHO Expert Committee. *World Health Organization Technical Report Series No. 331*. Geneva: WHO, 1966, p 19.
12. United Nations. Millennium Development Goals. New York: United Nations. 2000. Goal #4 related to child health and Goal #5 targeted the important role of midwives.
13. United Nations. Sustainable Development Goals. New York: UNDP, 2015. The Sustainable Development Goals (SDGs), also known as the Global Goals, were adopted by all United Nations Member States in 2015 as a universal call to action to end poverty, protect the planet and ensure that all people enjoy peace and prosperity by 2030. The 17 SDGs are integrated – that is, they recognise that action in one area will affect outcomes in others, and that development must balance social, economic, and environmental sustainability. The SDGs are designed to bring the world to several life-changing 'zeros', including zero poverty, hunger, AIDS and discrimination against women and girls. Goal #3, Health, contains the need for midwives and midwifery care and Goal #5 on Gender Equity reflects common interests of midwives and their ability to provide needed services for all women and girls.
14. Prior to the appointment of UK midwife Joan Bentley in the WHO post of Public Health Nurse Midwife, as WHO's official liaison with ICM, midwifery matters fell under the umbrella of the WHO Chief Nurse, who often was not a midwife and with limited knowledge or interest in midwifery as it was assumed that all midwives were nurses first.
15. Jelka Zapan was a paediatrician who emailed Petra ten Hoope-Bender, ICM Secretary General, 13 June 2001, informing Petra that she had just been 'nominated as Designated Technical Officer for the relation with ICM for the interim period (until a midwife is hired).'
16. SIDA secondment was time limited, and it took some time for another midwife liaison officer to be appointed by WHO to ICM, due in part to WHO lengthy recruitment processes.
17. WHO. *Work of WHO. 2nd 10 Year Review*. Geneva: WHO, 1967. Miss Lyle Creelman, Chief, Nursing Section WHO. *Letter to Miss M. Bayes, Executive Secretary, ICM, dated 8 February 1957*, congratulating ICM being granted official relationship with WHO. Miss Creelman notes, 'I am very glad of this and look forward to a continuance of the close co-operation we have had in the past.' (Letters retrieved from WHO archives).
18. Marjorie Bayes. *Letter to Dr Candau, Director-General, WHO, dated 6 January 1961*. In this letter Miss Bayes relays the unanimous resolutions of the ICM Triennial meeting in October 1960 for information and action. The second resolution read, 'The International Confederation of Midwives deplores the fact that there is no Midwifery Officer at WHO level and proposes that this Congress informs WHO to this effect.' In his response on 24 January 1961, Dr Candau wrote, 'The views expressed in the second resolution have been duly noted.' In a follow-up letter on 29 September 1975 to F Margaret Hardy, ICM Executive Secretary, related to WHO adopting the position that midwifery was a separate profession from nursing, the WHO Director General referred back to the Executive Board meeting at its 33rd session in 1964, 'when the proposal to appoint a midwife to the division of Public Health Services was found unacceptable and the post had to be changed to that of a public health nursing with midwifery training.' (Letters retrieved from WHO archives).
19. News Review. Third MIP [Meeting of Interested Parties] calls for more midwives. *Safe Motherhood Newsletter 4*: November 1990–February 1991, p 2.
20. ICM. *A Birthday for Midwives – Seventy-Five Years of International Collaboration*. Chiswick, London: ICM, 1994, pp 6, 8.
21. ICM and WHO. *Strengthening Midwifery Toolkit: Guidelines for Policy Maker and Planners to Strengthen the Regulation, Accreditation and Education of Midwives*. Geneva: WHO Department of Making Pregnancy Safer, 2006.
22. H Nakajima. 'Midwives: Guardian of the Future.' *World Health 2*: March–April 1997, p 3.
23. Joyce Thompson, a US nurse-midwife nominated by the Americas Region in 2000, served as Vice-Chair of GAGNM

from 2001-2007. Thompson was Director of the ICM Board of Management until 2005, so that she and the ICM Secretary General were present at all GAGNM meetings during that time. JE Thompson. The WHO Global Advisory Group on Nursing and Midwifery. *Journal of Nursing Scholarship*, 34:2, 111–113 (Second Quarter, 2002).

24 Marion Strachan. Nurse-midwifery in UNICEF. Bulletin Nurse-Midwives XVI:2, May 1971, p 10.

25 ICM. (SA/IC/R/4). Wellcome Collection. *Marjorie Bayes' History of ICM, first 50 years*. Bayes noted that consultative status with UNICEF and being on the special list of the International Labour Organization as a Non-Governmental Organisation was in place when the General Officers met in Geneva in 1962. Wellcome Institute Library document.

26 Marion Strachan. Nurse-midwifery in UNICEF. *Bulletin Nurse-Midwives* XVI:2, May 1971, p 12.

27 International News. ICM speaks out on breast feeding. *Midwifery* 1 (1985), p 47.

28 International News. ICM speaks out on breast feeding. *Midwifery* 1 (1985), p 47. Miss Margaret Peters, Director of the ICM Board of Management (1993–1999) was Australia's representative to UNICEF headquarters in New York City.

29 Janet Nelson. *Letter to Joyce E Thompson, President American College of Nurse-Midwives, 30 May 1991*. Miss Nelson was Chief, NGO Liaison Unit of UNICEF, and was confirming that two of ACNM members, Betty Carrington and Patricia Burkhardt, were accepted as official representatives for ICM to UNICEF [Joyce Thompson personal papers]

30 Joyce E Thompson. *Report of meeting with Dr France Donnay, UNICEF*. Joyce Thompson, ICM Deputy Director, January 23, 1997, at the UNICEF office in New York City. [Joyce Thompson personal papers]

31 Vincent Fauveau. Interview, 2017, noted, 'In 2000 when the work on EmONC [Emergency Obstetric & Neonatal Care] started with Deborah Maine, I realized the potential of midwives but didn't really connect until the meeting on Midwifery in the Community …' ICM President Bridget Lynch and Secretary General, Kathy Herschderfer and Vincent held several meetings in New York City to start new era of UNFPA-ICM collaboration.

32 Della R Sherratt and Karen Odberg-Pettersson. *Investing in Midwifery and Others with Midwifery Skills to Save the Lives of Mothers and Newborns and Improve Their Health: Policy and programme guidance for countries seeking to scale up midwifery services, especially at the community level*. New York: UNFPA & ICM, December 2006, p ii.

33 Nester T Moyo & Elizabeth Duff. Investing in midwives … to accelerate progress towards MDG5: ICM and UNPFA forge ahead. *International Midwifery: Journal of the International Confederation of Midwives* 21 (2), June 2008, pp 20–21.

34 UNFPA-ICM Midwives Programme 2008–2011. ICM-UNFPA announcement: *UNFPA investing in Midwifery and others with midwifery skills to accelerate progress towards MDG5*. 2008.

35 Vincent Fauveau. Interview 2017.

36 Interview with Anneka Knutsson, UNFPA Chief Reproductive Health Division, UNFPA, on 21 May 2021.

37 Luc de Bernis. Interview 2017.

38 UNFPA. *Global Midwifery Strategy 2018–2030*. New York: UNFPA, 2008.

39 Strengthening Midwifery Services with UNFPA. Downloaded from: www.internationalmidwives.org on 6 April 2021.

40 Downloaded from: www.internationalmidwives.org 6 April 2021.

41 ICM. *ICM Triennial Report 1993–1996*. Project: Dr Declercq was given £2,000 to seek funds to undertake a feasibility survey of midwifery personnel, p 23.

42 ICM. *Triennial Report 2011–2014*. The Hague: ICM, 2014, p 18.

43 ICM. *ICM Triennial Report 2008–2011*. The Hague: ICM, 2011, pp 18–19.

44 https://www.thelancet.com/series/midwifery

45 The Lancet Series on Midwifery announcement. 2016.

46 Family Care International, UNFPA-LACRO, ICM. *Strengthening Midwifery in Latin America and the Caribbean: A Report on the Collaboration between the Regional Office for Latin America and the Caribbean of the United Nations Fund for Population and the International Confederation of Midwives*. Panama: UNFPA, 2014.

47 Family Care International. *Making the Case for Midwifery: A toolkit for using evidence from the State of the World's Midwifery 2014 Report to create policy change at the country level*. New York: FCI, May 2014. UNFPA – LACRO. Annual workplan for Midwifery 2014. [Personal papers of Joyce Thompson]

48 ICM. *Letter to Member Associations. State of the World's Midwifery (SoWMy) 2021*, p 1. On ICM website: www.internationalmidwives.org

49 United Nations Joint News Release. *New report sounds the alarm on globally shortage of 900,000 midwives*. New York: United Nations, 5 May 2021.

50 The NHWA platform was the source of data for the Country profiles used in the 2020 *State of the World's Nursing* report which included a projection of shortages of nurses for 2030 considering 'density above threshold'. Sandra Land. *Briefing Note: SOWMy 2021 NHWA data-LAC*. Updated 5 August 2020.

51 JET personal information as UNFPA consultant in Latin America and the Caribbean through 2020.

52 ICM. *Letter to Member Associations. State of the World's Midwifery (SoWMy) 2021*. On ICM website: www.internationalmidwives.org

53 UNFPA, ICM, WHO. *The State of the World's Midwifery 2014. A Universal Pathway. A Women's Right to Health*. Geneva: Prographics, Inc, 2014.

54 ICM. *ICM Triennial Report 2011–2014*. The Hague: ICM, 2013, p 18.

55 Anneka Knutsson interview, 21 May 2021.

Chapter 16: *Health Professional Groups and the ICM*

'The International Federation of Gynaecology and Obstetrics and the International Confederation of Midwives have made a remarkable contribution to the existing knowledge of maternity care in the world ...'
MG Candau, Director-General WHO, 1966 Foreword, Maternity Care in the World, p ix.

INTRODUCTION

Much of the ICM's story is intertwined with other global health professional organisations concerned with the health of women, newborns, children, adolescents and families. Most ICM leaders realised that the tasks required to keep childbearing safe and to meet the sexual and reproductive health needs of adolescents, women and families was far too big for one organisation (ICM) or one group of health professionals (midwives). Three primary international health professional groups which partnered with the ICM from the early 1960s onward working together for healthy women, newborns and families are the International Federation of Gynecology and Obstetrics (FIGO)[1], the International Council of Nurses (ICN) and the International Pediatric Association (IPA). Each partnership was in keeping with the *Interorganisational Relationships Guidelines* agreed in 1996.[2] A brief history of these ICM partners, including networks and projects, are discussed in this chapter. Others are referenced in other chapters throughout the book.

INTERNATIONAL FEDERATION OF GYNECOLOGY AND OBSTETRICS (FIGO)
FIGO/ICM Joint Study Group (JSG): 1961–1979

FIGO during its third General Assembly in Vienna in 1961, set up a special committee to study the training and practice of midwives and maternity nurses throughout the world. Professor WCW Nixon, Professor of Obstetrics and Gynaecology at University College Hospital in London, UK, who chaired this committee until his death in February 1966, wrote:

'It was realized that such a study would only be feasible with the co-operation of the International Confederation of Midwives (I.C.M.), so I approached Miss Marjorie Bayes, Executive Secretary of the I.C.M. for help in this project. The I.C.M. readily agreed to assist.'[3]

Miss Bayes was a Secretary of the Royal College of Midwives (RCM) in London prior to being named Executive Secretary of the International Confederation of Midwives (ICM) in 1954. No doubt the RCM was well-known to Professor Nixon, and thus the ICM through Marjorie Bayes. It is important to note that Marjorie Bayes not only agreed to 'assist' with the survey, but also collected funds from midwives, midwifery associations and private organisations to cover most of the expenses, supplementing the small contribution from FIGO. As noted by Sir John Peel who succeeded Professor Nixon as Chair of the Study Group: 'The Study Group felt it was essential to have an obstetrician in London to work in close collaboration with the Secretary of the I.C.M.'[4]

The Joint Study Group (JSG) was the beginning of collaboration between the ICM and FIGO on a specific project, though midwives and obstetricians had worked with the WHO on various Expert Committees.[5] Sir John Peel in the Preface to the first *Maternity Care in the World*, wrote: 'This report is perhaps only the beginning of work that should be continued by both F.I.G.O. and I.C.M. in close association to elucidate further the many problems which it has served to highlight.'[6] He also noted that the JSG sought and received the cooperation of the WHO, the International Planned Parenthood Federation (IPPF)[7], the International Pediatric Association (IPA) and the United Nations Children's Fund (UNICEF).[8]

Purpose of the FIGO/ICM Joint Study Group – 1961–1976

The ICM and FIGO together formed the JSG to obtain better information on the practice and education of midwives throughout the world. This first global study of midwives and midwifery practice was undertaken, with a repeat survey completed ten years later that expanded content related to the professional midwife's roles as teacher and family planning counsellor.[9] The purpose of the JSG was reaffirmed in 1972 prior to the 1976 publication of the second edition of *Maternity Care in the World*.

Maternity Care in the World, 1st Edition 1966

A small working committee of the JSG (referred to as the Executive Committee), with support from various other agencies and individuals such as Margaret Thomas, a nurse-midwife consultant to the US Children's Bureau who worked with Dr Barnes at Johns Hopkins University, USA, developed a questionnaire/survey to be used to gather information. The survey went through many drafts with input from all the members of the JSG along with review by leaders of the British Perinatal Mortality Survey and the WHO. The final English version was edited by two British midwives on the staff of the Royal College of Midwives (RCM), Margaret Hardy and Margaret Sandover.[10] The English, French, Spanish and Russian questionnaires were sent out beginning in August 1963, with analysis of incoming data begun at the end of 1963.

The object of the survey questionnaire was to get the best view of midwifery practice and education from as many countries in the world as possible. The questionnaire was sent initially to those countries with more than one million population, approaching each country's Minister of Health and constituent societies of FIGO and the ICM. Though at least three questionnaires were sent to each country, the JSG asked that the various constituencies work together and submit just one report, similar to approach of the *State of the World's Midwifery Reports* in the 21st century. An additional questionnaire was sent to countries with less than one million population. As data started coming in, the Executive Committee realised that it was essential to invite national authorities to comment on how their country midwifery services should be developed in the future; hence the second questionnaire titled, the *Individual Country Report*, was part of the total report. Again, Professor Nixon wrote, 'without the enthusiastic support of Miss Marjorie Bayes, Executive Secretary of the I.C.M., and the generosity of the Royal College of Midwives, the success of this project would not have been assured.'[11]

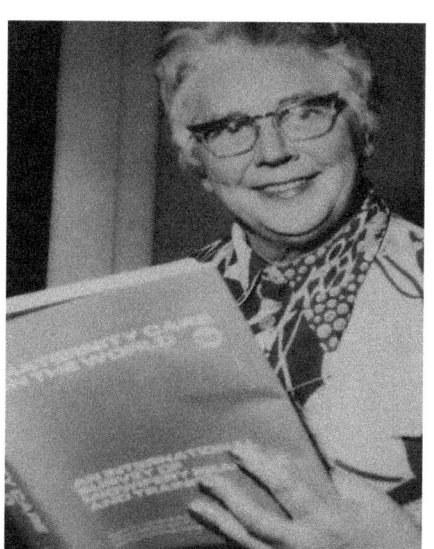

Marjorie Bayes holding Maternity Care in the World 1st Edition – ICM Archives at Wellcome Collection

The final report in February 1966 included data from 174 countries (90 confirmed reports by country officials and 84 other countries). The JSG was aware that the data provided came from governments and was not always accurate/complete as most governments did not have a register of midwives working in the field at the time. The results of the international survey of midwifery practices was published in 1969 in book form titled, *Maternity Care in the World: An International Survey of Midwifery Practice and Training*. Data on the number of midwives in practice was available from 153 countries (75 percent of the world's population) with missing data primarily from Mainland China with 23 percent of the world's population. It was estimated at the time of the report that approximately 700,000–800,000 professional and 'other' midwives were practicing in the world, albeit with great variation in the number of midwives per 1,000 population. For example, in Africa there were 8.2 professional midwives and 22 'other midwives' per 1,000 population and in Latin America, Mexico and Canada there were 18.1 professional midwives and 40 'other' midwives per 1,000 population.[12] The USSR had the lowest number of births per midwife at 21 and Latin America had the highest number at 339.[13]

Selected 1966 Outcomes Affecting ICM and Member Associations

The ICM learned that several of the life-saving skills, such as manual removal of placenta, starting intravenous infusions and giving blood transfusions, were only allowed in half or fewer of the countries reporting. In the majority of countries, the age of entry into midwifery education was 18 for professional midwives and lower for 'other' midwives. The length of preparation for professional midwives averaged 12 months post-nursing and 24–26 months direct entry. Most of the midwives were employed by governments with the exception of home-birth private practice midwives.

Recommendations from the JSG in the 1966 report of interest/importance to ICM in its ongoing work with MAs were:

1. Need to continue to gather data at set intervals on the midwifery workforce at national level in order to obtain more accurate data
2. International agencies are in the best position to advise on a common format for collecting data on midwives and midwifery practice
3. Although the Committee agreed it impossible to have an internationally agreed curriculum for the education of professional midwives, they did recommend:

a. Establishment of basic training requirement which would set a common minimum standard
   b. Uniformity of licensure regulations
   c. Development of local postgraduate training opportunities for midwives to balance out-of-country opportunities
   d. In general, midwives in collaboration with obstetricians should be responsible for the academic content of their education programmes.
4. All countries should be encouraged to maintain an accurate register of certificated midwives in practice
5. Every help and encouragement should be given to those developing countries with much to accomplish in maternity care
6. Everyone associated with I.C.M. and F.I.G.O. should bring the facts now available on midwives and midwifery training to the attention of appropriate government authorities
7. Attempts be made to obtain a greater country membership in ICM and FIGO and both should play an active role in improving standards, especially in those areas of the world most needing assistance
8. Having collaborated so well over a period of four years the ICM and FIGO should continue to work in close association on the many problems mutually shared, which this Report has served to identify.[14]

The ICM's efforts over the next 50 years addressed several of these recommendations, with, at times, limited success in the areas of education, regulation and advocacy. Prior content in this book illustrates many of those challenges and successes.

Continued Joint Study Group Efforts

The ICM/FIGO JSG that began in 1961 continued to meet sporadically depending on funds available, though the small Executive Committee, which included Miss Bayes, met at regular intervals. One of the recommendations from the 1966 report was that each continent should have a group of midwives and obstetricians meet to continue the discussions of the role of the midwife in maternity care and how to support the needs that were identified by region and country in the 1966 study.

European Working Party on Midwifery Training in European Countries – 1969

The European continent was the first to organise such a group, most likely because midwifery was well-established, travel was easier and both the Chair and Secretary were based in London. A three-day European Conference was convened in London in March 1969, attended by midwives, obstetricians and members of statutory bodies from 18 European countries. The conference attendants agreed that all European countries should adopt the 1965 WHO *Definition of the Midwife* (Chapter 11). This European group also recommended that professional associations of midwives in cooperation with the midwifery statutory body of their country should establish and maintain standards of training and practice of midwifery.[15]

One outcome of the European Conference was a Working Party with six midwives and six obstetricians representing each of the major language groups in Europe. It was important that each member of the Working Party had some role in the education of midwives. The Working Party was formed and met in Copenhagen 8–9 September 1969, under the chairmanship of Sir John Peel (FIGO) with Miss Marjorie Bayes (ICM) as Secretary. This Working Party made a minor edit of the WHO *Definition of the Midwife* (Chapter 11) and made several recommendations on midwifery practice and employment, midwifery education including postgraduate education and recommended that professional bodies in all countries consider possibilities of reciprocal recognition of the midwife based agreed standards.[16]

The *Report of a Working Party on Midwifery Training in European Countries* once published was presented at the triennial ICM Council meeting and the General Assembly of FIGO, with both groups approving the report.[17] Both the ICM and FIGO recommended continued research by the JSG. A full meeting of the JSG was held on 4–6 September 1972. The ICM President, Lucille Woodville (USA), was now Vice-Chair of the JSG and successfully solicited financial support for the meeting from the US Department of Health, Education and Welfare.[18]

Second FIGO/ICM Project Aim and Objectives – 1972

Members of the JSG meeting in London in 1972 agreed that the aim of continued study of midwifery training and practice in the world was: 'To continue the improvement of maternal and child care, and the quality of maternal and child life through the inclusion of Family Planning among the services provided by midwives of all categories in their expanding role.'[19] The objectives of the new study were related to identifying the present situation of maternity care and midwifery services in each country, suggesting practical improvements for the immediate future, and to 'agree intermediate and long term guidelines suitable to the particular groups of countries under survey'[20].

Outcomes: In order to carry out the aim and objectives, Marjorie Bayes and Lucille Woodville in 1972 convinced the United States Aid for International Development (USAID) to provide a substantial grant to the ICM, supported by the JSG. The USAID grant underwrote the last meeting of the JSG in July 1975 during which it was agreed to obtain updated data and publish the second edition of *Maternity Care in the World*. This publication included data on 209 countries including a brief description of the country; vital statistics available; medical and midwifery personnel; midwifery training and practice; hospital and other facilities and family planning services. Many countries did not have complete data, vital statistics were often not kept and/or unreliable and several had no data on midwifery. Though the focus of the Working Parties was on developing countries, the JSG agreed that information on midwifery was needed from developed countries as well. This same decision was made over 45 years later for the third *State of the World's Midwifery* report in 2021.

Maternity Care in the World, 2nd Edition 1976
The second edition of Maternity Care in the World was published in 1976 with a list of recommendations[21] that had been agreed by the JSG in July 1975. Those recommendations of particular interest to the ICM as an international organisation included:
1. Need to use internationally agreed definitions in vital statistics
2. Use of the agreed *International Definition of the Midwife* in designing educational programmes
3. Legislation to allow full scope midwifery practice, including family planning
4. Increase national member association memberships in ICM and FIGO
5. ICM and FIGO need to take an active part in helping to improve the standards of maternity care in those areas of the world needing assistance.

A final recommendation stated, 'Having collaborated so well over a period of years, the Joint Study Group of ICM and FIGO should continue to work in close association on the many problems – mutually shared – which this report has served to identify'[22] – a statement similar to the recommendations in the 1966 *Maternity Care in the World*.

Impact of the FIGO/ICM Joint Study Group on the ICM

The ICM gained an expanded knowledge of midwives and midwifery practice globally through its participation in the FIGO/ICM JSG at a time when it had limited knowledge of the status of midwives and midwifery in developing countries and few of those countries in membership. In the introduction to the 1976 second edition of *Maternity Care in the World*, the 1969 European Working Party recognised that, 'Good midwife doctor relationships depend on mutual recognition of and respect for each other's professional status and responsibilities.'[23] The JSG and the outcomes of the two editions of *Maternity Care in the World* offered the ICM member associations the opportunity to participate in country, regional and global activities and, in turn, receive international support for their demanding roles, especially in low resource countries. The results of the two global surveys also provided support for the ICM's role in defining standards for midwifery education and practice, beginning with a clear definition of the competencies needed by professional midwives wherever they lived and worked that were eventually adopted in 2002 (Chapter 12).

The FIGO/ICM/WHO *Definition of the Midwife*

One of the most notable outcomes of the FIGO/ICM JSG was the development and subsequent formal definition of the midwife and midwifery scope of practice in 1972. The first agreed definition of the midwife in 1965 came from the collective views of the members of the WHO Expert Committee on 'The Midwife in Maternity Care' who agreed they needed a clear definition of the midwife in order to carry out their task.[24] The second international definition of the midwife in 1969 came out of the ICM/FIGO Working Party on Midwifery Training in European Countries.[25] The third definition of the midwife was drafted by a sub-committee of the FIGO/ICM JSG in 1972 as members thought the WHO definition was out of date. The draft definition that was subsequently adopted by the ICM in 1972, FIGO in 1973, and the WHO shortly thereafter is discussed in detail in Chapter 11.

Ongoing ICM and FIGO collaboration

The JSG signalled an official relationship of mutual respect and collaborative work between midwives and obstetricians globally that has continued through the decades to the benefit of both the ICM and FIGO, midwives and obstetricians. In July 1982, the ICM Board of Management was considering the future of the JSG and its ongoing work with FIGO. It sent a letter to Professor Fairweather stating that it considered it was no longer appropriate to continue the JSG. However, the ICM wished to remain in good relationship with FIGO and other groups and for this reason suggested a FIGO action committee for maternal and child health which the ICM would support and collaborate with other groups.[26]

Several joint statements followed over the years as discussed later in this chapter. In addition, the ICM Secretary General (SG) was appointed as a full member of FIGO's Safe Motherhood Committee and the Obstetric Fistula Working Group.[27] Presidents (Directors) of the ICM and FIGO attend each other's global congresses, and often are plenary speakers, such as Dr Khama Rogo (MD, Co-chair PSMNH) at the ICM Manila Congress in 1999 and Joyce Thompson at the Washington, DC, XVI FIGO World Congress in September 2000. In 2017, ICM and FIGO signed a Memorandum of Understanding (MOU) to strengthen their collaboration well into the future. Ongoing collaboration between the ICM and FIGO has continued during each decade to the present time.

THE INTERNATIONAL PEDIATRIC ASSOCIATION (IPA)

The ICM relationship with the International Pediatric Association (IPA) began in the early 1970s.[28] It would appear that Thomas Stapleton, General Secretary of the IPA, often contacted Marjorie Bayes, ICM Executive Secretary, for contacts in various countries, such as Jamaica (31 July 1974) and Cuba (10 May 1979).[29] As a long-time partner, IPA sent representatives to most ICM Triennial Congresses. For example, Marjorie Bayes sent a letter to the IPA General Secretary Stapleton requesting that he ask Professor Nimrod O Bwibo of Kenya to represent the IPA and present a paper on 'Varieties of Malnutrition' at the ICM Congress in 1975 in Lausanne.[30] During the time of the Joint ICM/FIGO project, the IPA had representatives at each Working Party that followed in the various countries. The IPA continues to be an important part of the Partnership for Maternal, Newborn and Child Health (below) and continues to provide its expertise to the ICM on topics related to newborns and infants.

INTERNATIONAL COUNCIL OF NURSES (ICN)
Overview

Over the years the relationship between ICM and ICN can be characterised as going through periods of polite awareness (hands-off)[31], positive collaboration between the executives of each organisation during the early 2000s, to sharing and exchanging information that led to joint statements on issues of common interest, such as birth registration. The underlying contentious issue has always been discussion of whether midwifery is a profession separate/distinct from nursing. This question for midwives has always elicited a resounding 'yes' response going back as early as 1922, regardless of whether they were single qualified midwives or dual qualified nurse-midwives. Two significant meetings with the ICM at ICN headquarters in Geneva took place during the 1993–1996 triennium. The first was a 'Nurses and Midwifery Work Group' that considered the respective roles of midwives and nurses and the interaction of the two professions.

> 'The meeting was a cordial one although the two organizations maintained their independent, opposing views of midwifery as a specialty of nursing.'[32]

The ICN consulted with the ICM SG in a second meeting about needed guidelines for nurses and midwives involved in caring for HIV/AIDS patients. The ICM was not consulted further in the ICN's development of these guidelines, most likely because the ICM chose to ignore the request.

Decades of discussion with ICN leaders/consultants confirmed that the ICN's view was that midwifery was a specialty within nursing, though nearly half of the world's midwives were not nurses. In October 1996, the ICN adopted a position statement titled: *The Nature and Scope of Practice of Nurse-Midwives*.[33] The explanation given was that even though nurse-midwives have special skills and expertise in childbearing care, they do continue to practice within full-scope nursing, ending with: 'Therefore it is legitimate that the nursing profession participates appropriately in aspects of the education, standard setting and credentialing of nurse-midwives.'[34] This statement raised ongoing concerns/anger within some ICM MAs because ICN felt the need to become involved in international midwifery.[35] Other ICM leaders were concerned that the ICN's position on midwifery as a specialty within nursing resulted in the loss of separate midwifery regulation in many former British colonies by removing the term 'Midwives' from the Nurses and Midwives Councils.[36]

Margaretta Styles, President of the ICN in the 1980s, suggested that there was no need for an ICM since the ICN represented the world's midwives since they were all nurses (Refer to text box). The issue of professional status distinct from nursing was first recorded in 1923 in IMU documents (Chapter 3) and then again when debates occurred during the rebirth discussions in 1953 as to whether the IMU should join with the International Council of Nurses (ICN). Midwives at that meeting decided 'no' and renamed the organisation the International Council of Midwives.[37]

> *'I had the opportunity to talk with ICN President Dr Margretta Styles on several occasions as our paths crossed in different international meetings. I clearly remember her dedication to the nursing profession. On the day she expressed her view that 'since all midwives are also nurses, there was no need for ICM since ICN could speak and support midwives,' I countered with the results of a survey at the ICM Council meeting in which over ½ of the world's midwives were direct entry, without a nursing background. I was unable to change her mind, so we continued to disagree as colleagues.'*
>
> *Joyce Thompson, 2020*

The question of whether midwifery was a profession distinct from nursing was an important issue not only for the ICM/ICN relationship over time, but also for the ICM and the WHO. In July 1975, the ICM SG sent a letter to the Director General of the WHO with the ICM Council's request asking the WHO to recognise midwifery as a profession separate from nursing.[38]

Joint Efforts at the World Health Assembly (WHA)

ICM's work with the International Council of Nurses (ICN) over the years revolved around issues of human resource management and a joint approach to the WHO, as well as the important role of midwives and nurses in promoting Safe Motherhood.[39] In 1992 the WHO recognised that Nursing and Midwifery could contribute significantly to global health and established the Global Advisory Group on Nursing and Midwifery (GAGNM). Its mandate was to provide policy advice to the WHO Director-General and the WHO Cabinet to strategically enhance the contributions of midwifery and nursing within the context of all WHO priorities and programmes. Both the ICM and the ICN were key participants in this WHO initiative, gaining Observer status on the GAGNM.[40] Both the ICM and ICN worked closely together on World Health Assembly (WHA) resolutions on Midwifery and Nursing, including periodic progress reports requested by members of the World Health Assembly.[41]

In May 2006, the WHA endorsed Resolution WHA59.27 on *Strengthening Nursing and Midwifery* (one of several since the late 1980s) that reaffirmed the crucial contribution of the these professions to health systems and *Health for All*. This resolution prompted the Federal Minister of Health of Pakistan to host a high-level consultation on nursing and midwifery with a resulting joint declaration. *The Islamabad Declaration on Strengthening Nursing and Midwifery* called for scaling up nursing and midwifery capacity, the skill mix of existing and new cadres of workers and creating positive workplace environments.[42]

Triad Meetings

In 1999, collaboration with the ICN strengthened and the ICM became a member of the Triad meetings at the invitation of ICN. The Triad leadership organised biannual conferences for government chief nurses, chief midwives and WHO maternal health and health workforce departments to share, learn and adapt the development of midwifery and nursing to the needs of the day. Since the nursing and midwifery workforce was the largest health/illness workforce throughout the world, the WHO listened closely to their issues and World Health Assembly (WHA) members supported the joint WHA resolutions for strengthening nursing and midwifery to meet current and future health challenges.

Triad Communiqués were compiled prior to the WHA each year to address issues critical to the provision of safe, quality midwifery and nursing, including a focus on appropriate regulation. For example, government chief nursing and midwifery officers, representatives of national nursing and midwifery associations and regulatory bodies from 101 countries met in Geneva on 19–20 May 2006 along with the ICN, ICM and WHO leaders. Issues discussed related to the important role of midwives and nurses in addressing the Millennium Development Goals (MDGs); assuring competence and patient safety through regulatory mechanisms; ethical recruitment, retention and managed migration strategies; and providing equal access to equitable health care based on need rather than the ability to pay.

This group also supported a draft *Resolution on Nursing and Midwifery* to come forward during the WHA that year.[43] The ICN encouraged the ICM to continue as part of the Triad meetings following the Islamabad meeting in March 2007 but was disappointed that the ICM's attendance was inconsistent.[44]

Topics on the 2018 Triad agenda included: achieving the Sustainable Development Goals (SDGs) through decent work and health labour market analyses; leveraging the power of midwifery and nursing to deliver better health outcomes; nursing and midwifery development; youth, gender and migration needs; regulatory challenges in upskilling midwives and nurses in countries; and upscaling midwifery and nursing education and training. The theme of the June 2020 virtual Triad meeting was 'The nursing and midwifery workforces as essential to COVID-19 preparedness and response' in keeping with the global pandemic and the dire circumstances nurses and midwives, as frontline workers, were in caring for those infected with the virus and keeping those not infected safe.[45] These biannual meetings were well attended and presented an excellent opportunity to present midwifery, the ICM work on education, regulation and association development, and the importance of collaboration between the two professional groups, while respecting the differences in their areas of work.

Other ICM and ICN Collaboration
Despite the ongoing disparate views of the ICM and ICN leaders on the issue of professional status, the chief executive officers of both organisations began working together in earnest in early 2000. For example, they began collaborating on the role of regulators of midwives and nurses in 2004, with most of the meetings held during ICN meetings.[46] History demonstrated that lack of ICM representation at regulatory and other ICN meetings was due in part to the often-precarious financial status of the ICM in contrast to the fact that the ICN was well funded and located in Geneva. ICM representatives had to travel, often at their own expense, to attend such meetings. Both organisations also participated in drafting the Munich Declaration, 'Nurses and Midwives: A Force for Health', in June 2000.[47]

Judi Brown, the ICM's Deputy Director based in Australia, was well versed in regulatory issues and represented the ICM at several of the regulatory meetings when finances were available to fund her expenses. One outcome of these international meetings was the joint *News for Regulators* published by the

ICN. The second joint communiqué reported on the historic meeting held in Toronto, Canada, in October 2004. Participants identified 15 core activities they hoped to achieve globally, with the area of best practice most prolific in both the ICM and ICN. This area included standards, guidelines and competencies along with advocating for governmental, intergovernmental, midwifery and nursing regulatory agencies to support and exhibit best practice.[48] The ICM had adopted its first essential midwifery competencies in 2002, though such a task was much more complex for nursing and the ICN. The ICM had a place on the ICN international steering committee on midwifery regulation and contributed to the 7th International Regulation Conference in Taipei, Taiwan, May 2005.[49]

Both the ICM and the ICN were observers during meetings of the Global Advisory Group on Nursing and Midwifery as noted earlier and were participants in each version of the *Strategic Directions for Nursing and Midwifery* over the years. In addition, the ICN agreed the international education standards developed by Sigma Theta Tau International[50] and the WHO in 2009, *Global standards for the initial education of professional nurses and midwives*.[51] The ICM could not agree these WHO standards due to the basic requirement of a baccalaureate degree required upon completion of the basic nursing programme. The ICM was aware that many midwifery education programmes were not in institutions of higher learning nor did leading midwifery educators believe that a baccalaureate degree was necessary to prepare a competent midwife. The ICM finalised its own *Global Standards for Basic Midwifery Education* in 2010 (Chapter 12).

At times, the chief executives of global health professional associations with offices primarily in Geneva, Switzerland, get together in an informal group called the Chief Executive Officer (CEO) network.[52] The ICM Secretary General, Petra ten Hoope-Bender, became a part of this group during her tenure at the ICM.

PARTNERSHIPS FOR MATERNAL, NEWBORN AND CHILD HEALTH[53]

In 1999, the ICM and FIGO were invited to join the Safe Motherhood Inter-Agency Group (IAG)[54] to strengthen its capacity in addressing maternal and newborn health issues from a health care provider perspective. Representatives of the ICM (Joyce Thompson) and the World Bank (Dr Khama Rogo) were elected to chair the IAG[55] at the end of the November 2000 Tunis meeting on 'Skilled Attendance at Delivery', providing an excellent opportunity for the ICM to develop its role and influence in maternal and newborn health beyond midwifery alone. The ICM Director and SG (Petra ten Hoope-Bender) and the FIGO President (Pino Benajano) represented the two organisations. The Tunis conference resulted in seven countries being supported to implement their action plans for increasing skilled attendance at childbirth. Each country received support from one of the IAG member agencies. This dedicated country level support became one of the building blocks for a more extensive Partnership discussed below.

The Partnership for Safe Motherhood and Newborn Health – 2004

In subsequent IAG meetings suggestions were made to create a Partnership that would also include country delegations to report on their actions and results. A Transition Team was set up in December 2001[56] under the leadership of the IAG Co-Chairs initiating the discussions about a Partnership for Safe Motherhood and Newborn Health (PSMNH). Several meetings were needed to discuss the modus operandi of the PSMNH and how to ensure that both Safe Motherhood and Newborn Health would get enough attention and funding. Dr Khama Rogo (World Bank) and Petra ten Hoope-Bender (ICM SG) led the discussions with an ever-growing number of agencies interested to join and funders ready to financially support this Partnership. The WHO offered to house the PSMNH within its Reproductive Health and Research department. The PSMNH finally took off in early 2004. Petra ten Hoope-Bender was its first Executive Officer[57] and in charge of the day-to-day management of the PSMNH from its offices at the WHO in Geneva.

At the same time as the expanded PSMNH was developing, the World Bank in late 2003 set up the Healthy Newborn Partnership (HNP) and UNICEF established the Child Survival Partnership (CSP), both working with the same donors as PSMNH to secure funding for support to countries. To improve effectiveness, a merger was proposed and a transition team consisting of three agencies per partnership was convened by the WHO. It was tasked with developing a constitution, staffing arrangements, decision-making processes, communications and regular consultation with the leadership and members of the three partnerships.

The Partnership for Maternal, Newborn and Child Health – 2005

The transition team of the newly developing partnership gained from momentum from hosting the 'Lives in the Balance' conference in New Delhi, India, that was held on World Health Day, May 2005, bringing together government delegations from over ten countries to address their specific situation and needs with regard to reducing maternal and newborn deaths. The vision and goals laid out by delegates in the landmark Delhi Declaration[58] became the basis of the soon-to-be-formed Partnership for Maternal, Newborn and Child Health (PMNCH). The transition was completed by the end of July 2005. In September 2005, the PMNCH was launched at UNICEF House in New York.[59]

> 'The PMNCH represented an unprecedented collaboration between the world's leading maternal, newborn and child health professionals … uniting developing and donor countries, UN agencies, professional associations, academic and research institutions, foundations and NGOs to intensify and harmonise national, regional and global progress toward UN Millennium Development Goals 4 & 5.'[60]

At the time of the launch, there were 50 members. Its focus was on country-level activities aimed towards reduction of needless maternal, newborn and child deaths. Starting with a relatively small budget PMNCH had to find innovative ways to provide tailored country level support. At the Steering Committee meeting in September 2005, ICM Director (Joyce Thompson) explained the catalytic funding project of small grants ($10,000 or less) from the PMNCH to help countries strengthen their MNH capacity at country level. Countries were invited to develop creative proposals tailored to their specific needs, a mechanism that is still used today.

The Role of Health Professional Organisations in PMNCH

The ICM's Director spearheaded an initiative to define the role of Health Care Professional Organisations in the PMNCH, focused on increased effective collaboration between health care professional organisations (HCPOs) towards the achievement of the Millennium Development Goals (MDGs), specifically MDG 4 (reducing child mortality) and MDG 5 (reducing maternal mortality). The health professional organisations involved in the PMNCH included FIGO, IPA, ICM and the Council of International Neonatal Nurses (COINN). A joint statement[61] released on 12 September 2005, during the PMNCH launch in New York identified the crucial role health care providers play in reducing mortality and morbidity, but also in improving health professionals' education and regulation, leadership development, advocacy for maternal, newborn and child health and health system strengthening. The ICN endorsed the joint statement and later became a member of the PMNCH. The statement was used to support health professional groups at the international level in their efforts to guide and encourage their national societies/member associations to work with other key stakeholders in providing culturally appropriate, evidence-based skilled care.[62]

The ICM was part of the selection team for the new PMNCH Director. Petra ten Hoope-Bender remained Executive Officer until the new Director was selected. In September 2005, Dr Francisco Songane was appointed. Secretariat leadership has changed over time. Helga Fogstad was the Executive Director in 2021.[63]

The PMNCH Work Plan and Board Members

In the first PMNCH Work Plan (2006), the Partnership's added value of working together to improve MNH was proposed, including the continuum of care for maternal, newborn and child health. It also stressed the importance of working with global, regional and national health care professional associations in addressing barriers to implementation and promoting the acceptance and

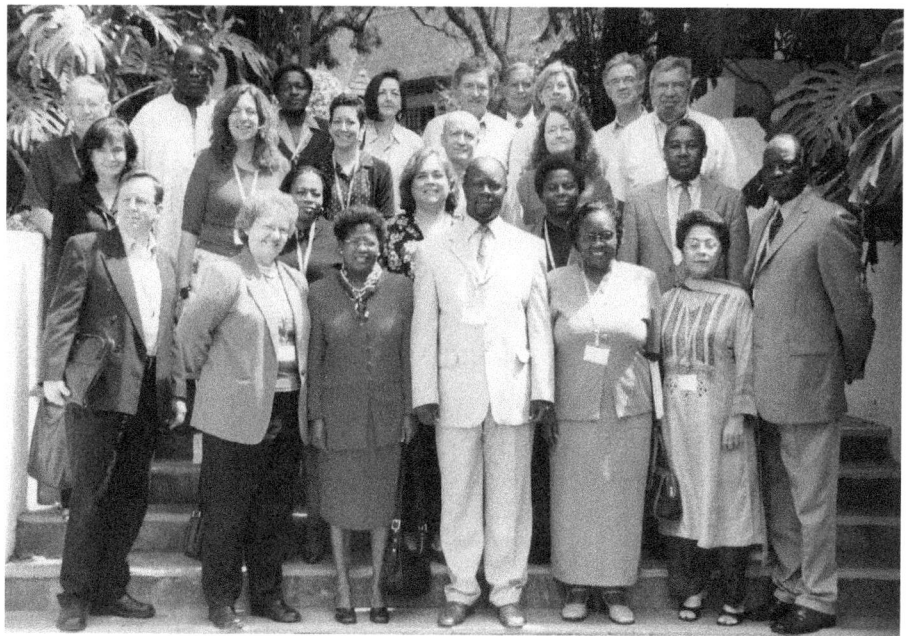

Board members of Partnership for Maternal, Newborn and Child Health – Courtesy of Joyce Thompson

implementation of an essential interventions package.[64] Of importance was the recognition by PMNCH members of the direct link between healthy pregnant women, births and healthy newborns – and the need to work together to keep the link in place.

Initially the ICM alternated with the other health professional groups for a seat on the PMNCH Board. In 2009 the ICM gained a permanent Board seat on the PMNCH.[65] This role has allowed for a stronger global presence of midwifery in the Sexual Reproductive Maternal Newborn Child and Adolescent Health discussions as well as better bonds with other health care professional organisations such as FIGO and the IPA.

In 2015, the PMNCH agreed the UN *Global Strategy for Women's, Children's, and Adolescents' Health* (2016–2030) and addressed its role in reaching the Sustainable Development Goals. Its new Vision in 2015 was, 'A world in which every woman, child and adolescent realises their right to health and well-being, leaving no one behind' and an updated Mission was 'To mobilise, align and amplify the voice of partners to advocate for women's, children's and adolescents' health and well-being, particularly for the most vulnerable.'[66] In 2021:

> 'Chaired by Rt Hon. Helen Clark, Former Prime Minister of New Zealand, PMNCH is the world's largest alliance for women's, children's and adolescents' health, bringing together partners from across the sexual, reproductive, maternal, newborn, child and adolescent health communities, as well as health-influencing sectors. The Partnership provides a platform for organizations to align objectives, strategies and resources, and agree on priority interventions to improve the health and well-being of women, children and adolescents.'[67]

Over the years, the ICM's ongoing leadership and involvement with the PMNCH has provided many opportunities to make the case for investing in midwifery and strengthening countries' continuum of care for the sexual and reproductive health and rights of adolescents and women, as well as newborn and child health.

ICM JOINT STATEMENTS

Several Joint Statements and joint Press Releases provide further evidence of the importance and shared value of the ICM's various partnerships in spite of some MAs at times questioning why the ICM entered into such partnerships and joint statements. This was evident in the Open Forum debate during the Brisbane

Council meeting in 2005 when one of the top three priorities of Council was 'transparent processes for signing joint statements'.[68] A key reminder to ICM leaders was the difficulty of entering into partnerships and joint statements that may be very important to midwives in one half of the world and not the other half, such as management of the third stage of labour, prevention of post-partum haemorrhage and how midwives were thought of as a skilled attendant. In spite of this difficulty, the ICM continued to participate actively in the development of joint statements in keeping with the mission of keeping all women safe and healthy.

A few of the joint statements are highlighted below.

The Midwife as Prototype Skilled Attendant

Perhaps the most important, yet controversial, of the joint statements came after several years' discussion of who is a 'skilled birth attendant' and what is meant by 'skilled care'. WHO Expert Committees began in the 1950s defining the difference between the trained midwife as a skilled birth attendant versus the traditional birth attendant (known under a variety of titles) practising in rural areas in many low resource countries (Chapter 4). The discussion of who was a midwife and how that person was prepared for the required scope of practice continued into the 1960s and 1970s, resulting in a 1972 updated definition of the midwife (Chapter 11).

In 1999, a joint WHO/UNFPA/UNICEF/World Bank statement called on countries to: 'ensure that all women and newborns have *skilled care* during pregnancy, childbirth and the immediate postnatal period.'[69] At that time, *skilled care* was defined as: 'care provided to a woman and her newborn during pregnancy, childbirth and immediately after birth by an accredited and competent health-care provider who has at her/his disposal the necessary equipment and the support of a functioning health system, including transport and referral facilities for emergency obstetric care.'[70] In 2000, both the ICM and FIGO decided there was a need to more clearly identify the skills needed to promote safe childbearing and good outcomes for mother and baby. Thus, they agreed on the following definition of skilled attendant:

> 'A skilled attendant is a health professional with midwifery skills, for example midwives, and those doctors and nurses who have been trained to proficiency in the skills to manage normal (uncomplicated) pregnancies, childbirth and the

immediate postnatal period and to identify, manage or refer complications in the woman and or newborn.'[71]

When the partners who initiated the global Safe Motherhood Initiative in 1987 (WHO/UNFPA/UNICEF/World Bank) noted that several accredited healthcare providers could fit the definition of skilled birth attendant, they decided it was important to define who those individuals were. The ICM and FIGO representatives were invited to join with the WHO Making Pregnancy Safer (MPS) team to accomplish this important task (See Text Box). Several discussions took place with agreement of the 2004 definition below:

> 'A skilled attendant is an accredited health professional – such as a midwife, doctor or nurse – who has been educated and trained to proficiency in the skills needed to manage normal (uncomplicated) pregnancies, childbirth and the immediate postnatal period, and in the identification, management and referral of complications in women and newborns.'[72]

Della Sherratt (WHO) and Petra ten Hoope-Bender (ICM) jointly struggled with writers of this document to get 'midwife' placed first in the list. 'The standard WHO way in published documents was to list "doctors – nurses – midwives", but we managed to change that to the new order because of the focus on normal (uncomplicated) pregnancies. Della fought this as the first defender, I backed her up.' PHB & DS 2020

Background on WHO's approach to use of term 'midwife'[73]

The issue for WHO referring to midwife, let alone licenced midwife, rather than referring to what was seen as a more generic term, 'health worker with Midwifery skills' has been the topic of long and often contentious debates within WHO for many years. The issue came to a head in 2004–5 during the writing of the World Health Report 2005. Recognising the stark fact that of all the MDGs, it was MDG5 that was most 'off track', WHO and its partners agreed that specific action was needed to intensify efforts in this area. Whilst there was consensus internationally that in order to reduce the numbers of avoidable deaths which occurred in and around pregnancy and childbirth there was the need to invest more in the provision of skilled care, there was far less agreement when it came to specific recommendations for how to achieve this, particularly when it came to issues of the providers of skilled care, commonly referred to as a Skilled Birth Attendant (SBA).

Although the main editors of the WHR-05 were convinced by and very supportive of the arguments and historical evidence that investing in a specialist cadre of licenced midwives, rather than a generic health provider who had been given some additional training, not only had merits, but was in the end cost-effective, others were anxious this was privileging, even promoting, a specific professional group and would be too difficult for many low-income countries. Eventually the need for specific competencies, and more specifically the need for these competencies to fit within a legal and regulatory framework which demonstrated not just competence at the point of training but ongoing and professional updating, won the day. Consequently, a compromise was agreed whereby the recommendation should be that a licenced midwife should be seen as 'the prototype' skilled birth attendant and as such, by implication, the best buy and countries should develop strategies to achieve this. It was pointed out that having a legal/regulatory framework had many benefits, not least the need for midwives to work in collaboration with physicians and other members of the wider maternity and child health community and therefore was not privileging any professional group. Moreover, this position would assist with Human Resource planning and predicting future workforce needs rather than just counting total health providers, many of whom may not even work in maternity areas let alone have kept the required midwifery competencies updated, even if they had them included in their initial pre-service programme.'

Throughout the years the ICM fought to have midwives recognised as the principal/primary skilled attendant along with the desire to use the title 'midwife' instead of skilled birth attendant in global and local documents. In fact, some members of the ICM were adamant that the ICM Board withdraw their support of the skilled attendant joint statement.[74] After due consideration of this request, the ICM Council decided that the consequences of withdrawal far outweighed letting the statement stand. These included the fact that the Joint Statement was in the public domain, and to withdraw ICM support would lead to withdrawal of the ICM midwifery competencies allowing UN agencies and others the freedom to alter core competencies for skilled attendants and eliminate any referral to midwives. In addition, if the ICM were to withdraw from the joint statement, it could be seen that the ICM is not trustworthy and would be excluded from future debates on maternal and newborn health.[75] Evidence of the importance of this statement for the WHO came in the form of Della Sherratt, WHO Designated Technical Officer to the ICM (see text below). She succeeded in having the final wording about skilled attendants in the World Health Report of 2005 on page 69 to read:

> 'The prototype for a skilled attendant is the licensed midwife. Less cost-effective options include nurse-midwives and doctors, assuming they have been specifically prepared to do this kind of work (most are not – or not sufficiently). Gynaecologists/obstetricians – of whom there is a large deficit in stagnating and reversal countries – are, as a rule, perfectly able to provide first-level care, although they are less cost-effective and more appropriate for back-up referral care.'[76]

Midwives and Nurses Call for Increased Skilled Attendance at Birth (2000)

Following on the heels of the Millennium Declaration and its Millennium Development Goals that recognised the important role that midwives and nurses with midwifery skills play in promoting Safe Motherhood, the ICM and ICN issued a joint press release on the 2 October 2000. The ICM SG Petra ten Hoope-Bender noted that the 'single most critical intervention for safe motherhood is to ensure that a health worker with midwifery skills is present at every birth.' Fadwa Affara, ICN consultant for Nursing and Health Policy, went on to state: 'Millions of women lack access to maternal health care that could save their lives.'[77] The press release went on to note that for the first time midwives and nurses are both represented as professions in international level debates on Safe Motherhood, working with the Inter-Agency Group (IAG) for Safe Motherhood. The two international organisations challenged their members to follow the recommendations of IAG to increase coverage and the quality of care for childbearing women.

In addition, the ICM and ICN participated in joint Press Releases in 2002 on the essential role of skilled attendance in childbirth and violence against health professionals.[78]

Birth Registration (2003)

The ICM and ICN joined together again to promote birth registration in June 2003 as a basic right of every child. The statement noted that almost two-fifths of the world's children (approximately 50 million babies in 2000) were born without being registered. 'Unregistered and undocumented children are extremely vulnerable to exploitation of every kind.'[79] The statement goes on to identify why birth registration is important for individuals and governments; the reasons births are not registered (e.g. rural site of birth, illiteracy, lack of facilities); the role of midwifery and nursing associations; and ending with a birth registration campaign. Both organisations collaborated again in 2007 on the Birth Registration Toolkit Identity: *Every Child's Right*.

Prevention of Post-partum Haemorrhage (2004 / 2006 / 2008)

The ICM and FIGO shared many common interests over the years, including addressing life-saving procedures such as prevention of post-partum haemorrhage. The joint statement of 2004 and its update in 2006 were important for midwives throughout the world as they struggled to prevent needless maternal deaths. In spite of an ICM Council mandate to the ICM Board to work with FIGO to agree such a statement, a few midwifery leaders in high resource countries were angry because they thought they were expected to carry out active management of the third stage of labour when they rarely used oxytocin (see Kim Campbell story in Chapter 5). In spite of some disagreement from high resource country midwives, the ICM continues to view the prevention of post-partum haemorrhage as an essential life-saving skill and midwives must have this competency no matter where they work. The latest update of the Prevention of Post-Partum Haemorrhage ICM/FIGO Joint statement occurred in 2008.[80]

Hammamet Call to Action: 'Scaling-up Midwifery in the Community' (2006)

The forum in Hammamet, Tunisia, brought together international agencies and organisations, midwives, nurses, physicians, health policymakers, professional associations, regulatory bodies and researchers from 23 countries around the world with the highest rates of maternal and neonatal mortality and morbidity.[81] The call to action called on governments, regulatory bodies, professional health care organisations, educators and communities to ensure the provision of midwifery services in the community by establishing or improving: 1) policies to ensure equitable access to midwifery services; 2) policies and regulatory systems to improve the number, deployment, status and conditions of work of midwives and others with midwifery skills; 3) competency-based education and training in midwifery skills; 4) peer and supportive supervision of providers in the field; 5) an enabling environment to support effective health care delivery, including infrastructure, communication, emergency transportation, adequate funding, equipment and supplies and 6) permanent monitoring and periodic evaluation of services. Of importance in this call to action was the recognition that the ICM had global essential competencies (2002) that were referenced and would be used to carry out this call.

A Global Call to Action (2010)

Midwives and other health professionals of the world along with development partners met prior to the June 2010 Women Deliver Conference in Washington, DC. One of the primary reasons for this meeting was to reinforce the key role that midwives and others with midwifery skills[82] play in addressing Millennium Development Goal 5 (maternal health) and Goal 4 (newborn component). This meeting was supported by UNFPA, Jhpiego, the WHO, the Global Health Workforce Alliance, UNICEF, FIGO, the ICM and International Association for Maternal and Neonatal Health (IAMANEH). The pledge made during this meeting was to join forces with governments, civil society and other partners to support WHA resolutions on midwifery and nursing to initiate a global movement to strengthen midwifery services. The participants called on governments and development partners to: 'invest in a midwifery workforce as a fundamental step towards a functioning primary health care system that can deliver for women and newborns, fostering a healthier future for all.'[83] Of importance in this joint statement was the number of ICM partners and their call for action by governments and development partners working at country level to make sure there are sufficient midwives available, deployed where needed most, within an enabling environment and with sufficient equipment and supplies. This statement also reinforced the expansion and importance of the ICM's partnerships going into the second decade of the 21st century.

WHO/UNFPA/UNICEF/ICM/ICN/FIGO/IPA Definition of Skilled Health Personnel Providing Care during Childbirth 2018

In order to measure progress towards the achievement of Sustainable Development Goal (SDG) #3: Ensure healthy lives and promote well-being for all at all ages, Target 3.1 (reduction of maternal deaths) and Target 3.2 (end preventable newborn deaths) and the aims of the UN's *Global Strategy for Women's, Children's and Adolescents' Health*, an updated definition of skilled health personnel for childbearing care was agreed. This statement replaced the 2004 Joint Statement by WHO, ICM and FIGO.[84] The agreed definition was:

> 'Skilled health personnel are competent maternal and newborn health professionals who are educated, trained, and regulated to national and international standards. They are competent in providing and promoting evidence-based, human-rights-based, quality, socio-culturally sensitive and dignified care to women and newborn infants. They are competent in managing labour and delivery to ensure a positive childbirth experience for women. In addition, they are competent in identifying and managing or referring women and/or newborn infants with health complications. As individuals, skilled health professionals are a part of an integrated team of maternal and newborn health professionals; these include midwives, nurses, obstetricians, paediatricians, and anaesthetists – together they perform all key life-saving services of maternal and newborn care.'[85]

FIGO noted that the 2018 definition and its supporting information were the first steps to informing data collection and measurement to clearly identify which health care providers can be counted as 'skilled health personnel providing care during childbirth' measured as the 'proportion of births delivered by skilled birth attendants', within the SDG indicator framework.[86] This definition of skilled health personnel will improve understanding of the proportion of births attended by competent maternal newborn health professionals. Their presence at childbirth is crucial towards reducing the likelihood of complications for women and their infants. It was also noted that ensuring that the person assisting the mother during childbirth is fully competent is critical for achieving progress towards the SDGs as well as the aims of the *UN's Global Strategy for Women's, Children's and Adolescents' Health*. It was noted by the writers of this book that this statement was not located on the ICM website in 2021 raising questions about whether the use of the term 'skilled attendant' for midwives as well as other health professionals is still being questioned by today's midwifery leaders and/or MAs.

THE LANCET SERIES ON MIDWIFERY – 2014[87]

The 2014 *Lancet Series on Midwifery* addressed the essential needs of childbearing women and their newborns in all countries with a thought-provoking series of international academic studies on midwifery practices, policies and outcomes. It was inspired by the awareness of unmet sexual and reproductive health needs around the world. It may also have been inspired in part by *Lancet* Editor Richard Horton's attendance at the 2011 ICM Triennial Congress in Durban, during which he was heard to remark, 'I wish I was a midwife!'[88]

The *Lancet Series on Midwifery* focuses on the essential needs of childbearing women, their newborns and families in all countries and 'provides a framework for quality maternal and newborn care that firmly places the needs of women and their newborn infants at its centre'[89]. The findings of this Series offer additional support for shifting from a fragmented system for maternal and newborn care that is focused on identification and treatment of pathology to a whole-system approach that provides the level of care needed at the time it is needed.

The full series can be found at: https://www.thelancet.com/series/midwifery/

SUMMARY

Evidence of the importance of ICM's role and importance in partnerships was offered at the end of this chapter addressing Joint Statements. Other Non-Governmental Organisations (NGOs) and donors have been important partners throughout the history of ICM and are addressed in various chapters in this book. The majority of these partnerships came about from the ICM's representation at various meetings hosted by these organisations since the early 1950s and ongoing efforts to provide the evidence that well-prepared midwives and appropriately regulated midwifery practice are essential to the health of women, newborns, adolescents and nations.

100 Years of the International Confederation of Midwives

1 The authors have tried to be consistent throughout this book in spelling of various organisations such as FIGO and IPA. We have used the website spelling without the 'a' in gynecology or pediatric when referring to the official organisations, and the 'ae' spelling in text, when used in quotations or when referring to the journals of each organisation.
2 ICM. *Interorganisational Relationships Guidelines*. Chiswick, London: ICM, 1996.
3 Joint FIGO/ICM Study Group. 'Introduction.' *Maternity Care in the World: An International Survey of Midwifery Practice and Training, First Edition*. Oxford: Pergamon Press, 1966 p xvii.
4 Joint FIGO/ICM Study Group. 'Introduction' in *Maternity Care in the World: An International Survey of Midwifery Practice and Training, First Edition*. Oxford: Pergamon Press, 1966, p xv.
5 Refer to Chapter 20 for details on ICM representation/observation on WHO Expert Committees during the 1950s.
6 Sir John Peel. 'Preface' in WHO. *Maternity Care in the World. Report of a Joint Study Group of the International Federation of Gynaecology and Obstetrics and the International Confederation of Midwives*. England: CM Printing Services, 1976.
7 IPPF was one of the NGOs present and participating in the 1987 Safe Motherhood conference in Nairobi, Kenya, and a founding partner in the SMIs.
8 WHO. *Maternity Care in the World. Report of a Joint Study Group of the International Federation of Gynaecology and Obstetrics and the International Confederation of Midwives*. England: CM Printing Services, 1976 p vi. MG Candau. 'Forward' in WHO. *Maternity Care in the World. Report of a Joint Study Group of the International Federation of Gynaecology and Obstetrics and the International Confederation of Midwives*. England: CM Printing Services, 1976, p ix, stated, 'It has been a privilege for the World Health Organization to be able to give some assistance to this survey, which has provided an excellent example of the valuable role that non-governmental organisations can play in the health field.'
9 Dr H Mahler. 'Foreword' in *Maternity Care in the World. 2nd edition*. England: CM Printing Services, 1976, p i.
10 MG Candau. 'Foreword.' *Maternity Care in the World: An International Survey of Midwifery Practice and Training*. Oxford: Pergamon Press 1966, p xvii.
11 Professor Nixon. 'Introduction.' *Maternity Care in the World: An International Survey of Midwifery Practice and Training*. Oxford: Pergamon Press, 1966, pp xix–xx. ICM. *Report of the 17th International Congress, Lausanne, Switzerland 21st–28th June 1975*. 'Report of Council Meeting and Other Reports' p 236. Miss Bayes reported that the Executive Committee of the ICM/FIGO Joint Study Group met at regular intervals during the 1972–1975 triennium, and would meet 7–9 July 1975, in London 'to discuss the new edition of Maternity Care in the world and the recommendations which should be included in it.' Miss Bayes also noted that 'Eight Working Parties had already been convened by the ICM for developing countries under the ICM/US-AID grant and with the co-operation of the ICM/FIGO Joint Study Group.'
12 The reader needs to be aware that use of overall 'country' statistics does not take into account remote and rural areas that exist in Latin America, Mexico and other areas of the world that do not include their numbers.
13 MG Candau. *Maternity Care in the World: An International Survey of Midwifery Practice and Training*. Oxford: Pergamon Press, 1966, 'The World Situation', p 3. The authors are aware that there was a greater ratio of doctors in the USSR at this time.
14 MG Candau. *Maternity Care in the World: An International Survey of Midwifery Practice and Training*. Oxford: Pergamon Press, 1966, 'The World Situation', p 18.
15 FIGO/ICM Joint Study Group. *Maternity Care in the World: International Survey of Midwifery Practice and Training 2nd Edition*. Great Britain: CM Printing Services, 1976, p vi.
16 FIGO/ICM Joint Study Group. *Maternity Care in the World: International Survey of Midwifery Practice and Training 2nd Edition*. Great Britain: CM Printing Services, 1976, pp vi–vii.
17 FIGO/ICM Joint Study Group. *Maternity Care in the World: International Survey of Midwifery Practice and Training 2nd Edition*. Great Britain: CM Printing Services, 1976 p ix.
18 FIGO/ICM Joint Study Group. *Maternity Care in the World: International Survey of Midwifery Practice and Training 2nd Edition*. Great Britain: CM Printing Services, 1976 p ix.
19 WHO. *Maternity Care in the World. Report of a Joint Study Group of the International Federation of Gynaecology and Obstetrics and the International Confederation of Midwives*. England: CM Printing Services, 1976, p x.
20 WHO. *Maternity Care in the World. Report of a Joint Study Group of the International Federation of Gynaecology and Obstetrics and the International Confederation of Midwives*. England: CM Printing Services, 1976, p x.
21 WHO. *Maternity Care in the World. Report of a Joint Study Group of the International Federation of Gynaecology and Obstetrics and the International Confederation of Midwives*. England: CM Printing Services, 1976, pp xiv–xv.
22 WHO. *Maternity Care in the World. Report of a Joint Study Group of the International Federation of Gynaecology and Obstetrics and the International Confederation of Midwives*. England: CM Printing Services, 1976, p xv.
23 WHO. *Maternity Care in the World. Report of a Joint Study Group of the International Federation of Gynaecology and Obstetrics and the International Confederation of Midwives*. England: CM Printing Services, 1976, p viii.
24 WHO. *The Midwife in Maternity Care: Report of a WHO Expert Committee*. Geneva: WHO Technical Report Series No 331, 1966, p 8.
25 WHO. *Maternity Care in the World. Report of a Joint Study Group of the International Federation of Gynaecology and Obstetrics and the International Confederation of Midwives*. England: CM Printing Services, 1976, p ix.

26 ICM/FIGO correspondence J Tomkinson 1975–80. Wellcome Institute Library document SA/ICM/M/2/2.
27 ICM. *ICM Council Meeting Minutes Vienna, Austria, 2002*. Agenda item 10: Board of Management Report May 1999–April 2002, p 2. 'Increased shared activities with FIGO, including efforts to address violence against women and obstetric fistula; ICM official membership on Steering Committee of the FIGO Save the Mothers' Fund'.
28 ICM. (SA/ICM/P/1/15/1). Wellcome Collection. *International Paediatric Association 1974–1979*.
29 ICM. (SA/ICM/P/1/15/1). Wellcome Collection. *International Paediatric Association 1974–1979*. Letters between Thomas Stapleton and Marjorie Bayes during 1974–1975, and between the IPA President Professor Dogramaci and Margaret Hardy during 1976–1977 indicated that IPA was asked to have paediatric representatives at all the FIGO/ICM Working parties in the various countries.
30 ICM. (SA/ICM/P/1/15/1). Wellcome Collection. *International Paediatric Association 1974–1979*. 3 March 1975 letter to Thomas Stapleton, General Secretary IPA.
31 Judith Oulton. Interview 2017.
32 ICM. *ICM Triennial Report 1993–1996*. Chiswick, London: ICM, p 23.
33 ICN. *Position Statement: The Nature and Scope of Practice of Nurse-Midwives*. Geneva: ICN, October 1996.
34 Fadwa A. Affara, Nurse Consultant. Memo to Presidents/Executive Directors, General Secretaries of ICN member Associations #5.2/B, dated January 1997. New Position Statements.
35 Catherine McCormick. Letter of 19 August 1997 to Joan Walker, ICM Secretary General, asking for appropriate action to take on this issue.
36 Personal experience of Joyce Thompson working in sub-Sahara Africa in 1990s, confirmed by ICM President Bridget Lynch during her term of office.
37 ICM. (SA/IC/R/4). Wellcome Collection. *Marjorie Bayes' Draft History of ICM, first 50 years*.
38 Margaret Hardy. Letter to WHO Director General dated 23 July 1975. On the 29 September 1975, the Director General responded by basically ignoring the question of professional status, then stating, 'As regards WHO personnel employed to assist national staff in the development of health programmes, the Organization must seek people with broad professional background and experience.' Marjorie Bayes had sent a similar letter to the WHO Director General on 6 January 1961 in which she sent an October 1960 ICM Council Resolution deploring WHO that there was no Midwifery Officer at WHO level.
39 News Review: Leading ladies in the initiative. *Safe Motherhood Newsletter 1*: November 1989–February 1990 pp 4–5.
40 Wellcome Institute Library uncatalogued material. Joyce E Thompson. The WHO Global Advisory Group on Nursing and Midwifery. *Journal of Nursing Scholarship*, 34:2, pp 111–113 (Second Quarter), 2002. Thompson was appointed by the US government to this group in 2000 and became vice-chair in 2001–2007. She worked with other midwife leaders to help WHO change their language from nursing/midwifery to nursing AND midwifery through her leadership of a WHO Collaborating Centre at the University of Pennsylvania beginning in 1993.
41 Petra ten Hoope-Bender. 'Report of ICM Representation, Partnerships and Projects in the International Health Arena.' ICM Council Agenda Item C-068, 2002, p 2.
42 Pakistan Ministry of Health, ICN, ICM, WHO. *Islamabad Declaration on Strengthening Nursing and Midwifery*, 4–6 March 2007.
43 ICN, WHO, ICM. *Triad Communique*, 19-20 May 2006, pp 1–2.
44 Interview with Judith Oulton, ICN Executive Director, 3 April 2017. Judith noted that 'ICM participation was limited and that wears on the relationships over time.
45 WHO, ICN, ICM. *The Eighth 'Triad Meeting' of the World Health Organization, the International council of Nurses, and the International Confederation of Midwives*. Agenda 16–28 June 2020. [Personal papers JET].
46 ICM & ICN. *Proposal for Creating New Mechanisms for Regulators within the International Confederation of Midwives and the International Council of Nurses*. November 2004.
47 Board of Management. *Report to the ICM Council 2002*, p 2: ICM President participated in drafting The Munich Declaration.
48 ICN, ICM. *News for Regulators*, Issue 3, February 2005.
49 ICM. *ICM Council Meeting Minutes, Brisbane, Australia, July 2005*. Agenda item 27.3.2.: Overview of Partnerships with Other (International) Organisations.
50 Sigma Theta Tau International is the global honour society for nurses and was chosen by the WHO to develop these standards. STTI recognises nurses prepared at the baccalaureate level and above, hence the requirement for a minimum of a baccalaureate degree.
51 WHO Department of Human Resources for Health. G*lobal standards for the initial education of professional nurses and midwives*. Geneva: WHO 2009.
52 Petra ten Hoope-Bender. 'Report of ICM Representation, Partnerships and Projects in the International Health Arena.' ICM Council Agenda Item C-068, 2002, p 3. In 2002, the CEO network included ICN, World Medical Association,

International Federation of Pharmacists, World Confederation for Physiotherapy, World Dental Federation, and the International Organisation of Occupational Therapists.
53 A major portion of this section on Partnerships for Safe Motherhood, etc., was contributed by Petra ten Hoope-Bender, former ICM Secretary General and then the first Executive Director of the PMNCH.
54 IAG members included: WHO, UNFPA, UNICEF, World Bank, IPPF, Population Council and Family Care International (secretariat), ICM and FIGO joined in 1999.
55 PSMNH Co-Chairs call, 3 May 2004: Dr Khama Rogo, World Bank, confirmed that financial support for ICM' role as co-chair throughout its tenure would be made available by the World Bank.
56 Minutes of IAG, 4 December 2001, Population Council, New York.
57 Petra resigned her position as Secretary General for ICM in 2003 and continued to work on the Transition team of the PSMNH.
58 https://www.who.int/pmnch/knowledge/publications/delhideclaration/en/
59 PMNCH Press Release. *Power of Partnership Highlighted at Global Launch.* New York, 12 September 2005.
60 PMNCH. *The Partnership for Maternal, Newborn & Child Health. Improving Health. Saving Lives.* Geneva: WHO, 2005. Pamphlet.
61 PMNCH. *Joint Statement: Health Professional Groups Key to Reaching MDGs 4 & 5.* Geneva: PMNCH, 12 September 2005.
62 PMNCH. *The Role of Health Care Professional Organisations in the PMNCH.* Geneva: PMNCH, 2007.
63 www.pmnch.org, downloaded 16 February 2021.
64 PMNCH Workplan 2006.
65 ICM. *Triennial Report 2008–2011.* The Hague: ICM, p 4: Global Partnerships: Midwifery essential to achieving MDGs 4, 5 and 6.
66 PMNCH. About the Partnership. 2015, p 2. www.pmnch.org
67 PMNCH eBlast. Downloaded from web 16 February 2021.
68 ICM. *ICM Council Minutes Brisbane, Australia 18–21 July 2005*. Min 05.24, p 22.
69 WHO. *Reducing maternal mortality. A joint statement by WHO/UNFPA/UNICEF/World Bank.* Geneva: WHO, 1999.
70 WHO. *Reducing maternal mortality. A joint statement by WHO/UNFPA/UNICEF/World Bank.* Geneva: WHO, 1999.
71 ICM and FIGO: *Definition of Skilled Attendant.* 2000.
72 WHO. *Making Pregnancy Safer: the critical role of the skilled attendant. A joint statement of WHO, ICM and FIGO.* Geneva: WHO/RHR/MPS Reference #WQ240 2004WO, 2004, p 1. This revised definition was endorsed by UNFPA and the World Bank.
73 This section was contributed by Della Sherratt, UK Midwife who had worked at the WHO. 2020.
74 ICM. *ICM Council Minutes Brisbane, Australia 18–21 July 2005*. Min 05.24 Motion that ICM withdraw its support from the joint WHO/ICM/FIGO statement 'Making Pregnancy Safer: the critical role of the skilled attendant' that originally passed (p 22), but was rescinded later after 'Kim Campbell, Canadian Association of Midwives, expressed concern that this decision was disrespectful, indicated a lack of support for members of the Board of Management and may have a negative impact on the position of the ICM internationally.' Min 05.25.3.6, p 29, 23.
75 ICM. *ICM Council Minutes Brisbane, Australia 18–21 July 2005*. Min 05.24 Motion that ICM withdraw its support from the joint WHO/ICM/FIGO statement 'Making Pregnancy Safer: the critical role of the skilled attendant' passed without full discussion, then later rescinded. Personal notes of J Thompson related to ICM Board Discussion in 2004.
76 WHO. *World Health Report 2005: Make Every Mother and Child Count.* Geneva: WHO, 2005, p. 69.
77 ICM and ICN. Press Release: *Midwives and Nurses Call for Increased Skilled Attendance at Birth.* Geneva: 3 October 2000, p 1.
78 ICM. *ICM Council Meeting Minutes Vienna, Austria, 2002.* Agenda 10: Board of Management Report, p 2, Joint Press Releases with ICN.
79 ICM and ICN. *Birth Registration: Every child has a right to a name and nationality. A Statement from the International Confederation of Midwifery and the International Council of Nurses.* June 2003.
80 ICM. *Triennial Report 2008–2011.* The Hague: ICM, p 23.
81 Hammamet Call to Action. *Scaling-up 'Midwifery in the community'.* 11–15 December 2006, Hammamet, Tunisia.
82 Vincent Fauveau, Della Sherratt, Luc de Bernis. Human Resources for maternal health: Multi-purpose or specialists? *Human Resources for Health* 6: 21 p 2008.
83 UNFPA, JHPIEGO, WHO, GHWA, UNICEF, FIGO, ICM, IMANEH. *A Global Call to Action: Strengthen Midwifery to Save Lives and Promote the Health of Women and Newborns.* Washington, DC, June 2010.
84 WHO. *Making Pregnancy Safer: the critical role of the skilled attendant. A Joint statement by WHO, ICM and FIGO.* Geneva: WHO 2004.
85 WHO. *Definition of skilled health personnel providing care during childbirth: the 2018 joint statement by WHO, UNFPA, UNICEF, ICM, ICN, FIGO and IPA.* Downloaded 26 April 2021 from: https://www.who.int/reproductivehealth/publications/statement-competent-mnh-professionals/en/.

86 https://www.figo.org/news/new-definition-skilled-health-personnel Downloaded 26 April 2021.
87 *Lancet Series on Midwifery*. Downloaded from www.internationalmidwives.org/collaborations on 26 April 2021. https://www.thelancet.com/series/midwifery.
88 Personal remembrance of ICM President Bridget Lynch.
89 ICM. *ICM Triennial Report 2014–2017*. The Hague: ICM, p 43.

Chapter 17: *ICM's Importance/Value to Midwives, Women and World Health*

'As we meet to celebrate the Fiftieth Anniversary of the Confederation, we are inspired to seek new horizons in our efforts to bring improved care to mothers and babies throughout the world. ... But let's not stand on our laurels. We must contemplate future goals for both the health of families around the globe, and for the growth of our Confederation. ... Decisions made at this Congress can help to promote healthful living, including the ability to plan one's family, reduce poverty, advance social and economic security, and be an influence for peace in the world.'

Lucille Woodville, ICM President 1972

INTRODUCTION

Beginning in 2011, the authors began talking with individuals who were strategically involved in the development and growth of the International Confederation of Midwives (ICM) over the years, including MAs throughout the Regions (Chapter 13). Formal interviews for this history book began in 2016. Of necessity, those interviews focused on selected individuals still alive since the 1960s. The interviews were conducted via email or in person with three major groups: 1) international midwife leaders; 2) ICM staff members of the Secretariat and 3) key non-midwife partners/representatives of partner organisations. Questions addressed in this chapter include:

1. What is your view of the importance/value of the ICM and its work to:
    a. midwives and midwifery associations,
    b. the health of women and childbearing families, and
    c other international associations?
2. What are the key challenges/lessons learned over the years?

The views of selected/key international midwives and obstetricians, donor agency representatives and other partners on the importance of the ICM in the global health arena are presented in this chapter. Specifically, the ICM's role in enhancing the sexual and reproductive health and rights of women, adolescents and childbearing families with well-prepared midwives providing high quality midwifery services. Many of the challenges faced and lessons learnt are summarised and, if remembered, will continue to guide its leaders and MAs to strengthen the ICM as a woman- and midwife-centred organisation into the next century (Chapter 18). It is hoped that in understanding the various views of the value of the ICM over the years, along with remembering ICM's pathway to both successes and challenges described throughout this book, the reader will celebrate the way forward for the ICM.

ICM's VALUE/IMPORTANCE TO THE HEALTH OF WOMEN
International Midwives' Perspectives

This chapter began with words from the 50th anniversary of the ICM. Lucille Woodville, ICM President in 1972, was addressing the midwives and friends attending the 16th ICM Congress in Washington, DC, USA.[1] Her comment was a fitting reminder of the past and moving forward.

Given the extraordinary number of international midwives who have contributed to the development and growth of the ICM during the past 100 years, it is impossible to include each one in this brief overview of midwives' perspectives of the importance of the ICM to the health of women, newborns and childbearing families. Edith M Pye (1934 President of IMU) and Marjorie Bayes (ICM SG) were instrumental in the rebirth of the ICM in the early 1950s as noted in Chapter 4. They followed the tradition of their foremothers, Frau De Graaf Van den Elst of the Netherlands, Mme Perneel of Ghent, Belgium, and Ellen Erup of Sweden. They were convinced that there was value in continuing an international organisation of midwifery associations with a remit to improve the health of women and childbearing families with midwives as the primary providers of services (Chapters 3, 4). The modern age of the ICM was led by elected and/or appointed officers who willingly volunteered their expertise, time and efforts; midwifery staff employed by the ICM; midwives working within the WHO and UNFPA; and midwives representing other ICM partner agencies. A summary of comments from several of these international midwives follows.

In 1987, Margaret Peters (Australia), immediate past-President of the ICM, provided a wake-up rally call to the midwives attending the 21st ICM Congress in the Hague as she reported on the need for global action, especially from

100 Years of the International Confederation of Midwives

midwives, to reduce high levels of maternal and newborn deaths, most notably in low resource countries.[2] This was preceded a few months earlier when the ICM Treasurer Dame Margaret Brain attended the 1987 Safe Motherhood meeting in Kenya that resulted in the global Safe Motherhood Initiatives (SMI) (Chapter 9). The resulting Collaborative Pre-Congress workshops contributed to upgrading the knowledge and skills of midwives to prevent needless deaths and disabilities of mothers and babies. The ICM was most willing to be a part of the solution for saving lives with well-prepared midwives in many countries.

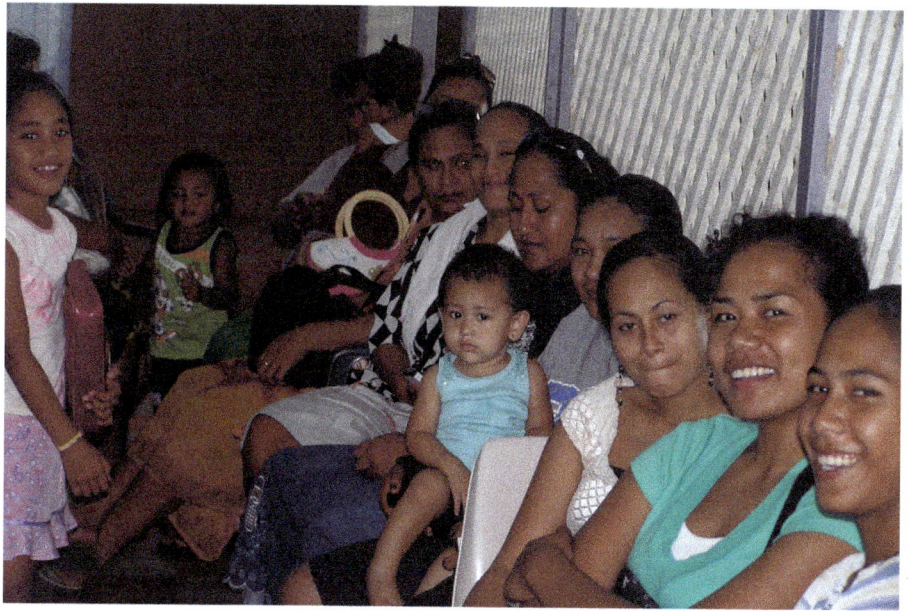

Mothers with children attending an ante-natal clinic in Samoa – Courtesy of Karen Gilliland

In 1995 at the 4th World Conference on Women in Beijing, China, the ICM issued a statement in support of improving the health and rights of women and childbearing families. It read, in part:

'The Confederation supports all national and international activities that promote women as persons, supports reproductive health targeting the reduction of maternal mortality, and lifelong women's health as an essential component of development. ... The Confederation pledges to work with women, with policy makers, and with governments to improve the status of women throughout the world.'[3]

The ICM's global commitment in support of women and their health continued when midwives and their philosophy and model of care were identified as essential interventions to keep women off the road to maternal disability and death[4] and improve the reproductive health and rights of adolescents, women and families. Key examples of midwives and their care have been recognised by the United Nations' agencies in the development of the 2000–2015 Millennium Development Goal #4 (Newborn Health) and Goal #5 (Maternal Health); the WHO's World Health Reports of 2005 and 2008; by UNFPA and others in the development of the 2015-2030 Sustainable Development Goal #3 (Good Health and Well-Being) and Goal #5 (Gender Equality) and in three State of the World's Midwifery Reports (2011, 2014, 2021). These examples reinforce former ICM President Frances Day-Stirk's statement that the ICM is vitally important to the health of women and childbearing families.[5]

A few selected quotations for this history book from international midwives' interviews during 2019–2020 illustrate the ongoing commitment/value of the ICM to the health of women and their families:[6]

> 'ICM protects women's and midwives' rights as human rights by issuing statements.' [Junko Kondo, Japan]
>
> 'ICM is very relevant to push the agenda and plight of women and childbearing families in a world of in-equality.' [Caroline Weaver, Australia]
>
> 'ICM is invaluable to the health of women due to its strengthening of midwives/ associations so they are better able to advocate for women and their families.' [Debrah Lewis, Trinidad & Tobago]
>
> 'I think ICM is crucial to the health of women and childbearing families because midwifery with its focus on physiological pregnancy and childbirth is crucial! "Physiology until proven pathology" is being trodden with large boots by those who want to "save lives" through interventions and think that's the only way.' [Petra ten Hoope-Bender, Netherlands]
>
> 'Because of the close relationship between the status of midwives and the status of women, ICM is important in profiling midwives and midwifery as valuable contributors to the health care team for the health of women and newborns. Women are proud when they see a female midwife leading a process and giving advice to their government officials. So are midwives. This makes women and childbearing families see what is possible for women.' [Nester Moyo, Zimbabwe]

International Obstetricians' Perspectives

There were several international obstetricians/gynaecologists who played a major role in the development of the ICM and in carrying out its Aims over the past 100 years, beginning with Professor Frans Daels who pushed for the formalisation of the IMU in 1922 (Chapter 3). When asked their perspective during interviews in 2019–2020 on the value/importance of ICM to the health of women, a few of ICM's current obstetric colleagues' responses follow.

> 'Where the midwives were empowered to take more responsibility, the changes in maternal and newborn health were more visible. For example, in some parts of India, Tanzania and Kenya the midwives are involved in delivering postpartum (PP) contraception services; in Tanzania TAMA (ICM MA) is leading the institutionalisation of Postpartum IUD services and working with FIGO.' [Sabaratnam Arulkumaran, FIGO]
>
> 'The advocacy and communications that came through the ICM and others and the role of the midwives in Maternal Newborn Health (MNH) at country level led to improvement in MNH. It was the start of an international movement that helped reduce maternal and newborn mortality and strengthened the role of the midwife at the decision-making table.' [Vincent Fauveau, UNFPA]
>
> '… but we forgot the "care" elements like birth-preparedness, quality of care as experienced by women and the non-medical aspects needed to deliver the Essential Interventions in RMNCH[7]. The ICM contributed to that part of the agenda.' [Luc de Bernis, WHO]

Luc de Bernis also commented that during the time that Vincent Fauveau was with UNFPA, midwives from the ICM were involved in several activities, e.g. the Hammamet meeting (Chapter 16) and the start of the *State of the World's Midwifery* reports (Chapter 15). He also said that Vincent really saw the key role that midwives play in reducing maternal and neonatal mortality and morbidity. Della Sherratt (UK midwife) who worked alongside Vincent also commented on his role in supporting and pushing the ICM and midwives to take an active role in keeping motherhood safe for all women.[8]

VALUE OF THE ICM TO MIDWIVES AND MIDWIFERY ASSOCIATIONS
International Midwives' Perspectives

Most of the midwives who responded to this question identified the ICM's development of core documents (Chapter 11), global competencies and standards (Chapter 12), selected Position Statements and tools (Chapter 10) as vitally important to Member Associations (MAs) (Chapter 13). These provided essential support for midwifery associations and midwives themselves as they advocated for professional status and legal recognition in many countries and promoted the midwifery philosophy and model of care in all countries. These ICM core documents and standards were also essential to validating midwives' evidence-based practice (EBP). Midwifery EBP supported the vital role of the midwifery workforce in the prevention of maternal and neonatal mortality and morbidity and the promotion of the sexual and reproductive health and rights for girls, adolescents, women and families. Thus, the ICM's core documents, global competencies, standards and tools (e.g. the Midwifery Association Capacity Assessment Tool discussed in Chapter 9) helped MAs strengthen their roles in advocacy, education, research and regulation of the midwifery workforce. As noted by Judith Brown[9] from Australia:

> 'ICM is absolutely vital as it connects midwives and the work and expertise of midwives globally & assists them to be able to articulate the work which needs to be undertaken and sustained with major stakeholders in maternal and newborn health. ICM gives midwives a voice for midwives' and women's health.'

In addition, Nester T Moyo (Zimbabwe), ICM Programme Manager for several years, noted:

> 'The ICM is invaluable for the survival and identity of midwives globally. The ICM sustains midwifery and midwifery services as a viable area of study where intelligent and well-educated women can be developed into highly qualified professionals who can stand shoulder to shoulder with other professions.'

The value of the ICM Collaborative Pre-Congress workshops (Chapter 9) and materials published afterward was referenced by Valerie Tickner, a UK midwife who worked with Barbara Kwast, a WHO midwife from the Netherlands, on these workshops. Materials developed in these workshops were frequently shared with governments and professional bodies (where they existed). The materials continue to be used by MAs and midwives to upgrade, maintain and improve the quality and cost-effectiveness of respectful maternity care throughout the world, though the initial focus was on midwives working in countries with the highest levels of maternal and newborn deaths and morbidities.

> 'The changes were significant in midwives, especially post Kobe ICM Collaborative Pre-Congress Workshop in 1990. Midwife educators became deeply involved in the approach to learning about the 5 major causes of maternal death, integrating this content into their education programmes.' [Valerie Tickner, UK]

A few other quotations further illustrate the value/importance of the ICM to midwives and its MAs follow.

> 'The visibility and increasing respect for, and recognition of, midwives through the ICM has allowed the same for midwives in many countries. … Midwifery associations are able to utilise the ICM documents such as the Standards, Position Papers, Calls for Action to negotiate with governments and other national organizations.' [Debrah Lewis, Trinidad & Tobago]
>
> 'The ICM is indispensable to midwives and midwifery associations.' [Bridget Lynch, Canada]
>
> 'The ICM is the key to its Member Associations, particularly those emerging and less established.' [Frances Day-Stirk, UK]
>
> 'The ICM is essential to support midwife colleagues as they seek professional status in many countries, to strengthen midwifery associations so they can be a strong voice for sexual and reproductive health, and to promote the midwifery philosophy and model of care in all countries.' [Joyce Thompson, USA]
>
> 'As the only international organisation that speaks for midwives and about midwifery in the global arena, ICM's work and role are central. The ICM is the only organization/NGO/Health Care Professional organization that can speak with legitimacy for and about midwives/midwifery in the international health arena.' [Petra ten Hoope-Bender, The Netherlands]
>
> 'The ICM provides guiding principles to develop or review [the midwifery association's] own standards and statement of midwives.' [Junko Kondo, Japan]

International Obstetricians' Perspectives

As noted earlier in this book, several international obstetricians/gynaecologists were instrumental in the ICM's development as a global leader in midwifery. They included Professor WCW Nixon and Sir John Peel of the ICM/FIGO Joint Study Group (Chapter 16); Nicholson J Eastman (Johns Hopkins University); Khama Rogo (World Bank); Andre Lalonde (FIGO, Canada), Luc de Bernis (FIGO and WHO) and Vincent Fauveau (UNFPA). A few of their comments follow.

Sir John Peel, representing FIGO, brought greetings to the 1972 ICM Congress with the following words focusing on the relationships between midwives and obstetricians:

> 'For centuries male and female midwives have been conducting a sort of clandestine war over the bodies of their patients as to who should take possession of them. I think the fact that we are where we are today is an indication of the fact that, in most places throughout the world, the hatchets have been buried and we realize that we are members of a team and cannot do our jobs without one another. We have learned to respect and admire one another's functions and activities.'[10]

Other partner obstetricians spoke of the importance of the ICM to midwives and midwifery associations:

> 'If there hadn't been an ICM, the tasks of UNFPA and the WHO would be much harder. It represents the voice of midwives in all the maternal health aspects and dynamics, though that voice could be louder. FIGO is interesting, but the ICM is very strong and they both need each other. The international arena has grown from the strength of the ICM and vice versa, especially with regard to the standards and competencies for midwives.' [Luc de Bernis, WHO]

Sabaratnam Arulkumaran[11] noted:

> 'Initially I paved the path for closer interaction between the ICM and FIGO by exploring joint projects and ICM/FIGO conference reciprocal joint sessions. The ICM emphasised the need for team working and to build trust and respect for each other to the benefit of mothers and babies.'

International Partners' Perspectives

Barbara Kwast, WHO Designated Technical Officer to the ICM 1986–1991, and leader of the ICM/WHO collaborative Pre-Congress Workshops in Safe

Motherhood (Chapter 9), noted:

> 'The ICM strengthened midwifery, but the international organizations [WHO, UNFPA] put the midwives onto their tasks at country level. If midwives were not in those programmes at country level, it was often due to a weak national midwives' association.'[12]

Dr Paul Van Look, Director of Reproductive Health Research Department at the WHO where maternal health was housed, noted:

> 'I believe interaction with the WHO may have strengthened some of the ICM's normative work and the increased international profile of the ICM. The ICM logo is on WHO publications, for instance, the midwifery education modules.'

Anneka Knutsson, Chief, Reproductive Health Branch, UNFPA, and former Programme Director at SIDA, guided the funding of the UNFPA/ICM 'Investing in Midwives Programme' launched in Ghana in 2009. She became closely engaged with the ICM in 2005 when she was stationed in Bangladesh with UNFPA who wanted midwives in country offices and worked to upgrade the preparation of community-based skilled attendants to midwives. Anneka worked with consultant Della Sherratt at the time on faculty training of trainers in midwifery. She met Nester Moyo from Zimbabwe at the Tunisia meeting and learned more about the ICM and its role in strengthening midwives and reducing maternal and newborn deaths and disabilities. This was also the meeting where the foundation for the partnership programme between the ICM and UNFPA on 'Investing in Midwives' began. She closed her interview with:

> 'ICM is not only a global professional association for Midwives. The ICM is a voice for the rights and empowerment of women to demand information, quality of care and services, be they the women or adolescents that seek midwifery care and services or midwives themselves.'[13]

Anneka's lifetime goal given her early childhood in Ethiopia was to do something meaningful, to do good in the world, to make a difference! With her background as a nurse, a midwife, and with a PhD in pedagogics, she became a strong proponent of midwives, midwifery and sexual and reproductive health. Most recently in her role within UNFPA, she is leading efforts to fund some ICM core activities in leadership and education and projects within the Strengthening Midwifery Globally programme since 2017.

IMPORTANCE/VALUE OF THE ICM TO ITS GLOBAL PARTNERS

Partnerships attract key groups, finances and resources which might not be available to a single association. Positive partnerships are built upon common areas of interest/concern, based on mutual respect and trust, and strengthened through information sharing, understanding and continuous communication. Throughout this book there are several discussions of the importance of the ICM's partners to the work and status of the ICM. Here are some examples of the ICM's value to several of its partners.

As noted in Chapter 16, Professor WCW Nixon, Professor of Obstetrics and Gynaecology at University College Hospital in London, UK, was the chair of the FIGO committee to study the training and practice of midwives and maternity nurses throughout the world in 1961. He wrote:

> 'It was realized that such a study would only be feasible with the co-operation of the International Confederation of Midwives (I.C.M.), so I approached Miss Marjorie Bayes, Executive Secretary of the I.C.M. for help in this project. The I.C.M. readily agreed to assist.'[14]

This was the beginning of the ICM/FIGO Joint Study Group and led to a continued strong relationship between the two health professional groups to the present time, acknowledging the fact that each organisation benefited from its relationship with the other. This was also a watershed moment for the ICM and midwives as through the country-level workshops that were held, governments realised and acknowledged the midwives' leadership of these country projects. Indeed, the partnership with FIGO opened many doors for midwives and the ICM activities, internationally and locally. And through its MAs, the ICM opened many doors for regional and local FIGO activities.

The ICM's presence and partnership with the WHO was deemed essential, beginning in the early 1950s, and strengthened with the ICM's involvement in the global Safe Motherhood Initiatives. Barbara Kwast promoted midwives as the lynchpin[15] in any Safe Motherhood activity and helped the ICM personnel prepare triennial Pre-Congress Collaborative Workshops, introducing the ICM leaders to other UN agencies including UNICEF and UNFPA (Chapter 15).

In addition, the ICM's partnership with the WHO afforded midwives' entry into many low resource countries (LRCs) welcomed by most WHO country offices. The ICM staff and officers also became known by government representatives to the World Health Assembly each year as they presented many statements, especially during the 1990s, when women, children, newborns and/or health issues were high on the agenda. Paul Van Look, WHO, noted that:

> 'The beginning of the 21st century saw the emergence of a global convergence on the complementary roles of skilled attendance at delivery which was and is almost exclusively provided by midwives, and emergency obstetric care. Until that time, opinions on the value of these two approaches had often been at loggerheads.'[16]

During the 1960s and 1970s, the ICM efforts were key in working with many governments to gather the details needed for the publication of two editions of *Maternity Care in the World* (Chapter 16). These efforts demonstrated again the ICM's effective working relationship with another international organisation, the Federation International of Gynecology and Obstetrics (FIGO). Dr Jerker Liljestrand, former Treasurer of FIGO, noted that, as chairperson of the FIGO Safe Motherhood Working Group, he brought the ICM onto that committee represented by the Secretary General, Kathy Herschderfer. He went on to note:

> 'When the ICM started to engage on strengthening midwifery, it gave voice and re-balanced the relationship between the two professions. Better with the two professions together ... The role of the midwife in the former Soviet Union and Lithuania resulted in obstetricians starting to work more closely with midwives which helped change maternal newborn health there.'[17]

Della Sherratt (UK midwife) who worked at the WHO towards the end of the 1990s, recalled her experiences of knowing and working with the ICM below:

> 'From 1980, Maternal and Child Health became more visible globally, midwives in wealthier countries became more active globally and outraged about the plight of midwives and women and babies. I have to say there have always been some midwives voicing concerns, but there were big events for raising funds to support safe motherhood initiatives. Midwives were now being asked to give opinions, not always listened to, I may add, and Medical doctors still seen as "the experts".'[18]

Others commented on the importance of the ICM to its global partners.

> 'The ICM informs and educates other organisations about the competency of midwives and the value of midwifery in the health care systems for effective

quality maternal and newborn health services.' [Nester Moyo, Zimbabwe]

'In the 1980s–1990s, the WHO had an important role to play in strengthening midwifery (led by with Barbara Kwast), including publishing the WHO Midwifery Modules based on outcomes of the 1990 Kobe Pre-Congress Workshop. In the 1990s and beyond, ICM has been a positive influence/partner on WHO activities surrounding education standards (the WHO Essential Competencies for Midwifery Educators 2014) and tools for strengthening midwifery globally (the WHO Strengthening Midwifery Toolkit, updated 2013).' [Joyce Thompson, USA]

'The advocacy and communications that came through the ICM and others and the role of the midwife in Maternal Neonatal Health (MNH) at country level was important. It was the start of an international movement that helped reduce maternal and newborn mortality and strengthened the role of the midwife (and the UNFPA Country Office Midwives) at the decision-making table. ... MDG5[19] also helped profile midwives. There wasn't really a clear picture on how to achieve this MDG before.' [Vincent Fauveau, UNFPA]

'The international arena has grown from the strength of the ICM and vice versa, especially with regard to the standards and competencies for midwives.' [Luc de Bernis, WHO]

Vincent Fauveau confirmed that the UNFPA started using the ICM standards once available. The ICM's involvement and strong leadership within the Interagency Group on Safe Motherhood that transitioned to the Partnership for Safe Motherhood and Newborn Health (PSMNH) and finally the Partnerships for Maternal, Newborn and Child Health (PMNCH) reflects the value/importance of the ICM to its partner organisations (Chapter 16). Paul Van Look, the WHO, responded:

'With formal establishment in September 2005 of the Partnership on Maternal, Newborn and Child Health (PMNCH) based at WHO, Petra (former ICM SG) became PMNCH's first Director.'

In a keynote address to the 2005 ICM Congress in Brisbane, Australia, Dr Khama Rogo, representing the World Bank and co-chair of the PSMNH, said:

'The world needs midwives, now more than ever. The world recognizes that without midwives, there can be no safe motherhood. And ... every obstetrician will accept that without the midwife, obstetric practice is dead ... After all, we need each other and the women whose health we are trained to preserve, need us ... together.' [Khama Rogo, Co-Chair PSMNH, Kenya]

Ann Starrs from Family Care International, the Secretariat for the PSMNH and PMNCH, responded with:

'ICM's impact [on IAG and PSMNH] was enormous (specifically on increasing awareness of the importance of health care professionals and their associations at global and country levels for reducing mortality and morbidity). However, it depended heavily on who was the representative (both for ICM and FIGO).'[20] [Ann Starrs, FCI]

LESSONS LEARNT FROM HISTORY

Lessons learnt along one's journey through life are essential for not only understanding the present but also planning for the future without repeating the mistakes of the past. Throughout the past 100 years the ICM has been on a learning curve, changing and adapting to meet the global demands and needs of midwives, women and communities in countries. As noted in the earlier part of this chapter, the ICM and its activities are now valued throughout the world and midwives well-respected in most countries. However, along with successes come many lessons learnt along the way that, when remembered, can lead to a very bright future for the organisation.

Perhaps Della Sherratt's[21] words a few years ago can highlight some lessons needing attention in order for the ICM to move forward successfully in the 21st century:

'I have become rather disheartened of later years in midwives both at home and abroad. I am seeing a lack of sisterhood. There is a rise of professionalism in international work (now paid) which is good, but the downside is an apparent lack of willingness in volunteerism, collaboration, willing to share and try to find common solutions. In some countries where professional midwifery is just taking off, I see a lack of willingness to foster and nurture younger midwives which leads to no succession building, which, in turn, is having a negative impact on how the ICM is perceived – not so much seen as the place to go for help/advice. A key factor is ICM's not able to be a true partner (only work if they have funds) that leads to no capacity to make changes at country level. ... There appears to be a lack of possibilities and sometimes even unwillingness to help midwives in low-income countries (unless it brings funding or research publication possibilities). … Maybe it's about having the right personality at the helm/in visible places both in countries and in ICM.'

Nester Moyo, long-time ICM Programme Manager, noted another lesson for the ICM and its leaders:

'One of the most effective ways the ICM can demonstrate the value of midwives to health care team and health of women and newborns is by running projects in countries. It is not only the impact of the said projects that will raise the profile of midwifery and midwives but the fact that governments will see midwives leading and running projects that are useful to their populations. Advocacy alone does not do this as it could be seen as a voice in the wilderness. People are more convinced with things they can see and touch.'

Judith Brown, former ICM Deputy Director and Director, spoke of an important factor that has influenced ICM over time:

'I think sometimes midwives and others don't fully understand how much of themselves volunteer midwives have given to the ICM, e.g., Margaret Peters and others over many years personally financially supporting the ICM. When finances were tight many Board members covered expenses of attending meetings themselves, and many midwives gave up their vacation entitlements and long service leave to attend. Many midwifery leaders would not want to be given accolades for this. They felt privileged to contribute, but we should remember the sacrifices the leaders have made and still continue to make to keep ICM strong. Without them there might not be an ICM. Also, the work of the Secretary Generals – their true value has never really been documented.'

Barbara Kwast, Dutch midwife at the WHO and long-time supporter of the ICM, noted:

'The ICM started to focus more on the role of the midwife and collaboration with the UN agencies at the start of the Safe Motherhood Initiative (SMI). The Board at that time didn't really understand why international collaboration was important and it was hard to "pull" them into the international arena. … The change in the role and presence of midwifery was heavily dependent on the midwives themselves wanting to raise their profile in countries.'

As noted earlier, Luc de Bernis (WHO) commented that without the ICM, the tasks of UNFPA and the WHO would have been much harder. However, he added that '*ICM represents the voice of midwives in all the maternal health aspects and dynamics, though that voice could be louder.*'

The ICM has learned many lessons from the midwives and the women they serve, along with ICM's interactions with a variety of global, regional and national partners. Principal among these lessons has been:
1. The need for ICM leaders and midwife representatives to speak with strong voices based on a solid knowledge base in decisions about women's health and rights and at policy tables
2. A willingness to work with partners sharing a common vision
3. Sensitivity and a willingness to learn from others about the diversity of population needs throughout the world that affect the needs and services of midwives.

ICM'S CHALLENGES MOVING FORWARD

Challenges moving forward based on key lessons learnt were highlighted by Bridget Lynch, former President of the ICM. These included:
- Invisibility and lack of autonomy of midwives
- Regional development – development of strong regional associations to support networking and similar education and regulation across the region – providing reciprocity to work across borders in the regions
- Developing high quality midwifery educators and policy leaders in country through external programs
- Clear strategic directions process at Council/Governance level with continuity from one triennium to the next
- Stable financing of the organization – beyond relying on solely on membership fees and Congress profit.[22]

When Anneka Knutsson, Chief Reproductive Health Branch, UNFPA, was asked her view of ICM's future, she responded with the following challenges:

> 'I think ICM is moving toward an increased presence in the global health arena. However, it needs to continue, strengthen, and/or push its member associations and midwives to:

- Strengthen their view of women at the centre of all ICM efforts
- Have leaders with strong, clear, internationally knowledgeable, evidence-based voices
- Create positive inter-professional collaboration at all levels
- Advocate for midwife-led continuity of care
- Provide quality care at all times in all places
- Demand an enabling environment for all the work of the midwife
- Advocate for an evidence-based body of midwifery knowledge & share with the world
- View of the work of the midwife beyond childbearing care
- Avoid "victim" speak.'[23]

The ICM's ongoing challenges facing the organisation, its member associations and the profession of midwifery are summarised below, building on the insights offered throughout this chapter along with comments from the ICM Regions who responded to the survey (Chapter 13).

1. **Purpose**: Need to stay focused on the vision and mission of the organisation which may change over time.
2. **Autonomy**: Need to increase the visibility and autonomy of midwives in many countries, avoiding 'victim speak' at all times.
3. **Leadership**: Need to have committed international midwife leaders with knowledge and strong voices and the skills to balance the diverse needs of its member associations.
4. **Member Services**: Need to develop strong regional networks of midwifery associations to support working together in the region to establish education, regulation and evidence-based practise based on global standards.
5. **Member Services**: Need to continue to develop senior midwifery policy leaders and young midwifery leaders at country level (succession planning).
6. **Governance**: Need to continue the clear strategic direction process during Council meetings with continuity from one triennium to the next.
7. **Financial Viability**: Need to have stable financing of the organisation beyond membership fees and Congress profit, led by knowledgeable financial experts.

8. **Global Partners**: Need to continue to maintain and expand <u>mutually beneficial, positive partnerships</u> committed to the health of women, newborns and childbearing families.

SUMMARY

The content of this chapter is focused on a variety of perspectives on the value/importance of the ICM to women, to its Member Associations and the midwives they represent, and to its international partners and donors. Taken together with regional MA views, there is no question that the ICM as a global health professional organisation has made a positive difference in the health of many women, newborns, adolescents and families over the past 100 years as well as empowering the midwives its serves. However, in order to move forward, the ICM, its leaders and its MAs need to consider lessons learnt over the past 100 years and challenges that need to be addressed in order to move forward in 2023 and beyond. With these in mind, the story moves to Chapter 18 and the immediate future of this predominantly woman-led, woman-oriented organisation serving and empowering midwives and women throughout the world!

100 Years of the International Confederation of Midwives

1 Lucille Woodville. President's address, p 1. In New Horizons in Midwifery edited by Alice M Forman, Susan H Fischman, Lucille Woodville. Baltimore, MD: Waverly Press, 1973.
2 Margaret H Peters. A Challenge for Midwives, the reduction of maternal mortality and morbidity rates throughout the world. Midwifery 4:1 (March 1988) pp 3–8. https://doi.org/10.1016/S0266-6138(88)80051-2.
3 ICM. Statement to the 4th World Conference on Women September 1995, Beijing, China: Women and Their Health: Midwives in Partnership. Chiswick, London: ICM, 1995.
4 Mahmoud Fatalla. The Maternal Death Road (video). Geneva: WHO.
5 Interview with Frances Day-Stirk, 2021.
6 The names were attached to each quote to emphasise the global reach of the ICM.
7 This abbreviation stands for Reproductive Maternal, Newborn and Child Health.
8 Vincent Fauveau noted in his interview that in 2007 UNFPA, ICM and SIDA started the 'Investing in Midwives and Others with Midwifery Skills (MOMS) partnership.
9 Judith Brown was elected Deputy Director, then Director of the ICM Board of Management 1999–2008, and also filled in as Chief Executive for a short period in 2013. Interview in 2019.
10 Sir John Peel. Greetings from the International Federation of Gynaecology and Obstetrics. New Horizons in Midwifery: Proceedings of the 16th Triennial Congress of the International Confederation of Midwives October 28–November 3, 1972, Washington, DC Baltimore, MD: Waverly Press, 1973, p 4.
11 Dr Arulkumaran is a Sri Lankan Tamil physician, former president of the Royal College of Obstetricians and Gynaecologists and the International Federation of Gynaecology and Obstetrics and president-elect of the British Medical Association. Interview in 2020.
12 Interview with Barbara Kwast, 2017.
13 Interview with Nester Moyo, 2020.
14 Joint FIGO/ICM Study Group. 'Introduction.' Maternity Care in the World: An International Survey of Midwifery Practice and Training, First Edition. Oxford: Pergamon Press, 1966, p xvii.
15 Barbara E Kwast, Joan Bentley. Introducing confident midwives: Midwifery education – action for safe motherhood. Midwifery 7:1 (March 1991), pp 8–19. https://doi.org/10.1016/S0266-6138(05)80129-9
16 Interview with Paul Van Look, 2017.
17 Interview with Jerker Liljestrand, 2017.
18 Interview with Della Sherratt, 2020.
19 MDG 5 refers to Millennium Development Goal #5 that addressed maternal health and the need to reduce maternal mortality and morbidity with midwives as the strategic intervention needed.
20 Interview with Ann Starrs, 2019.
21 Della Sherratt, a midwife from the UK, was deeply involved in ICM, first as an international consultant in Bangladesh, then in her role as the WHO designated Technical Officer for ICM. She was also a consultant for UNFPA and WHO. Interview in 2020.
22 Interview from Bridget Lynch, March 2021.
23 Interview with Anneka Knutsson in May 2021.

Chapter 18: A Vision for the Future of the ICM and Midwifery[1]

'Midwives have stood by women and stood by midwifery throughout the ages. It is an honour to be a part of this ancient, wise, diverse, and versatile community. To support the next generation of women to attain their sexual and reproductive health and rights, midwives will need to foster cross-generational as well as cross-national and global learning. Midwives will also need to build on their joint global midwife knowledge and trust the power of the new generation of midwives to lead ICM forward!'

Franka Cadée, ICM President 2022

INTRODUCTION

The 100-year history of the International Confederation of Midwives' (ICM) is preceded by many centuries of the work of midwives in their communities with women and their families across the globe. Midwifery is one of the oldest professions on earth and has evolved through time. It is still evolving as a current wind of change allows midwives to stand up and be seen and heard again, supported by rigorous evidence showing the positive impact of midwives.

It is essential to realise that a vision for the future is shaped by all the midwives who have come before and on whose broad shoulders midwives have had the privilege to stand. The ICM honours all midwives globally who led the way before us, with whatever name given by their communities. To mention but a few:[2]

> midwife, قابلة, partera/matrona, 助产士, babica, porodní asistentka, jordemoder, vroedvrouw, hebamme, mami, emaginak, акушерка, эх барич, သားဖွားဆရာမ, सुडेनी, ਧਾਈ, दाई, ਘੋਲ, පවුල් සෞඛ්‍ය සේවිකාවන්ගේ, акушерка, llevadora, levatrice, primalja, ämmaemand, kätilö, Sage-femme, μαία, bába, Ljósmóður, cnáimhseach, ostetrica, մանկաբարձուհի, ধাত্রী, 助產士, ಬಾಣಂತಿ, દાયણ, மருத்துவச்சி, మంత్రసాని, ผดุงครรภ์, ebe, akuşer, قابلئ نسا, توغۇت ئانىسى, مڈوائف, Bà mụ, מְיַלֶּדֶת, pîrik, ماما, vroedvrou, አዋላጅ, mzamba, ungozoma, ndi a, umubyaza, nyamukuta, umulisadaada, mkunga, umbelekisi, agbębi, Zumbelethisi, mananabang, hilot, palekeiki, mpampivelona, दाई, 助産婦,

357

> ಸೂಲಗಿತ್ತಿ, акушер, धाப, 산파, акушерка, ບາງແະດງຮັບ, മിഡൈഫ്, बाळंत,
> kaiwhakawhanau, faatosaga, vecmāte, akušerė, mammenfra, акушерка, qabla, jordmor,
> położna, moaşă, акушерка, barnmorska, акушер, акушерка, bydwraig, אָקושעריןי"

As noted in the text at the beginning of this chapter, midwives are needed to empower and assist women to attain their sexual and reproductive health and rights. In order to achieve these aims, the ICM will put their trust in the new generation of empowered midwives and member associations to lead the ICM forward!

STRENGTHENING MIDWIFE ASSOCIATIONS IS ICM'S CORE BUSINESS

The ICM has been an organisation of Midwife Member Associations (MAs) since 1922. And even though midwives' primary reason for being is to support women, other people and their families within the community to attain their sexual and reproductive health and rights, it is ICM's core business to position every national MA to be the "go to" organisation that enables and strengthens the profession of midwifery.

The ICM is a collective of MAs and, as such, all midwives in one of the 143 associations in membership in 2022 form a part of the ICM, representing around one million midwives globally. The ICM is growing steadily and as more midwives unite in MAs, the ICM could double its membership and thereby represent more than two million midwives globally. *The State of the World Midwifery Report 2021* highlighted a current shortage of 900,000 midwives.[3] If governments follow the data and invest in midwives so that each country achieved universal coverage of midwife-led continuity of care by 2035, this could mean that midwifery care for all women everywhere could be optimised, averting 67 per cent of maternal deaths, 64 per cent of newborn deaths and 65 per cent of stillbirths.[4] This would also mean that ICM's membership could grow and thus represent the needed three million midwives globally.

The ICM is transforming to become a global *'movement for midwifery with women at the centre'*, as envisioned in ICM's Triennial Strategy 2020–2023.[5] To attain this the ICM will need to continuously respond to the needs of its MAs, using all creative ways and with the right balance of the human touch as well as digital means. The ICM continues its development into a robust, reliable and agile learning organisation, with operational, financial and governance processes befitting its aims and strategic objectives. By implementing ICM's 2020–2023 Strategy, in co-creation with its members, Head Office, Board and partners, the ICM will become the global movement needed to change the paradigm to a world where women everywhere have a midwife by their side for themselves, their newborn and community.

AUTONOMY OF WOMEN, MIDWIVES AND THE ICM
Women

Autonomy of women and adolescent girls means they have the right to decide if, when and with whom they want to become pregnant as well as where, how and with whom they want to give birth. This is a great good and a human right. In 2019, the White Ribbon Alliance collected 1.2 million demands from women and girls for quality reproductive and maternal health care in 114 countries. Respectful and dignified care was at the top of the 20 demands collected. This was followed by access to medicines and supplies, clean water and more and better supported midwives. The report concludes with the following words:

> 'Listening to women is a radical act. But acting on what we hear is revolutionary.'[6]

Midwives

As for midwives who are predominantly women, doing women's work for and with women is not much different. It will be interesting to see outcomes of a forthcoming new campaign that will tell us 'what midwives want'. Systemic bias including gender bias is part and parcel of midwifery. The profession has been institutionalised in many countries within a bio-medical model in which midwifery does not sit comfortably, even though midwives have adapted very capably. By adapting, midwives have also had to make compromises to the distinct philosophy and approach to midwives' care.

Midwives have been marginalised for many centuries through inadequate education, regulation and leadership. Let the global community be brave and bold and listen to midwives' voices and act upon what midwives have to say and need. This will support midwives to empower themselves and heal, which will in turn support midwives to reach their potential and take up their key role in securing optimal midwifery care for all women and families everywhere.

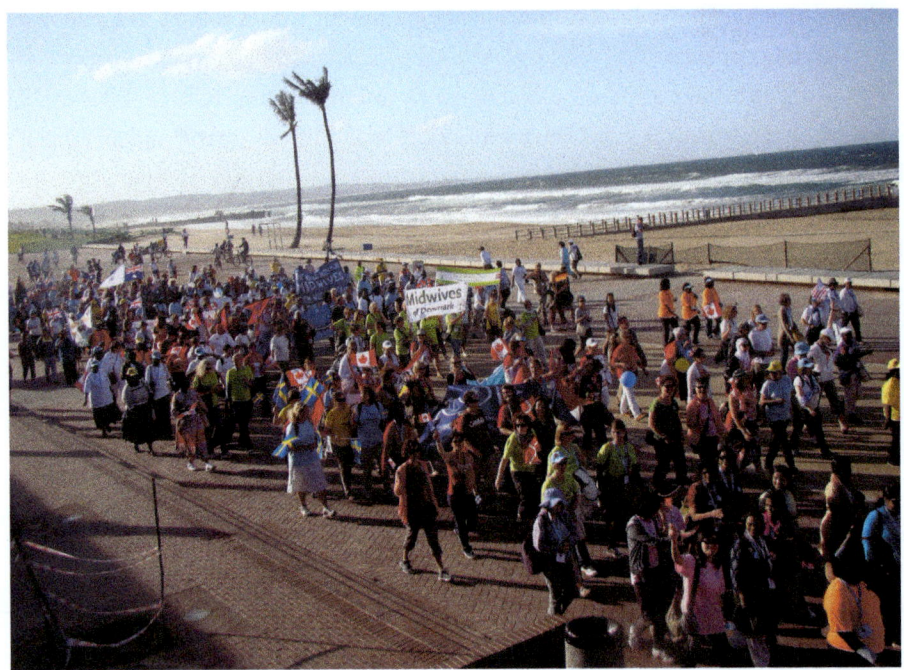

Durban walk for midwives (2011) – ICM Archives at Wellcome Collection

Evidence of the boldness of the global community to address what women and midwives need is reflected in the growing number of partners who have joined with the ICM in a 10-year effort called *PUSH for Midwives*. This campaign will push for more funding for more midwives, improved education, better pay and working conditions, more gender equality and increased respect and autonomy for the profession. Ten years sounds long, but ICM's leadership understands that it will take a concerted effort and investment to achieve the changes required to meet the campaign's goals. It is also timed specifically to end as the Sustainable Development Goals are targeted to be met by 2030:

> 'PUSH will accelerate progress on reducing maternal and neonatal mortality, advance SRHR, address key barriers to women's leadership in the global health workforce, and shift underlying gender norms that undervalue women's rights, lives and work.'[7]

ICM'S GLOBAL STRATEGY 2020–2023: THE WAY FORWARD

The 2021–2023 ICM strategy describes its main goal of *'positioning ICM as an expert in creating, advising, influencing and enabling the profession of midwifery globally'*. The ICM's autonomy is crucial to achieving this goal. Governance and operational reform is underway and as a learning organisation the ICM will need to remain agile. A shift to a smaller and less hierarchical competency-based Board, in addition to expanded regional support from the ICM Head Office, will help ICM's leaders to better respond to the context and needs of its MAs in each of its six Regions. Supporting MAs to strengthen themselves as well as diversifying ICM's income, including securing core funding and working in equal partnership with other stakeholders, is crucial for ICM's sustainability. Current core funding through the generous support of the Swedish International Development Cooperation Agency (SIDA) to implement ICM's 2020–2023 strategy has given the organisation breathing room and time to enable the necessary transformation of the ICM.

Even though direct entry midwifery education is the preferred path, there are also other paths to becoming a midwife in some countries, and what they all have in common is that midwifery is practised only by midwives. Midwives have a wide scope of practice, with pregnancy and birth at the core. Midwives' scope of practice differs globally, but the basic essential competencies are the same.[8] Midwifery has a specific philosophy and model of care.[9] This model of care is based on a perfect combination of head and heart. By facilitating an enabling environment for midwives, developing a new professional framework, working in a team with other health care professionals and partners and building on the current evidence while encouraging further research using gender disaggregated data that answers the questions that women and midwives want answered, the ICM will foster a stronger movement for midwifery, hand in hand with women.

SUMMARY[10]

Throughout its 100-year history, the International Confederation of Midwives has gone through many growth spurts with a few stumbles along the way. With perseverance, leadership and collaboration with other international health organisations, the ICM has not only survived but developed into a global organisation with a strong voice for and with women, midwives and global health.

100 Years of the International Confederation of Midwives

The ICM's mandate for the past 100 years has been to strengthen midwives and as a consequence the ICM has, through its members, improved the health of women and families and will continue to do so in the next 100 years. From direct entry midwifery programmes to nurse to midwife bridging programmes, most ICM regions have a mixed model, combining elements of multiple pathways in order to serve women and childbearing families. It is only with appreciation of the complex myriad factors that have shaped each region both past and present that midwifery can continue to progress. Autonomous midwifery guided by excellence in guidelines with the support of key partners MUST be the way forward if the Confederation hopes to make actual gains in the size, composition and diversity of the midwifery workforce and in improving health outcomes in all countries while strengthening the ICM as a strong voice for midwives and women's health.

As well-known author George Santayana wrote, 'Those who cannot remember the past are condemned to repeat it.'[11] Winston Churchill, in a speech before the British House of Commons in 1948, built upon Santayana's quote, noting, 'Those who fail to learn from History are condemned to repeat it.'[12]

Whatever reason for studying the history of the ICM one may have, it is hoped that the way forward for the ICM will build upon the successes of the past and lessons learnt while addressing the challenges identified. ICM's efforts to move forward as an international organisation filled with strong midwifery associations led by visionary international midwives, healthy women, men and other people and long-term collaborative partners is vital. No one organisation's efforts will result in Health for All – it takes everyone working together to achieve the best health outcomes for children, adolescents, women and men throughout the world.

100 Years of the International Confederation of Midwives

1 This chapter was contributed by the 2022 ICM President, Franka Cadée from the Netherlands.
2 'Midwife in Different Languages.' https://www.indifferentlanguages.com/words/midwife Accessed 4 May 2021.
3 UNFPA, ICM, WHO. *State of the World Midwifery report 2021*. https://www.unfpa.org/publications/sowmy-2021 Accessed 5 May 2021.
4 A Nove, IK Friberg, L de Bernis, F McConville, AC Moran, M Najjemba, ... and CS Homer. Potential impact of midwives in preventing and reducing maternal and neonatal mortality and stillbirths: a Lives Saved Tool modelling study. The Lancet Global Health, 9(1), 2021 e24–e32.
5 ICM. *ICM Triennial Strategy 2020-2023*. https://www.internationalmidwives.org/assets/files/general-files/2021/01/20212023-icm-strategic-plan-eng-ext_final.pdf , accessed 4 May 2021.
6 What women want. Whatwomenwant.org https://static1.squarespace.com/static/5aa813dd3917ee6dd2a0e09e/t/5d1120ccdf7cbc0001b99c57/1561403606693/What-Women-Want_Global-Findings.pdf , accessed 4 May 2021.
7 PUSH for Midwives. https://www.pushcampaign.org.
8 Essential Competencies for Midwifery Practice, 2019. https://www.internationalmidwives.org/our-work/policy-and-practice/essential-competencies-for-midwifery-practice.html, accessed 4 May 2021.
9 Philosophy and Model of Midwifery Care, ICM core document. Revised and adopted at Prague Council meeting, 2014. https://www.internationalmidwives.org/assets/files/general-files/2020/07/cd0005_v201406_en_philosophy-and-model-of-midwifery-care.pdf, accessed 4 May 2021.
10 The summary was written by the authors of the book, taking into account the entire 100-year story of the ICM.
11 George Santayana. *The Life of Reason: Reason in Common Sense*. New York: Scribner's, 1905, p 284.
12 Winston Churchill. Speech before House of Commons, 1948. Downloaded from Google.com – famous quotes from history, 8 June 2020.

Annex A

Member Association Issues and Resulting ICM Position Statements / Documents[1]

Time Period	Member Association Issue	ICM Position Statements, Core Document or Standard[2] Dates[3]
1920s–1930s	Safe birth practices Status of Midwives Protection of Motherhood Safety of Humanity Maternal Mortality	Protection of midwife from other professions – 1922 Discussion on length of midwifery programme – 1923 with no agreement Protection of maternity and protection of the families with many children, is the centre of all social questions – 1935 The Midwife in the Service of Peace – 1938 First paper on Maternal Mortality – 1938
1950s–1960s		
1970s–1980s	LRC Midwives unable to pay fees – twinning Length of MW education Safe Motherhood themes	*ICM Definition of the Midwife – 1972* Resolution on Breastfeeding – 1984

1990–1999[4]	Scope of practice Education and Regulation of Midwives Support of Mothers & Babies Partnerships with women and others sharing same vision and mission	Professional Accountability of the Midwife – 1990 Continuing Professional Education – 1990 Appropriate Education for Midwives – 1990 Appropriate Legislation for Midwives – 1990 Childbirth Practices – 1990 Planned Pregnancies & Parenthood – 1990 The Role of the Midwife in Research – 1990 Trade Displays – 1990 World Alliance for Breastfeeding Action Statement – 1992 ***ICM International Code of Ethics for Midwives – 1993*** ***ICM Mission Statement – 1993*** Appropriate Intervention in Childbirth – 1993 Home Birth – 1993 Women, Children & Midwives in Situations of War & Civil Unrest, HIV/AIDS – 1993 Policy-Making and Resource Allocation – 1993 Rights of Indigenous Women & Their Families – 1993 The Midwifery Partnership with Women – 1993 Breast Feeding – 1993 ***Global Vision for Women and Midwives – 1996*** Care of the Newborn – 1996 Care of Women Post Abortion – 1996 Trade Displays, Sponsorships – 1996 Consumer Consultation in Midwifery Legislation – 1999 Midwives, Women and Human rights – 1999 Protecting the Heritage of Indigenous People – 1999 The Role of the Midwife in Research – 1999 Women, Children and Midwives in Situations of War and Civil Unrest – 1999 Female Genital Mutilation – 1999 Sexually Transmitted Diseases – 1999 Human Immunodeficiency Virus/Acquired Immunodeficiency Syndrome (HIV/AIDS) – 1999 Prenatal Screening and Diagnosis –1999 Establishment of Networks or Advisory Panels on Aspects of Midwifery Practice, Education or Service Management – 1999
		Development of and Resource Allocation for Midwifery and Reproductive Health – 1999

2000–2010	MW education, regulation Autonomy of profession Continuity of MW care Balancing needs of HRC and LRC midwives to reduce MMR Promotion of Normal Birth Human Rights	***ICM Essential Competencies for Basic Midwifery Practice 2002*** Framework for Midwifery Legislation and Regulation – 2002 Ethical Recruitment of Midwives – 2002 The Promotion of Vaginal Birth in Preference to Caesarean Section in the Absence of Evidence-Based Clinical Criteria – 2002 Exclusive Breastfeeding and HIV Infection – 2002 Appropriate Maternity Services for Normal Pregnancy, Childbirth, and the Postnatal Period – 2002 Midwives and the Abuse of Women and Children – 2002 Positive Action to Reduce Smoking and Passive Smoking in Pregnancy – 2002 Qualifications and Competencies of Midwifery Teachers – 2002 Debt Cancellation and Other Economic Policies that Affect Health and Especially Safe Motherhood – 2002 Partnership between Women and Midwives – 2005 ***ICM Midwifery Philosophy and Model of Care – 2005*** Midwifery: An Autonomous Profession – 2005 ***ICM Vision and Mission – 2008*** Collaboration and Partnerships for Healthy Women and Infants – 2008 The Midwife is the First Choice Health Professional for Childbearing Women – 2008 Qualifications and Competencies of Midwifery Educators – 2008 ***ICM Global Standards for Midwifery Education with Guidelines, 2010***

2011–2020	Education, regulation, Association Strengthening MDGs 4,5,6 and SDGs Keeping birth normal Autonomy of Profession	***ICM Global Standards for Midwifery Regulation 2011*** *** ICM Glossary of Terms for Education – 2011 ICM Bill of Rights for Women and Midwives – 2011***
		Birth Registration, Impact of Climate Change – 2014 Partnerships Between Professional Midwives and Traditional Caregivers with Midwifery Skills – 2014 ICM Physiological Management of the Third Stage of Labour – 2017
		Migrants and Refugee Women and Their Families – 2017 Midwives and the Human Rights of Lesbian, Gay, Bisexual, Transgender, and Intersex People – 2017
		Role of Community Health Worker in Maternity Care – 2017 Use of Intermittent Auscultation for Assessment of Foetal Wellbeing during Labour – 2017
		ICM Definition of Midwifery – 2017

1 The dates given on the table reflect the first time MAs agreed the statement or document.
2 Core documents and/or standards are **bolded** in the table. Position statements are not bolded.
3 Attempts were made to list only the first date when a given position statement and Core Document was adopted by the ICM Council so that the ready could see the evolution of Member Association Issues by decade as reflected in the document of the time.
4 Wellcome Institute Library Uncatalogued Box 3. Not all position statements retained the historical sequence of when first adopted. Many of the later revisions eliminated any dates prior to 2000 and/or changed the name of the original document, making it somewhat difficult to trace the origins of each statement.

Annex B

Countries represented at each Conference / Congress / Meeting 1921–1938

(1921)[1] Bruges	1922 Ghent	1923 Antwerp	1925 Prague	1928[2] Vienna
Flanders	Belgium	Flanders Wallonia	Belgium	Belgium
England	England	England	England	England
Holland	Holland	Holland	Holland	Holland
		Czechoslovakia	Czechoslovakia	
	Switzerland*			
	Italy*		Italy	
			Bulgaria	Bulgaria
			Germany	Germany
			Austria	Austria
			Latvia	
			Poland	Poland
			Denmark	
				Hungary
				Prussia [b]
				Moravian[b]

1 1921 was the planning meeting for establishing the IMU.
2 Communications 1932, p 30. Countries in membership in 1928 England, Germany, Holland, Flemish, Poland, Hungarian, Denmark,
Yugoslavia, Latvia, Austria, Czechoslovakia.
3 Communications 7, 1935, p 34. Russia not in list of those being represented but they are reported to have asked a govt minister to
communicate with IMU.
  * sent apologies
  a 'unofficial'
  b asked to join IMU, Moravian organisation included Silezian and Slovakian midwives

100 Years of the International Confederation of Midwives

1932 Ghent	1934 London 300	1936 Berlin 200 + 1,000 German Midwives	1938 Paris 650/700
Belgium	Belgium	Belgium	Belgium
England	England	England	England
Holland	Holland	Holland	
Czechoslovakia	Czechoslovakia*	Czechoslovakia	Czechoslovakia
		Switzerland	Switzerland
	Italy	Italy	Italy
Bulgaria*		Bulgaria	Bulgaria
Germany	Germany	Germany	Germany
Austria	Austria	Austria	Austria*
Poland	Poland*	Poland	
Denmark*	Denmark	Denmark	Denmark
Yugoslavia*	Yugoslavia*	Yugoslavia	Yugoslavia
Hungary	Hungary	Hungary	
	Sweden	Sweden	Sweden
France[a]	France	France	France
	India (British)		
	Lithuania		
Lettland		Luxembourg	Luxembourg
Russia[3]		Estonia	Estonia
		Danzig	Danzig
		Finland	Finland*
		Spain*	Spain*
		Algeria	
		Ireland	
		Lithuania	Lithuania
		Roumania	

Annex C

Table of ICM Congresses and Themes 1954–2021

Location	Year	Theme
London, UK[1] (10th)	1954	**The Midwife – Her Education and Responsibilities**
Stockholm, Sweden (11th)	1957	**Theme: The Role of Midwives in Relation to Maternity Care**[2] <u>Sub-themes</u>: Psychological Aspects of Childbearing; Care of the Newborn; Pre-Natal and Post-Natal Exercises[3]
Rome, Italy (12th)	1960	**The Midwife in the World of the Future**[4]
Madrid, Spain (13th)	1963	**The Function of the Midwife in the World Today**[5]
Berlin, Germany (14th)	1966	**The Midwife — Her Education and Responsibilities**[6]
Santiago, Chile[7] (15th)	1969 3–7 November	**The Midwife's Role in a National Programme for Maternity and Child Care**[8]
Washington DC, USA (16th) 50th Anniversary of ICM	1972 October 28–November 3 $70,000 profit	**New Horizons in Midwifery**[9] <u>Sub-themes</u>: Midwife's role in Family Planning; care of mother during labour and birth; infant nutrition including breastfeeding
Lausanne, Switzerland (17th)	1975 21–28 June	**The Midwife and the Family in the World Today**
Jerusalem, Israel (18th)	1978 3–8 September	**Midwives: The Key to Human Prosperity**

Brighton, England (19th)	1981	**Today's Midwife Tomorrow** Sub-themes: The midwife as clinician; the midwife as educator; the midwives as counsellor
Sydney, Australia (20th)	1984	**Midwives, Families, Nations, and the World** Sub-Themes: Midwifery in the Western Pacific; Educating a Nation's Midwives; Choices of Practice; The Search for Knowledge; and Towards the Year 2000
The Hague, The Netherlands (21st)	1987	**Midwives Hold the Key to Healthy Families**
Kobe, Japan (22nd)	1990 $150,000 profit	**A Midwife's Gift Love, Skill and Knowledge** Sub-Themes: Midwifery Practice in the World; Midwives and Bio-ethics; Midwives and technology; Midwifery education and research
Vancouver, British Columbia, Canada (23rd)	1993	**Midwives Hear the Heartbeat of the Future** Sub-Themes: New visions of midwifery, knowledge, research; Safe Motherhood Initiatives
Oslo, Norway (24th)	1996	**The Art and Science of Midwifery gives Birth to a Better Future** Sub-Themes: Reproductive and Infant Health; Cultural differences in childbirth practice and midwifery; Psychological aspects of childbirth; Midwifery education, research and leadership
Manila, Philippines[10] (25th)	1999	**Safe Motherhood: Beyond the Year 2000** Sub-Themes: Women's health promotion; Infants & children's health promotion; Safe Motherhood; Communicable diseases; Midwifery education; Counselling

Location	Year	Theme
Vienna, Austria (26th)	2002	**Midwives and Women together for the Family of the World.** Sub-themes: Research; Education; Care for the Caregiver; Special Issues
Brisbane, Australia (27th)	2005	**Midwifery: Pathways to Healthy Nations** Sub-themes: History; Professionalisation; Current ways of Knowing, Diversity of Thought; Future-Healthy Nations, SM Partnerships, Multi-dimensional Aspects of Health
Glasgow, Scotland (28th)	2008	**Midwifery: a worldwide commitment to women & newborns:** Sub-themes: Women's voices; Appropriate use of reproductive & birth technology in maternal & newborn health; Strengthening midwifery; Promoting the health of women and families; Ethics & philosophy daily
Durban, South Africa[11] (29th)	2011	**Midwives Tackling the 'Big 5' Globally** Sub-themes: Globalisation; Listening to Women and their Partners; the Continuum of Care; Strengthening Midwives and Midwifery Practice; Culture, Society and Traditions
Prague, Czech Republic (30th)	2014	**Midwives: Improving Women's Health Globally** Sub-Themes: Bridging midwifery and women's health rights; Access: bridging the gap to improving care and outcomes for women and their families; Education: The bridge to midwifery and women's autonomy; Midwifery: bridging culture and practice
Toronto, Canada (31st)	2017	**Midwives – Making a difference in the world** Sub-themes: Midwives as Partners; Teachers; Researchers; Leaders

100 Years of the International Confederation of Midwives

Bali, Indonesia (32nd)	2020[12] Pandemic resulted in postponement until 2023 in person; held as a virtual Congress in June 2021	**Midwives of the World: Delivering the Future.** Sub-themes: Midwives protect the future through up to date competencies; Midwives invest in the future through women and family centred quality care; Midwives advocate for the future through effective empowerment; Midwives secure the future through strong regulatory mechanisms
Bali, Indonesia (33rd)	2023	**Together again from evidence to reality**

1 First ICM Congress after WWII. The decision to have triennial congresses was taken in 1936 but was not activated until 1954.
2 Ruth Coates & Marion Strachan. The Eleventh International Congress of Midwives. *Bulletin Nurse-Midwives* 2:3, September 1957, p 41. Lucille Woodville. Historical Background on International Confederation of Midwives. *Bulletin Nurse-Midwives* XVI: 2, May 1971, p 27.
3 'Hattie Hemschemeyer Represents U.S. Nurse-Midwives at Congress.' *Bulletin Nurse-Midwives* 2: 2 April 1957, p 24, list the Professional Programme of International Confederation of Midwives 11th International Congress, Stockholm, 23–28 June 1957. ICM (SA/ICM/R/4). Wellcome Collection. Marjorie Bayes. *History of Midwifery 1st 50 years*.
4 ICM (SA/ICM/R/4). Wellcome Collection. Marjorie Bayes. *History of Midwifery 1st 50 years*. Lucille Woodville. Historical Background on International Confederation of Midwives. *Bulletin Nurse-Midwives* XVI: 2, May 1971, p 27.
5 Lucille Woodville. Historical Background on International Confederation of Midwives. *Bulletin Nurse-Midwives* XVI: 2, May 1971, p 27.
6 Lucille Woodville. Historical Background on International Confederation of Midwives. *Bulletin Nurse-Midwives* XVI: 2, May 1971, p 27.
7 First ICM Congress outside of Europe.
8 Lucille Woodville. Historical Background on International Confederation of Midwives. *Bulletin Nurse-Midwives* XVI: 2, May 1971, p 27.
9 ICM (SA/ICM/M1-1). Wellcome Collection. *Joint Study Group 1970–1980*. Katherine Kendall. Sixteenth International Confederation of Midwives Congress. *Journal of Nurse-Midwifery* XVIII:1, Spring 1973, pp 26–27.
10 This was the first time an ICM Council and Triennial Congress was held in a Low Resource Country (LRC).
11 This was the first time an ICM Council and Triennial Congress was held on African continent.
12 Bali Congress 2020 postponed due to COVID-19 pandemic; was held virtually in June 2021.

Annex D

Table of ICM Partners and Projects 1951–2022

Organisation	Areas of Interest	Date Began
Long-Term Partners		
World Health Organization (WHO)	Maternal, Child Health & Primary Care Midwifery education Pre-Congress Workshops (1987–2005) Triennial workplan with WHO Liaison (1981–2023) *State of the World's Midwifery* Reports (2011, 2014, 2021) *Midwives' Voices, Midwives' Realities* (2016) *Framework for Action: Strengthening Quality Midwifery Education for Universal Health Coverage 2030* (2019)	1951
International Federation of Gynecology and Obstetrics (FIGO)	Women's health FIGO/ICM Joint Study Group Pre-Congress Workshops Fistula repair, Prevention PP Haemorrhage, Non-medical gender-based sex selection joint statements Emergency Obstetric Care; Life Saving Skills	1961
International Pediatric Association[1]	Offered advisers to working parties 'Ten Steps' as IPA/FIGO/ICM principles for maternal & infant care[2] (May 1992) (Complemented breast-feeding 10 steps) PMNCH Health Professional Group (2005–present)	1974
International Council of Nurses (ICN)	ICM welcomed ICN statement on Family Planning policy[3] Nursing and nurses[4] (1995) CEO Network – Petra (2000) Joint Statements Triad & Regulation Meetings WHA Resolutions on Nursing & Midwifery Global Advisory Group on Nursing & Midwifery	1974

United Nations Children's Fund (UNICEF)	Child and Maternal Health support Breastfeeding Joint statement Pre-Congress Workshops *Midwifery Education for Universal Health Coverage 2030* (2019)	1984
United Nations Fund for Population Assistance (UNFPA)	Midwives and Safe Motherhood Pre-Congress Workshops (1993–2005) Support for LRC midwives at 1972 Congress Investing in Midwives Project (2009–2013) State of the World's Midwifery Reports (2011, 2014, 2021) Strengthening Midwifery Services (2017–2018) ICM Mentoring Guidelines for Midwives 2020[5] (2019) Annual Workplan with ICM (2018) *Midwifery Education for Universal Health Coverage 2030* (2019)	1993
Governmental International Aid Organisations		
United States	USAID funding ICM/FIGO Joint Study Group Working Parties (1972–1979) USAID sub-contracts to Jhpiego – MNH (2001) Meeting of the Minds Midwives Voices, Midwives' Realities (2016)	1972
United Kingdom	Charity Status (1983–1999) DFID funding of Anglophone African workshops	1983
Australia	AUSAID funding New Delhi Mid-Triennium Meeting	1998
The Netherlands	Dutch Ministry of Foreign Affairs (2002–2007)	2002
Sweden	The Swedish International Development Cooperation Agency (SIDA) funded strengthening midwives and midwifery globally for the achievement of MDGs 4 & 5; 2020–2023 for support of ICM's core activities	2009

Germany	Federal Ministry for Economic Cooperation and Development Shifted the venue of activities to Tanzania, another GIZ priority country to help facilitate south-to-south collaboration between the associations in the two countries	2014
Project Specific Partners		
International Planned Parenthood Federation (IPPF)	Close contact, observers at our working parties and officers visited HQ; paid for midwives from several Caribbean territories to working party in Barbados; Miss Bayes Brighton conference 1973, Mr Fenney attending meeting in Bucharest[6] Family Planning services	1974
International Association for Maternal and Neonatal Health (IAMANEH)	Supported FIGO/ICM/IAMANEH workshop[7] 26 Feb 1992	1991
The Rockefeller Foundation	Mid-Triennium Workshop in Ghana	1989
White Ribbon Alliance	Launched at ICM Congress in Manila, Philippines Shared Board members Memorandum of Collaboration (2006/2010)[8] *Midwives' Voices, Midwives' Realities* publication with WHO and ICM (2016)	1999
American Academy of Paediatrics	'Helping Babies Survive'[9]	
United Nations AIDS Programme (UNAIDS)	Women and family health Pre-Congress Workshop on HIV/AIDS	1999
Family Care International (FCI)	IAG-Safe Motherhood secretariat Skilled Birth Attendance – Tunisia meeting Regional SM workshops	1999

Interagency Group on Safe Motherhood (IAG-SM) Partnership for Safe Motherhood & Newborn Health (PSMNH) Partnership for Maternal, Newborn, Child Health (PMNCH)	Maternal, Newborn and Child Health Supported ICM representative to meetings Joint Statement: 'Health Professional Groups Key to Reaching MDGs 4 & 5' (2005) 'Essential Interventions Project' with FIGO, WHO and ICM (2013)	1999
Johnson & Johnson: Consumer, Inc.; Baby; J&J International	Gold sponsor Triennial Congresses (2002–2021) Workshops held during Triennial Congresses ICM research education and leadership awards (2016) Young Midwifery Leaders programme (2016–2018)	1999
Johns Hopkins Programme for International Education of Gynaecology and Obstetrics (JHPIEGO) Maternal and Neonatal Health (MNH)	Maternal and Neonatal Health Midwifery education Field-testing of Essential Competencies (2000) Meeting of the Minds (2001) Funding midwives to Zimbabwe mid-Triennium workshop (2001) 'Helping Mothers Survive' training modules[10]	2000
United Nations Commission for Human Rights (UNCHR)	Women's rights and women's health Pre-Congress Workshop on Violence Against Women	2002
Sanofi Espoir Foundation [France]	Small grants programme: **A Midwife for Every Mother and Baby** Strengthening Midwifery Education in French-speaking Africa (2015–2019) CBE Workshops, Mentoring educators	2013
Direct Relief	ICM/Direct Relief Mapping Tool Distribution of Midwives Kits (2013–2019)	2013

Laerdal Global Health	Prepared Trainers Helping Mothers Survive Bleeding after Birth (HMS-BAB), and Helping Babies Breathe (HBB) (2013) 10,000 Happy Birthdays (2014–2017) 50,000 Happy Birthdays program[11] (2018–2020) Congress sponsor	2013
Bill & Melinda Gates Foundation	Subcontract with Integrare – *SoWMY Report 2014* Expanding Quality Midwifery Services (2015–2017) Development & testing MEAP In-country testing of Midwifery Services Framework Strengthening Midwifery Services (SMS) (2018–2021) MSF Phase 2; Update MACAT; MEAP; MEDPath; ICM's *Global Midwifery Competency Assessment Tool*	2013
MacArthur Foundation	Strengthening Midwifery Associations in Mexico (11/2016–5/2018) Raising profile of Midwifery through advocacy and multi-stakeholder collaboration (2018–2020)	2016
New Venture Fund	Respectful Care by and for midwives (with UNFPA) Advocacy skills for midwives (with UNFPA)	2017

1 ICM (SA/ICM/C/1/18/1). Wellcome Collection. Secretaries report: Executive *Committee, Helsinki, Finland, 10–13 March 1974*.
2 ICM (SA/ICM/H7-10 (2 of 3). Wellcome Collection. *Joan Walker letter to Board of Management*, 30 October 1992.
3 ICM (SA/ICM/C/1/18/1). Wellcome Collection. S*ecretaries report: Executive Committee, Helsinki, Finland, 10–13 March 1974*.
4 ICM (SA/ICM/C/1/22). Wellcome Collection. *Executive Committee*, Uganda, 11 January 1995. ICN invited ICM to meet for two days in March 1995 to discuss nursing and midwifery related subjects. Invitation accepted.
5 ICM & UNFPA. *Mentoring Guidelines for Midwives 2020*. The Hague: ICM, 2019.
6 ICM (SA/ICM/C/1/18/1). Wellcome Collection. *Secretaries report, Executive Committee, Helsinki, Finland*, 10–13 March 1974.
7 ICM (SA/ICM/H-7-8). Wellcome Collection. *Joan Walker Correspondence for workshop*.
8 *Letter to Theresa Shaver, President WRA from Agneta Bridges, ICM SG, dated 2 February 2010*. The letter stated that the ICM Executive Committee approved the Memorandum of Collaboration with White Ribbon Alliance in December 2009; The attach MOC was signed 4 February 2010, but the Duration section stated that the Memorandum would take effect December 2006 when the discussions began originally. It is possible that the final MOC was not checked for dates.
9 Helping Babies Survive (HBS) is a suite of programmes developed by the America Academy of Pediatrics and based on the latest WHO Guidelines. The training programmes include Helping Babies Breathe, Essential Care for Every Baby and Essential Care for Small Babies.
10 Helping Mothers Survive (HMS) is a suite of programmes developed by Jhpiego, in line with the latest WHO guidelines and endorsed by global professional organisation such as ICM, FIGO, AAP, ICN and UNFPA.
11 ICM Website: downloaded 9 February 2021. Laerdal supported the ICM directed project with other partners in Ethiopia, Rwanda and Tanzania led by the national midwifery associations. Used the Jhpiego programme Helping Mothers Survive (HMS), the American Academy of Pediatrics simulation programs of Helping Babies Survive (HBS) and Helping Babies Breathe (HBB) and Low Dose High Frequency (LDHF) approach for skills development.

Annex E
Wording of Objects/Aims in Constitutions of the IMU/ICM 1925–2022

Year	Wording of Aims/Objectives[1]
1925 1928	'contribution to the appropriate institution of the protection of <u>maternity and baby nursing</u>, by means of the scientifical, ethical and social elevation of the standing of the midwife.'[2]
1934	'The International Federation of Midwives has for its object the protection of the <u>mother</u> and <u>child</u>. With this object in view the efforts and activities of the Federation shall at the same time be directed towards the scientific, moral, social and economic improvement of the profession of the midwife.'[3]
1954	'The purpose of the Confederation shall be to assist the National Groups in working together for the purpose of promoting <u>family</u> health, improving the standard of maternal care and advancing the training and professional status of midwives.'[4]
1981	'aims to advance education in midwifery and spread knowledge of the art and science of midwifery with the aim of improving the standard of care provided to <u>mothers</u> and <u>babies</u> and the family, throughout the countries of the world.'[5]
1993	'will advance worldwide the aims and aspirations of midwives in the attainment of improved outcomes for <u>women</u> in their childbearing years, <u>their newborn</u> and their families wherever they reside.'[6]
1996	'to advance education in midwifery and spread knowledge of the art and science of midwifery with the aim of improving the standard of care provided to <u>mothers</u> and <u>babies</u> and the family, throughout the countries of the world; to support and advise, when required, associations of midwives in liaison with their governments; to advance the provision of maternity care and to develop the role of the midwife as a professional practitioner in her own right.'[7]

1999[8]	'to advance education in midwifery, to promote world-wide the aims and aspirations of midwives and to attain improved outcomes for <u>women</u> in their childbearing years, their <u>newborn</u> and their families, wherever they reside.'[9]
2005[10]–2022	'to advance worldwide the goals and aspirations of midwives in the attainment of improved outcomes for <u>women</u>, their <u>newborns</u> and families during the <u>childbearing cycle</u>, using the ICM midwifery philosophy and model of care.'[11]

1. The terms 'mothers, women, child, babies' and 'newborns' are underlined to illustrate the change in thinking of ICM Council members over the years about the focus of ICM activities. 'Family' was initially in 1954 and added back in 1981.
2. IMU. *Communications of the International Midwives' Union*, 8, 1936, p 61
3. IMU. *Communications of the International Union of Midwives*, 8, 1936, p 61.
4. ICM. *The International Confederation of Midwives Constitution Agreed by Council on September 10th, 1954*. [Personal papers of Helen Varney Burst] To be sent to the Wellcome Library ICM archives.
5. ICM. Margaret Peters noted that the 1981 Constitution was redrafted as a key action taken to address the financial crisis. In addition, it more clearly identified the lines of authority and responsibilities of a smaller decision-body in between Triennial Council meetings, notably a three-member Board of Management. 'It introduced the reduced size of the Board and led to the relocation of the HQ from the palatial sized one to the attic of Sloane Street [London]. Plus, of course, the part time employee to keep it ticking over so bankruptcy was averted and charity status retained.' Written note to J Thompson, 4 April 2020.
6. Nester M Moyo. *International Young Midwifery Leaders Programme proposal*. December 2003. [Personal papers of Joyce Thompson]
7. ICM. *Constitution of the International Confederation of Midwives*. Registered Charity No. 326297; ICM: 10 Barley Mow, Chiswick, London, 1996, Article 3, p 1. ICM. *Notice to Member Associations from ICM HQ reported on the four resolutions withdrawn at the May 1996 Council meeting*. During the 1996 council meeting, it was noted that minor amendments were made to the ICM Constitution in 1987, 1990 and 1993 (notes at end of 1993 Constitution), and that the 1996 Council asked and the BOM agreed that a major review and redrafting of the Constitution was needed to represent the aims and global strategy more accurately. The 1996–1999 triennium resulted in a major exchange of ideas and suggested redrafts, and a full day was given during the 1999 Council meeting to further discuss and agree the changes to the ICM Constitution at the same time the decision on moving ICM HQ to the Netherlands was made. However, the UK Constitution remained active for an additional time until the Dutch government accepted ICM as an official organisation.
8. This was first Constitution considered under Dutch law as the move to the Netherlands occurred end of 1999. However, this Constitution was actually approved under UK charity status as the Dutch government had yet to officially approve ICM as an organisation. The Charity Commissioners agreed to continue to support ICM until such time as the organisation was approved by the Dutch government (2004).
9. ICM. *Constitution*. Eisenhowerlaan 138, 2517 KN The Hague, The Netherlands, 1999, 3, p 1.
10. ICM. *Minutes of ICM Council, Brisbane, Australia*. 18–21 July 2005. MIN 05.23 ICM Legal Issues p 20.
11. ICM. *Final draft Constitution* (11-03), approved with revision 4/20/04. Translated Deed of Recording of the ICM Constitution under Dutch law. No change in aims and objects noted throughout next decade.

Annex F

Table of ICM Appointed and Elected Officers 1954–2023

Triennium[1]	Appointed Presidents	Appointed Vice Presidents	Appointed Treasurers
1954	Miss Nora B Deane (UK)	Miss Ellen Erup (Sweden)	
1957	Miss Ellen Erup (Sweden)	Madame Luzzi (Italy)	
1960	Madame Jay[2] (France)	Srta Maria Garcia Martin (Spain)	
1963	Srta Maria Garcia Martin (Spain)	Frau Anne Springborn (Germany)	
1966	Frau Anne Springborn (Germany)	Olga Julio de Mellado (Chile)	
1969	Olga Julio de Mellado (Chile)	Lucille Woodville (USA)	Miss N B Deane (UK)
1972	Lucille Woodville (USA)	Georgette Grossenbacher (Switzerland)	
1974	Georgette Grossenbacher (Switzerland)	Rachel Reches (Israel)	
1978	Rachel Reches (Israel)	Winfred A Andrews (UK)	Betty Knox (UK) Margaret Brain (UK) August 1977–1981
1981[3]	Winfred A Andrews (UK)	Margaret H Peters (Australia)	As of 1981, the Treasurer was elected as part of the Board of Management.

381

1981–1984	Margaret H Peters (Australia)	Filippa Lugtenburg (Netherlands)	
1984–1987	Filippa Lugtenburg (Netherlands)	Sumiko Maehara (Japan)	
1987–1990	Sumiko Maehara (Japan)	Carol Hird (British Colombia)	
1990–1993	Carol Hird (British Colombia)	Sonja Irene Sjøli (Norway)	
1993–1996	Sonja Irene Sjøli (Norway)	Alice Sanz de la Gente (Philippines)	
1996–1999	Alice Sanz de la Gente (Philippines)	Maria Spernbauer (Austria)	
1999–2002	Maria Spernbauer (Austria)	Caroline Weaver (Australia)	
2002–2005	Caroline Weaver (Australia)	Dame Karlene Davis (UK)	
2005–2008[4]	Dame Karlene Davis (UK)	As of 2008, the ICM managed Congresses with Host Association, but no appointed Vice President	

	Elected Directors[5]	Elected Deputy Directors	Elected Treasurers
1981–1984	Karin Christiani (Sweden)	Georgette Grossenbacher (Switzerland)	Margaret Brain (UK)
1984–1987	Karin Christiani (Sweden)	Margaret Peters (Australia)	Margaret Brain (UK)
1987–1990	Karin Christiani (Sweden)	Helga Schweitzer (Germany)	Margaret Brain (UK)
1990–1993	Margaret Peters (Australia)	Helga Schweitzer (Germany)	Sr Anne Thompson (UK)
1993–1996	Margaret Peters (Australia)	Joyce Thompson (USA)	Sr Anne Thompson[6] – 12/94 (UK) V Ruth Bennett 9/94–96

1996–1999	Margaret Peters (Australia)	Joyce Thompson (USA)	Julia Allison (UK)[7] Ruth Ashton (UK) 19 Oct 1997–May 1999
1999–2002	Joyce Thompson (USA)	Judith Brown (Australia)	Ruth Ashton (UK)
2002–2005	Joyce Thompson (USA)	Judith Brown (Australia)	Franka Cadée (Netherlands)
2005–2008	Judith Brown (Australia)	Bridget Lynch (Canada)	Franka Cadée (Netherlands)
	Elected President	Elected Vice President	Elected Treasurer
2008–2011	Bridget Lynch (Canada)	Frances Day-Stirk (UK)	Marian van Huis (Netherlands)
2011–2014	Frances Day-Stirk (UK)	Debrah Lewis (Trinidad)	Marian van Huis (Netherlands)
2014–2017	Frances Day-Stirk (UK)	Address Malata (Malawi)	Myrte de Geus[8] (Netherlands) Ingela Wiklund (Sweden)
2017–2020	Franka Cadée (Netherlands)	Mary Kirk (Australia)	Ingela Wiklund (Sweden)
2020–2023	Franka Cadée (Netherlands)	Sandra Oyarzo (Chile)	Vitor Varela (Portugal)

The dates of early officers were those found in the Wellcome Institute Library

100 Years of the International Confederation of Midwives

1 The decision to have triennial congresses was taken in 1936 but was not activated until 1954 reflected in Constitutional revisions.
2 ICM Vice-President Madame Jay covered the 1990 Rome Congress as Madame Luzzi was ill and dying.
3 The ICM Constitution of 1981 changed from honorary Officers to Council-elected individuals in the roles of Director, Deputy Director and Treasurer (Board of Management). The Association hosting the congress 6 years out became the Honorary Vice-President for 3 years, then President for three years, ending her term as the Congress host.
4 During the 2005 ICM Council, the positions of Director and Deputy Director were re-titled to an elected President and Vice President. At this time, the positions of appointed ICM President and Vice President related to hosting a Congress were eliminated.
5 Under the Constitutional revision in 1981, the Board of Management was established, with those three midwives elected by the entire ICM Council every triennium. Those individuals served from the end of the Triennial Congress when elected until the end of the next Triennial Congress, unless re-elected. See Table of ICM Congresses and Presidents for complete list of Honorary Presidents from 1987 to 2008, when the elected President, Vice-President and Treasurer replaced the Director, Deputy Director and Treasurer. The Honorary President role as host of the Triennial Congress was eliminated in 2008.
6 ICM. *Letter from Miss Joan Walker to All Member Associations 9 June 1994*, announcing that Sister Anne Thompson, Treasurer of the Confederation since 1990, is resigning as Treasurer in order to take up a post with the World Health Organization.
7 Margaret Peters. *Letter to All Member Associations. 20 June 1997*, pp 1–2. This letter informed ICM MAs that Julia Allison, who was elected Treasurer of ICM in Oslo in May 1996, resigned her position in June 1997 as 'she has resigned from the midwifery association of which she was a member, which makes her ineligible to continue in the position of Treasurer of the Confederation.' In accord with the ICM Constitution clause 38(i)b, the vacancy was to be filled by the candidate who polled the next highest number votes at the last election, and that was Miss V Ruth Bennett. Because of other commitments Miss Bennett could not take up the Treasurer position in June, so nominations for this position were requested from Member Associations. Ruth Ashton was nominated and voted in on October 1997.
8 Myrte de Geus was elected treasurer in 2014 and resigned for personal reasons. Ingela Wiklund was appointed Interim Treasurer April 2016-June 2017.

Annex G

Tables of ICM Member Associations by Region
1954–2021
ICM Anglophone Africa Region
Country, Name and Year Midwifery Associations Accepted for ICM Membership

Country	Name of Association	Year
Ghana	Gold Coast Midwives Association (GCMA)[1] Ghana Registered Midwives Association (GRMA)	1954 1982*
Nigeria	National Association of Nigerian Nurses and Midwives (NANNM)	1957; 2014*
Sierra Leone	Sierra Leone Midwives Association	1969; 1982*
Nigeria	Professional Association of Midwives of Nigeria (PAMON)	1981
Zimbabwe	Zimbabwe Midwives Group	1981
Liberia	Liberian Midwives Association	1982*
Ethiopia	The Ethiopian Midwives Association	1990*
Uganda	Uganda Private Midwives Association	1990*
Tanzania	Tanzania Registered Midwives Association (TAMA)	1992*
Gambia	The Gambia Midwives' Association	1993*
South Africa	Genootskap vir Vroedvroue in Suidelike Afrika [The Society for Midwives of South Africa]	1994*
Zimbabwe	Zimbabwe Confederation of Midwives	1997*
Malawi	The Association of Malawian Midwives (AMAMI)	1998*
Kenya	Midwives' Chapter of National Nurses Association of Kenya	2008

100 Years of the International Confederation of Midwives

Country	Name of Association	Year
Uganda	Uganda National Association for Nurses & Midwives (UNANM); now Uganda Nurses and Midwives Union (UNMU)	2008*
Zambia	Midwives Association of Zambia (MAZ)	2011*
Lesotho	Independent Midwives Association Lesotho	2011*
Rwanda	Rwanda Association of Midwives (RAM)	2014*
Namibia	Independent Midwives Association of Namibia	2015*
Kenya	Midwives Association of Kenya (MAK)	2016*
South Sudan	South Sudan Nurses and Midwives Association	2019*

* ICM members in 2021; where two dates given = membership lapse.

ICM Francophone Africa Region
Country, Name and Year Midwifery Associations Accepted for ICM Membership

Country	Name of Association	Year
Burkina Faso	Association Burkinabé des Sages-Femmes et Maïeuticiens (ABSF/M) [Burkina Association of Midwives]	1982*
Benin	Association des Sages-Femmes du Bénin [Association of Midwives of Benin]	1992*
Mali	Association des Sages-Femmes du Mali (ASFM) [Association of Midwives of Mali]	2001*
Mozambique	Associaçao de Parteiras de Moçambique [Association of Midwives of Mozambique]	2006*
Senegal	Association Nationale des Sages-Femmes du Sénégal [National Association of Midwives of Senegal]	2007*
Gabon	Association des Sages-femmes du Gabon [Association of Midwives of Gabon]	2010*
Cameroun	Association des Sages Femmes et Assimilés du Cameroun ASFAC	2010*

Burundi	Association Burundaise des Sages-Femmes d'Etat (ABUSAFE) [Burundian Association of State Midwives]	2011*
Madagascar	Fédération Nationale des Sages-Femmes de Madagascar	2011*
Ivory Coast	Association des Sages-Femmes Ivoiriennes (ASFI) [Association of Ivorian Midwives]	2012*
Chad	Association Tchadienne des Sages-Femmes	2013*
Togo	Association de Sages-Femmes du Togo (ASSAFETO)	2013*
Comoros	Fédération Nationale des Associations des Sages-Femmes et Accoucheurs aux Comores	2014*
Niger	Association des Sages-Femmes du Niger (ASFN) [Midwives Association of Niger]	2014*
Dem. Republic of the Congo	Société Congolaise de Pratique de Sages-Femme	2015*
Dem. Republic of the Congo	Association Nationale des Sages-Femmes du Congo	2017*
Guinea Republic	Association Nationale des Sages-Femmes de Guinée (ASFEGUI)	2015*
Central Africa	Association des Sages-Femmes et Infirmiers accoucheurs de Centrafrique (ASFIACA)	2020
Burundi	The Midwife in Action's Association (MAA)	2021

*= ICM members in 2021; where two dates are given = membership lapse.

ICM North America & Caribbean Region of Americas
Country, Name and Year Midwifery Associations Accepted for ICM Membership

Country	Name of Association	Year
United States of America (USA)	American College of Nurse-Midwifery (ACNM) American Association of Nurse-Midwives (AANM)	1956 1956
Jamaica	Jamaica Midwives' Association (JMA)	1966; 1981*
USA	American College of Nurse-Midwives (ACNM)[2]	1969*
USA	Midwives Alliance of North America (MANA): International Section	1981*
Canada	Midwifery Association of British Colombia (MABC)	1982
Canada	Association of Ontario Midwives (AOM)	1984
Trinidad & Tobago	Trinidad & Tobago Association of Midwives (TTAM)	1990
Canada	Association des Sages-Femmes Diplômés du Québec Regroupement Les Sages-Femmes du Québec (RSFQ) [Group of Midwives of Quebec]	1990
Canada	Alberta Association of Midwives (AAM)	1991
Barbados	Barbados Nurses Association: Midwives Group	(1998)2002*
Canada	Canadian Association of Midwives (CAM)[3]	2002*
Haiti	Association des Infirmières Sages-Femmes d'Haïti (AISFH) [Association of Nurse Midwives of Haiti]	2006*
Suriname	Suriname Organization of Midwives (SOM)	2006–2019*
Guyana	Midwives Association of Guyana (MAG)	2012*
USA	National Association of Certified Professional Midwives (NACPM)	2014*

*= ICM members in 2021; where two dates are given = membership lapse.

ICM Latin America & Mexico Region of Americas
Country, Name and Year Midwifery Associations Accepted for ICM Membership

Country	Name of Association	Year
Chile	Colegio de Matronas de Chile AG [College of Midwives of Chile]	1969; 1982*
Paraguay	Federación Paraquaya de Obstetras Name change: Asociación de Obstetras del Paraguay (A.O.P.) [Midwives Association of Paraguay]	1981*
Brazil	Associação Brasileira de Obstetrizes e Enfermeiros Obstetras (ABENFO) [Association of Nurses & Midwives of Brazil]	1982; 2010*
Ecuador	Asociación de Obstetrices de Salud Pública [Association of Public Health Midwives]	1996
Argentina	Colegio De Obstétricas De La Provincia De Buenos Aires (COPBA) [College of Midwives of the Province of Buenos Aires]	1999*
Peru	Colegio de Obstetras del Peru [College of Midwives of Peru (CMP)]	2003; 2005*
Ecuador	Federación Nacional de Obstétricas y Obstetras del Ecuador (FENOE) [National Federation of Midwives of Ecuador]	2005*
Uruguay	Asociación Obstétrica del Uruguay (AOU) [Midwives Association of Uruguay]	2010*
Costa Rica	Asociación de Profesionales de Enfermería Obstétrica de Costa Rica (APEOCR) [Association of Nurse-Midwives of Costa Rica]	2019*
Mexico	Asociación de Parteras Profesionales (APP) [Association of Professional Midwives]	2019*

*=ICM members in 2021; where two dates given = membership lapse.

100 Years of the International Confederation of Midwives

ICM Asia–Pacific Region
Country, Name and Year Midwifery Associations Accepted for ICM Membership

Country	Name of Association	Year
Australia	Australian College of Midwives, Inc (ACMI)	1972*
Indonesia	Indonesian Midwives Association	1979*
Sarawak	Sarawak Midwives Association (SMA)	1980*
Hong Kong	Hong Kong Midwives Association (HKMA)	1981*
Japan	Japanese Midwives Association (JMA)	1966; 1981*
Japan	Midwives Division, Japanese Nursing Association, (JNA)	1981*
New Zealand	New Zealand College of Midwives (NZCOM)	1981*
Philippines	Integrated Midwives' Association of the Philippines, Inc (IMAP)	1981*
Taiwan	Midwives' Association of the Republic of China (MARC) as of 1999 Name change: Taiwan Midwives Association	1982*
Korea	Korean Midwives Association	1982*
Japan	Japan Academy of Midwives (JAM)	1989*
Sri Lanka	Government Midwifery Service Union of Sri Lanka Government Midwifery Service Association in 1999 Sri Lanka Nurse Midwives Association (SLNMA) 2021	1992*
Cambodia	Cambodia Midwives Association (CMA)	1995*
Philippines	National Capital Region Midwives Association, Inc. (NCRMA)	1996*
Vietnam	Vietnam Association of Midwives (VAM)	1996
India	Society of Midwives of India (SMI)	2003*
Papua New Guinea	Papua New Guinea Midwifery Society (PNGMS)	2006*
China	Zhenjiang Midwives' Association	2009

Mongolia	Mongolian Midwives Association (MMA)	2010*
Philippines	Philippine League of Government & Private Midwives, Inc (PLGPMI)	2011*
Sri Lanka	Sri Lanka Nurse Midwives Association Government	2011*
Bangladesh	Bangladesh Midwifery Society	2011*
Kyrgyzstan Republic	Kyrgyz Alliance of Midwives (KAM)	2014*
Tajikistan	Tajikistan National Association (TNA)	2014*
Timor Leste	Associação das Parteiras de Timor-Leste Midwives Association of Timor-Leste	2015*
Nepal	Midwifery Society of Nepal	2016*
Brunei Darussalam	Brunei Darussalam Nurses Association	2016
Myanmar	Myanmar Nurse & Midwives Association (MNMA)	2019*

*=ICM members in 2021; where two dates given = membership lapse.

ICM Eastern Mediterranean Region
Country, Name and Year Midwifery Associations Accepted for ICM Membership

Country	Name of Association	Year
Lebanon	Association des Sages-Femmes Diplomées de la Faculté Française de Médecine [Midwives Association of the Faculty of Medicine]	1982
Iran	Iran Midwifery Population Iranian Midwives Association	1984*
Morocco	Association Marocaine de Sages-Femmes (AMFSF) [Moroccan Association of Midwives]	1991*
Afghanistan	Afghan Midwives Association	2005*
Pakistan	Midwifery Association of Pakistan	2007*
United Arab Emirates	Midwives Emirates National Nursing Association	2010*
Yemen	National Yemeni Midwives Association (NYMA)	2010 (11)*
Somaliland	Somaliland Nursing & Midwifery Association	2014 (3)*
Lebanon	Association des sages-femmes universitaires (ASFU)	2014*
Somalia Puntland	Puntland Association of Midwives	2014*
Somalia Somaliland	Somaliland Nursing and Midwifery Association (SLNMA)	2014*
Tunisia	Association Tunisienne des Sages-Femmes Tunisian Association of Midwives	2014*
Palestine	Midwifery Section of the Palestinian Nursing and Midwifery Association (PNMA)	2104*
Morocco	Association Nationale des Sages-Femmes au Maroc	2015*
Somali	Somali Midwives Association (SOMA)	2016*
Saudi Arabia	Saudi Midwifery Group (SMG)	2018 *
Iran	Iran Scientific Association of Midwifery (ISAM)	2019) *
Iraq	Iraqi Midwives Association	2019*

Lebanon	Ordre des Sages-Femmes du Liban [Lebanese Order of Midwives]	2019*
Morocco	Arab State Midwifery Network	2017; suspended 2019

*ICM members in 2021; where two dates given = membership lapse; dates in parentheses are from ICM records.

ICM European Region[4]
Country, Name and Year Midwifery Associations Accepted for ICM Membership

Country	Name of Association	Year
Belgium (French speaking)	Comité de Concertation des Accoucheuses Belges [Consultation Committee of Belgium Midwives]	Pre 1990
United Kingdom	Royal College of Midwives (RCM)	1954*
Malta	The Midwives' Association of Malta	1975*
France	Organisation Nationale des Syndicates de Sages-Femmes [National Union Organization of Midwives]	1981
Ireland	Midwives' Section Irish Nurses Organization and National Council of Nurses of Ireland	1981*
Israel	Israel Midwives' Association	1981; 2020*
Norway	Den Norske Jordmorforening [The Norwegian Association of Midwives]	1981*
Spain	Asociación Española de Matronas Midwifery Association of Spain	1981*
Switzerland	Schweizerischer Hebammenverband [Swiss Midwifery Association]	1981
Austria	Österreichisches Hebammengremium [Austrian Midwifery Association]	1981; 1996*
Norway	Jordmorforbundet - NSF Norwegian Nurses' Association National Midwifery Section	1982*
Czech Republic	Czech Association of Midwives	1982; 1992*
Denmark	Den Almindelige Danske Jordemoderforening [Danish Association of Midwives]	1982*
Finland	Suomen Kätöilliitto [Finish Midwifery Association]	1982*
Germany	Bund Deutscher Hebammen E. V. [Association of German Midwives, Reg.]	1982*

Greece	The Hellenick Midwives Association	1982*
Iceland	Icelandic Midwives' Association	1982*
Italy	Associazione Italiana di Ostetricia (AIO) Renamed Italian Association of Midwives for Cultural Contacts Abroad (AIORCE)	1982*
Malta	The Midwives' Association of Malta	1982*
Netherlands	Nederlandse Organisatie van Verloskundigen [Royal Organisation of Dutch Midwives (KNOV)]	1982*
Sweden	Svenska Barnmorskeförbundet [Swedish Association of Midwives]	1983*
Switzerland	Federation Suisse des Sages-Femmes [Swiss Federation of Midwives]	198?
United Kingdom	Association of Supervisor Midwives	1985
United Kingdom	Association of Radical Midwives	1986
Luxembourg	Association Luxembourgeoises des Sages-Femmes [Luxembourg Association of Midwives]	1987*
Spain	Consejo General de Enfermería Sección Matronas Renamed Consejo General de Enfermería, (Vocalía Matrona)	1987*
Spain	Federación de Asociaciones de Matronas de España (FAME)	1991*
Spain	Asociación Catalana de Llevadores [Catalán Association of Midwives]	1991*
United Kingdom	Independent Midwives Association	1992
Czech Republic	Czech Midwives Association (CAS) Renamed Czech Association of Midwives	1992*
United Kingdom	Midwifery Society of the Royal College of Nursing	1995*
Latvia	Association of Midwives of Latvia	1996*
Poland	Midwives Section, Polish Gynaecologist Association Renamed Polish Midwives Association	1997*
Estonia	Estonian Midwives' Association	1997*
Belgium	Belgian Midwives Association (BMA)	1998*

Russia	Lique Midwives of Russia [League of Midwives of Russia]	1999
Belgium (English speaking)	Vlaamse Organisatie van vroedrouwen[5] [Flemish Association of Midwives]	1999
Slovenia	Zbornica Zdravstvenenege-Slovenija-Sekcija Medicinskih Sester-Babic [Nurse and Midwives Association of Slovenia]	1998*
Bosnia-Hercegovina	Udruzenje Babica u Bosni i Hercegovini [Association of Midwives in Bosnia and Herzegovina]	2004
Portugal	Associacao Portuguesa Dos Enfermeiros Obstetras (APEO) [Association of Portuguese Nurse Midwives]	2004*
Romania	Romanian Midwives Association	2005
Cyprus	Cyprus Nurses and Midwives Association	2005*
Azerbaijan	Azerbaijan Midwives Association	2007
France	Collège National des Sages-Femmes (CNSF)	2009*
Georgia	Midwives Association of Georgia	2010*
Croatia	Croatian Chamber of Midwives	2010*
Turkey	Midwives Association of Turkey	2010*
France	Collectif des Associations & Syndicats des Sages-Femmes (SFMa) Renamed Société Française de Maïeutique (SFMa) in 2014	2011*
Bulgaria	Alliance of Bulgarian Midwives	2016*
Czech Republic	Czech Union of Midwives	2017*
Romania	Independent Midwives Association of Romania	2017*
Kosovo	Midwifery Association of Kosovo	2018*
Iran	Iran Scientific Association of Midwifery (ISAM)	2019*
Hungary	Hungary Midwives Association	2019*
Iraq	Iraqi Midwives Association	2019*
Serbia-Bosnia	Balkan Midwives Association	2019*

*= ICM members in 2021; where two dates are given = membership lapse.

1 The original Ghana midwives' association was named the Gold Coast Midwives Association. The name changed to Ghana Registered Midwives Association (GRMA) in 1957 when Ghana changed its name from Gold Coast to Ghana at independence.
2 The two nurse-midwifery associations that became members of ICM in 1956 merged to become the American College of Nurse-Midwives in 1969, continuing as an ICM Member Association without a break in membership.
3 The four Provincial midwifery associations in Canada with ICM membership since the 1980s merged into one in 2002, becoming the Canadian Association of Midwives without a lapse in ICM membership.
4 It is unfortunate that records from the 1950s are lacking and none of the European Associations responded to the survey in Chapter 13. Thus, it is impossible to know which MAs in Western Europe were members of the ICM in 1954.
5 There is a question whether the Belgian midwives' associations merged under one association as dates for this one cannot be found in current ICM records.

Annex H

Geographical Location of ICM Headquarters 1939–2022

Geographical Location	Time Frame
France[1]	1939–1954
15 Mansfield Street London (within RCM HQs)	October 1954–December 1974
47 Victoria Street, London, UK	1974–1981
Lower Belgrave Street, London, UK[2]	1981–1987
Barley Mow, Chiswick, London, UK	1987–December 1999
Eisenhowerlaan 138, 2517 KN, The Hague, The Netherlands	January 2000–2006
Laan van Meerdervoort 70, 2517 AN, The Hague, The Netherlands	2006–April 2018
Koninginnegracht 60, 2513 AE, The Hague, The Netherlands	May 2018–present

1 ICM (SA/ICM/C1/18/2). Wellcome Collection. *Minutes of Executive Committee 18th September 1954*. Minutes noted move of the secretariat from France to England in 1954 when it 'became a worldwide organisation and that the running costs were subsidised by RCM.'
2 Margaret Peters. Written notes to JT on 4 April 2020. MP wrote that during the 1981 Brighton Council a new Constitution was adopted. 'I think it is the key action taken to address the financial crisis [loss of USAID grant and extremely low registration at Congress). It introduced the reduced size of the Board and led to the relocation of the HQ from the palatial sized one (Victoria Street) to the attic of Lower Belgrave Street. Plus of course the part-time employee to keep it ticking over, so bankruptcy was averted, and charity status retained.' She went on to say she was Deputy Director in 1984 and remembers meeting in the attic. ICM. *ICM Council Minutes 1987*, p 4. Lease of 57 Lower Belgrave Street expired December 1987, and board was to investigate a move outside of London proper.

Annex I:

Winners of the Marie Goubran Memorial Leadership Award 1993–2020

Year	Awardees	Country	Project
1993	Ren Neang	Cambodia	Established Cambodia Midwives Association (1994)
1993	Vivian Donkor	Ghana	Obtain advanced degree in midwifery
1996	Feddy Mwanga	Tanzania	Her service to midwifery and her future aspirations
1996	Rosaline Lapan	Papua New Guinea	Midwifery services to women in Papua New Guinea
1999	Nester T Moyo	Zimbabwe	Strengthen Midwifery Education in Zimbabwe
1999	Lennie Kamwendo	Malawi	Strengthen Midwifery Education in Malawi
2002	Cecilia Anna Asare	Ghana	Senior Midwife of the Koforidua Regional Hospital
2005	Amoateng-Boahen	Ghana	Midwife in-charge of the Maranatha Maternity Clinic in Kumasi
2008	Ghislaine Francoeur	Haiti	Posthumous – Founding Director of Haiti's first national Midwifery School
2011	Christina Mudokwenyu-Rawdon	Zimbabwe	Leadership in Midwifery Education
2014	Kingsley Musama	Zambia	Exemplary care in a rural setting. First male midwife to receive the award.
2016	Yoana Strancheva	Bulgaria	Introduction of newborn examination skills
2017	Kiran Mubeen	Pakistan	Capacity building for community midwives in Helping Babies Breathe

2018	Kusmayra Ambarwati	Indonesia	Mom to Baby programme: MOMMY MOMBI
2019	Veroncia Oduro-Kwarteng	Ghana	Capacity Building in Helping Babies Breathe
2020	Manju Chhugani	India	Study of safe delivery application with nursing students

Index

Page numbers in *italic* font are used for illustrations.

Ababio, Kathryn *294*
abortions and related care 170–1, 224
abuse of women 43–4, 190–1
accreditation programme *see* Midwifery Education Accreditation Programme
Addo, Fredrica Kwarley Aba 53
advocacy tools 191–2, 228, 265, 284, 303
Affara, Fadwa 330
affiliated associations and other groups 60–1
  see also member associations
affiliations, of regional groups 244, 251
African American midwives 250
African regions *see* Anglophone Africa
American Association of Nurse-Midwives (AANM) 43
American College of Nurse-Midwives (ACNM) 138, 162, 190, 247, 250, 252, 271 n.11, 278, 283, 388
American regions *see* Latin America and Mexico; North America/Caribbean
  Anglophone Africa region 238–45
  historical background 238–9
  impact on ICM 244–5
  member associations 239, 385–6
  value of ICM membership 239–44
Arulkumaran, Sabaratnam 32, 343, 346
Ashton, Ruth 163, 199, 220, 383
Asia-Pacific/Western Pacific region 257–63
  historical background 257–8
  impact on ICM 261–3
  member associations 258–60, 390–1
  value of ICM membership 260–1
association development 240, 254–5, 260, 265
associations of midwives 50–2
Australia 41, 42, 109, 258
Australian College of Midwives Inc. (ACMI) 165, 262, 274
Austrian Midwives' Association 51

autonomy of midwives 205–6, 359–60
awards for midwives 181–3

Bayes, Marjorie
  and FIGO Joint Study Group 310, 311, *311*, 315
  ICM Executive Secretary 72, 77, 118, 132, 291
  and other organisations 71, 79
Belgium 41, 52, 53
beliefs of midwives 213, 214
Bernis, Luc de 290, 299–300, 343, 346, 350, 353
Bill and Melinda Gates Foundation 172, 185, 190
Bill of Rights for Women and Midwives 215–16, 280–1
birth registration 331
Black Sash campaign 249
Brain, Margaret 117, 341
breastfeeding 297–8
Brown, Judith 127, 187–8, *189*, 196, 321, 344, 352
Burkina Faso 169

Cadée, Franka 112–13, 122, 301, 357
calls to action 331–2
Campbell, Kim 95
Canada 246, 249–50, 250–1
capacity building 242–3, 249, 299
Capitation Assistance Fund 107
Caribbean Islands 245
  see also Trinidad
Central Midwives Board 42
chain of office 155–6
challenges for the future 353–5
charity status 88, 105, 106–7, 118
Chief Executives 119–24
Child Survival Partnership (CSP) 323
China 258
Code of Ethics 44, 96, 138, 140, 144, 147,

166, 205, 210–16, 231, 252, 276, 279–80, 365
Collaboration and Partnerships for Healthy Women and Infants position statement 283–4
collaborations and donors 184–6
Columbia University Award 182–3
communication with member associations 124–30
competencies 37–8, 195, 221–5
Competency-Based Education (CBE) workshops 171–2
conferences *see* regional meetings and conferences; United Nations World Conference on Women (1995); Women Deliver (WD) global conferences
Congress Interpretation Fund 107
congresses 155–8
    pre-1954 55–7, 63–5
    1954 London 75–6
    1957 Stockholm 80
    1960 Rome 155
    1963 Spain 155–6
    1999 Manila 156
    finances 104–5
    hosts 96–7
    locations 155–6
    management 156
    regional participation 250–1, 255–6
    remote access 127
    Safe Motherhood workshops 158–64, 298
    structure 156–8
consultants, use of 145, 148
consumer representation 94, 274–5, 278
Conti, Nanna 62, 65
COVID-19 pandemic 123, 301
Cowper-Smith, Frances 120, 252

Daels, Frans 52, 53, 55, 65–6
Dawley, Katherine 40
Day of the Midwife *see* International Day of the Midwife
Day-Stirk, Frances 88, 345
Deane, Nora B 56, 75, 77
Decade of the Midwife campaign 106
definitions
    midwife 37, 54, 74, 206–9, 281, 292, 316
    midwifery 216–17
    midwifery competence 37–8, 221
    profession 204–5
    skilled birth attendants 327–8

skilled care 327
skilled health personnel 333
Dennis-Antwi, Jemima 241, 243
Direct Relief 185
domains of midwifery practice 222–3, 224
donors and donations 102–3, 106, 109, 184–6, 242–3
Downe, Soo 130
Duff, Elizabeth 129

Eastern Mediterranean region 263–7
    historical background 263
    impact on ICM 267
    member associations 263–4, 392–3
    value of ICM membership 264–6
Eastman, Nicholson J 73, 76, 346
education for midwives 154–74
    congresses 155–8
    country workshops 169–71
    Expert Committee on Midwifery Training 73–4
    ICM focus 38
    leadership training 187–8, *189*
    for midwifery teachers 171–3
    regional meetings and conferences 167–9
    Safe Motherhood workshops 158–64, 298
    standards and guidelines 225–30, 242, 248, 260, 322
    symposia and workshops 164–7, 171–2
    UNFPA and 300–1
Education Standards Task Force (TF) 226
Education Standing Committee (ESC) 194–6, 227, 230
Elst, Frau De Graaf Van den 53
empowerment 277–8, 286
England 40–1, 42, 158
Erup, Ellen 56, 77, 80
Essential Competencies for Basic Midwifery Practice 195, 221–5, 300
ethical treatment, standards for 44–5
ethics, code of [see Code of Ethics]
European Region, member associations 394–7
European Working Party on Midwifery Training 314
expectations for the future of ICM 267–70

Family Care International (FCI) 191, 303
family planning 142
Fauveau, Vincent 299, 343, 350
feminism 40–2, 48

finances of the ICM 101–14
  core funding 105–6
  financial ups and downs 86–7, 110–14
  overview 101–2
  recurring expenditures 109–10
  regional meetings and conferences 261–2
  sources of income 102–7
  support for associations and midwives 107–9
France 41, 42, 75
French-speaking midwifery 169, 172, 185
funds for associations and midwives 107–9
  see also donors and donations

Ganges, Frances 120, 122, 163, 252
Gates Foundation 172, 185, 190
Gebour, Olga 50, 51, *52*
gender-based decision making 46–7
gender empowerment 277–8, 286
Germany 51, 105
Ghana 53, 169–70, 241
Global Goodwill Ambassadors 192
Global Standards for Midwifery Education and *Companion Guidelines* 195, 227–30, 242, 248, 266, 300
Global Standards for Midwifery Regulation 230–3, 241, 248–9, 262–3, 266
Global standards for the initial education of professional nurses and midwives 322
Global Strategy document 143, 147, 151, 177
global trends 47, 261
goals of the ICM 144, 147
Gold Coast Midwives' Association (GCMA) 53, 238
Goubran, Marie 117, 120, 128, 181–2, *181*
Guilliland, Karen 257, 263, 276

Hague, The, Netherlands 88, 105, 115 n.29
Hammamet meeting and Call to Action 298, 331–2
Happy Birthdays projects 185, 242
Hardy, Margaret 101, 119, 311, 336 n.38
headquarters of ICM 87, 88, 110, 118, 398
health professional groups 309
  International Council of Nurses (ICN) 318–22
  International Federation of Gynecology and Obstetrics (FIGO) 309–17
  International Pediatric Association (IPA) 317

  Partnership for Maternal, Newborn and Child Health (PMNCH) 324–5
  Healthy Newborn Partnership (HNP) 323
  Helping Babies Breathe (HBB) workshops 242
  Helping Mothers Survive (HMS) workshops 242
Hemschemeyer, Hattie 250
Herschderfer, Kathy 112, 349
Hird, Carol 108, 252, 382
historical background 33–4, 40–1
Hong Kong 258, 260
Hoope-Bender, Petra ten 119, 122, 322–3, 325, 328, 330, 342, 345, 350
Hubbard, Louisa 42
Huis, Marian van 113, 383
human rights 44, 48, 137, 170–1, 279, 280–1, 359
importance of ICM
  to global partners 348–51
  to the health of women 340–3
  to midwives and midwifery associations 344–7

India 53, 165, 166, *168*
indigenous midwives 246, 262
International Association for Maternal and Neonatal Health (IAMANEH) 332
International Code of Ethics for Midwives 210–13, 279
International Confederation of Midwives (ICM)
  aims of the ICM 34–5, 84–5, 96, 177
  Board of Management (BoM) 87, *87*, 89–90
  Byelaws 88–9
  chain of office 155–6
  challenges for the future 353–5
  charity status 88, 105, 106–7, 118
  Code of Ethics 44, 96, 138, 140, 144, 147, 166, 205, 210–16, 231, 252, 276, 279, 280, 365
  Constitution 77, 85–7, 92–3, 285
  core documents 204–17, 218 n.5
  Council 38, 41, 46–7, 58, 72, 75–8, 82 n.41, 85–98, 99 n.6–9, 102–3, 105–9, 111–3, 115, 117–21, 127–8, 130, 132–3, 138, 141–4, 147–8, 156, 158, 164–8, 171–2, 176 n.25, 178–9, 181, 186–7, 189–90, 193–9, 206–11, 213–7,

222–7, 231, 233, 236 n.44, 250, 257, 261, 263, 266, 274–5, 277–8, 280–1, 285–6, 289, 297, 314, 319, 327, 329, 331, 353–4, 380 n.7–8
Executive Committee 77, 77, 85–6, 86, 90–2
Executive Secretary 77, 78
Foundation (Stitching) 88
headquarters 87, 88, 110, 118, 398
joint statements 326–32
lessons learnt 351–2
logo of the ICM 35
membership categories 94–5, 275
membership criteria 93–4, 274
membership fees 103–4, 112
mission statements 142–3
name of the organisation 76
Non-governmental organisation 79, 80
objectives and goals 143–4, 146, 147, 152 n.2
position statements 73, 180, 276, 278, 279, 280, 283–4, 318
Presidents, elected 88
Regional Representatives 87, 87, 90–1, 92
Secretariat 97–8, 117–24
Secretary General 59, 90, 97, 102, 119–20, 349, 352
standing committees 192–7
Strategic Plan 2021–2023 285–6, 361
strategy documents 143–51
strengths and weaknesses 45–6, 46–7, 145
vision statements 138–42, 277–8
International Council of Midwives (ICM) 72, 75–6
International Council of Nurses (ICN) 318–22
joint efforts at the WHA 319–20
joint statements 330–1
other collaborations with ICM 321–2
triad meetings (ICM, ICN & WHO) 320–1
International Day of the Midwife (IDM) 197–200, 241, 261, 284
International Federation of Gynecology and Obstetrics (FIGO) 309–17
definition of midwife 206–8, 316
early partnership with 36, 80, 110, 120, 125–6, 348, 349
European Working Party 314
joint statements 331

Joint Study Group (JSG) 309–10, 313, 316
Maternity Care in the World (1969 & 1972) 311–13, 314–16
ongoing collaboration 317
Safe Motherhood Inter-Agency Group (IAG) 322–3
International Federation of Midwives Organization (IFMO) 71–2
International Journal of Childbirth (IJCB) 130–1
International Midwifery (IM) 129
International Midwifery Journal 308
International Midwifery Matters (IMM) 128–9
International Midwives' Union (IMU)
affiliated associations and other groups 60–1
aim of Union 85
associations before 1922 50–2
finances 61–2
foundation of 40, 43, 52–3
name of the association 53–4
obstetricians, involvement of 65–6
officers 56, 59–60
purpose of 54–5
regulations 57–9
secretariat 57
war, effects of 65–7
International Pediatric Association (IPA) 36, 317
Investing in Midwives project 124, 243, 298–9
Islamabad Declaration on Strengthening Nursing and Midwifery 282, 320
Italy 42, 51

Jamaica 249
Japan 104, 257–8, 260
Jay, M. 56, 77
Johns Hopkins Programme for International Education of Gynecology and Obstetrics (Jhpiego) 112, 146, 184–5, 303
Johnson and Johnson International (J&J) 18, 105, 157, 175 n.11, 182, 184, 188, 244, 262, 377
joint statements 326–32
on birth registration 331
calls to action 331–2
on prevention of post-partum haemorrhage 331
on skilled birth attendants and care 327–30

Kamara, Angela 226
kits for midwives 185
Knutsson, Anneka 299, 301, 347, 353–4
Kondo, Junko 342, 345
Kwast, Barbara 108, 159, *294*, 346–7, 348, 352

Laerdal Global Health 185
Lancet Series on Midwifery 334
Lang, Dorothea 106, 109, 116 n.35, 116 n.47
Latin America and Mexico region 253–7
    impact on ICM 256–7
    member associations 253–4, 389
    value of ICM membership 254–6
leadership building 243, 252–3, 255, 261, 266
leadership training 187–8, *189*
legacy of the ICM 38–9
lessons learnt 351–2
Lewinsky, Thomas 148
Lewis, Debrah 342, 345
Liljestrand, Jerker 349
'Listen to Women' campaign 278
Look, Paul van 347, 349, 350
low resource countries (LRCs)
    attendance at congresses 78
    congresses in 156
    difficulties in 158
    membership of ICM 104, 180–1
    Safe Motherhood Initiative (SMI) 158, 159
    twinning of 187
Luzzi, V 56, 77
Lynch, Bridget 88, 220, 226, 232, 345, 353

MacArthur Foundation 186
male midwives 46, 182
Marie Goubran Memorial Award 181–2, 399–400
Maternal and Neonatal Health (MNH) 191
Maternal Mortality Rate (MMR) 158, 165
maternal, newborn and child health partnerships (PSMNH/PMNCH) 322–6, 350–1
Maternity Care in the World (1969 & 1972) 302, 311–13, 314–16
McLeod, Ian 75
'Meeting of the Minds' (2001) 146, *146*, 187
Member Association Capacity Assessment Tool (MACAT) 189–90
Member Associations (MA) 177–200
    activities of the ICM 177–9

awards for midwives 181–3
financial support of 261–2
future of 358
International Day of the Midwife 197–200, 241, 261
issues, addressing of 179–81
membership numbers 78, 80, 104, 256, 262
standing committees 192–7
support for country activities 183–6
tools for strengthening 186–92
see also regional perspectives
membership categories 94–5, 275
membership criteria 93–4, 274
membership fees 103–4, 112
Midwifery: An Autonomous Profession position statement 280
Midwifery in the Community meeting 298
midwifery, definitions of 216–17
Midwifery Education Accreditation Programme (MEAP) 172, 230
Midwifery Education Development Pathway (MEDPath) 300
Midwifery Partnership with Women position statement 276, 278
Midwifery Regulation Toolkit 233
Midwifery Services Framework (MSF) 190, 241
midwives
    definitions 37, 54, 74, 206–9, 281, 292
    historical background 33–4
    scope of role 141–2, 209
    words for 357–8
Midwives Association of British Columbia, Canada (MABC) 104, 107–8
Midwives Institute 42
Midwives' Kits 185
Midwives, Women and Human Rights position statement 279
mission statements 142–3
model of care 37–8, 213–15, 280
Mossé, Mme 60, *61*, 65, 75
Moyo, Nester
    lessons for the ICM 352
    Marie Goubran Award 182
    Member Association Capacity Assessment Tool (MACAT) 189–90
    on member associations 177
    philosophy and model of care 213
    on value of ICM 342, 344, 349–50
    Young Midwifery Leaders Programme

(YML) 187–8, *189*
Murray, Michelle 130–1
Musama, Kingsley 182

Nature and Scope of Practice of Nurse-Midwives position statement 318
Neonatal Mortality Rate (NMR) 158
Netherlands 88, 105
New Venture Fund 186
New Zealand 41, 42, 258, 276
New Zealand College of Midwives (NZCOM) 94, 272, 274–5, 276, 285
newsletters 128–30
Nixon, WCW 309–11, 346, 348
North America/Caribbean region 245–53
    historical background 245–6
    impact on ICM 251–3
    member associations 247–8, 388
    value of ICM membership 248–51
nurses *see* International Council of Nurses (ICN)
nursing and midwifery 42, 318

objectives of the ICM 143–4, 146, 147
obstetricians
    IMU, involvement in 65–6
    views on ICM 343, 346
office equipment 125, 126, 127
outreach 132–3

Paget, Rosalind 42
Pairman, Sally 123–4, *123*, 232, 233
papers, preparation of 127
partnerships
    for maternal, newborn and child health (PSMNH/PMNCH) 322–6, 350–1
    with organisations 36–7, 79–80, 279–80, 281–4, 289–90, 305–6 *see also* health professional groups
    of regional associations 244, 251
    value of ICM to partners 348–51
    with women 274–5, 276–7, 278–9
    see also twinning of member associations; United Nations Population Fund (UNFPA); World Health Organization (WHO)
Pearse, Jackie 273
Peel, Sir John 310, 314, 346
Peters, Margaret
    ICM board 89, 99 n.18
    ICM constitution 86

ICM finances 87, 101, 110–11
    and low resource countries 154, 156
    on status of midwives 152 n.16
    WHO and ICM 289
Philippines 258
Philosophy and Model of Midwifery Care 213–15, 280
position statements 73, 180
    Collaboration and Partnerships for Healthy Women and Infants 283–4
    Midwifery: An Autonomous Profession 280
    Midwifery Partnership with Women 276, 278
    Midwives, Women and Human Rights 279
    Nature and Scope of Practice of Nurse-Midwives 318
post-partum haemorrhage 331
pre-congress workshops (PCW) 158–64
Presidential Chain of Office 155–6
profession, midwifery as 204–5
Professional Practice Committee (PPC) 193
project management 127–8
Pye, Edith M
    on 1949 meeting of midwives 71
    1954 ICM Congress 75, 76
    on Frans Daels, disappearance of 65, 66
    motion against war 67
    on need for IMU after WWII 70
    photographs *56, 70*

Rathbone, William 42
recognition for midwifery/midwives 240–1, 248, 254, 265
regional meetings and conferences 167–9, 261–2, 266
regional perspectives 237–70
    Anglophone Africa 238–44
    Asia-Pacific/Western Pacific region 257–63
    Eastern Mediterranean region 263–7
    expectations for the future of ICM 267–70
    Latin America and Mexico region 253–7
    North America/Caribbean region 245–53
    survey 238
registration of births 331
regulation of midwives 42, 230–3, 241, 248–9, 262–3
Regulation Standing Committee (RegSC) 196–7, 231–2
representation of the ICM 132–3
Research Standing Committee (RSC) 193–4

Respectful Maternity Care (RMC) 190–1, 284, 300
Ribbens, Geoff 45, 137, 145
Riede, Frieda 71–2
right to vote 40–1
rights *see* Bill of Rights for Women and Midwives; human rights
Rogo, Khama 350–1
Royal College of Midwives (RCM)
    1954 ICM Congress 75–6
    and the ICM 43, 101, 118
    and IFMO 71
    International Day of the Midwife 199
    see also Bayes, Marjorie; Pye, Edith M

Safe Motherhood Fund (SMF) 108–9
Safe Motherhood Initiative (SMI) 43, 158–64, 220–1, 296, 298, 330
Safe Motherhood Inter-Agency Group (IAG) 322–3
Sanofi Espoir Foundation 172, 185
Saraki, Toyin Ojora 192
Save the Children Award 183
Saving Newborn Lives Award 183
Schuiling, Kerri 130
scope of role of midwives 141–2, 209, 266
Secretary Generals/Chief Executives 119–24
Seguranyes Guillot, Gloria 237
sexual and reproductive health (SRH) 142, 190, 217, 243, 255, 326, 360
Sherratt, Della 328, 330, 349, 351–2
skilled birth attendants 327–8, 329
skilled care 327
skilled health personnel 333
Smith, Zepherina 42
social context 40, 43–6
social status of women 141
Sosanya, RO 84
Sponsor a Midwife (SAM) Programme 107–9
staffing 124
    see also Secretary Generals/Chief Executives
standards and guidelines for midwifery education 225–30, 242, 248, 260, 266, 322
standards for ethical treatment 44–5
standards for regulation of midwives 230–3, 266
standing committees 192–7
Starrs, Ann 351
State of the World's Midwifery (SoWMy) reports 302–5

Strachan, Marion 297
strategy documents 143–51
Strengthening Midwifery Services (SMS) 186, 300–1, 331–2
Strengthening Midwives Associations programme 282
Strengthening Nursing and Midwifery resolution 282, 320
strengths and weaknesses of ICM 45–6, 46–7, 145
Strid, Judi 274–5
Styles, Margaretta 319
suffrage 40–1
Sustainable Development Goals (SDG) 215, 281, 293
Swedish Association of Midwives 71, 81 n.2
Swedish International Development Agency (SIDA) 105–6, 115 n.30, 186, 361
symposia and workshops 164–7

themes 38
Thomson Ann 29
Thompson, Anne Sr 89, 109, 117, 163–66, 220, 294, 296, 382
Thompson, Henry 210, 219 n.26
Thompson, Joyce
    code of ethics and 210, 219 n.26
    ICM website and 131
    ICN and 319
    photograph *189*
    standards and guidelines and 226, 236 n.44
    on value of ICM 345
    workshops by 166
Tickner, Valerie 345
toolkits 190–3, 233
tools 186–92
    see also advocacy tools
Traditional Birth Attendants (TBA) 73, 74, 327
Trained Midwives Registration Society 42
training *see* education
translation, problem of 62, 95, 107
trends, global 47
Trinidad 165, 166, 188, 245
Trinidad and Tobago Association of Midwives (TTAM) 249
twinning of member associations 187, 252–3, 262, 282

Uganda 164, 165
United Kingdom 46, 88, 105

see also England
United Nations Children's Fund (UNICEF) 36, 79, 297–8, 323, 324
United Nations Global Strategy for Women's, Children's, and Adolescents' Health 326
United Nations Millennium Development Goals 242, 293, 303, 324, 332
United Nations Population Fund (UNFPA) 3 6, 124, 186, 298–302, 302–3, 305
United Nations Sustainable Development Goals 215, 281, 293
United Nations World Conference on Women (1995) 277, 341
United States Agency for International Development (USAID) 86, 110, 183
United States of America 245–6
universal suffrage 40–1
Updegrove, Kim 131

value of ICM
    to global partners 348–51
    to the health of women 340–3
    to midwives and midwifery associations 344–7
Varela, Vitor 46
visibility of midwives 240, 260, 265
vision for the future 357–62
vision statements 138–42, 277–8
voice of women 274

Walker, Joan 109, 117, 119, 120–1, *121*, 126, 204
Walsh, Denis 130
weaknesses of ICM see strengths and weaknesses of ICM
Weaver, Caroline 342
websites 131–2
What Women Want Campaign 284
White Ribbon Alliance 186, 282, 359
Wiklund, Ingela 102
WithWomen Charity 106–7, 114
women and the ICM 272–86
    constitution review 285
    consumer representation 274–5
    organisations as partners 281–4
    vision for women and midwives 276–8
    women as partners 278–81
    women's work 273–4
Women Deliver (WD) global conferences 280
women, status of 141

women's suffrage 40–1
Woodville, Lucille 252, 314–5, 339–40, 381
work of women 273–4
working parties 183–4
workshops 158–64, 164–7, 169–71, 171–2, 242, 298
World Bank 323
world conference on women see United Nations World Conference on Women (1995)
World Health Organization (WHO)
    first partner of ICM 290
    definitions of midwife 206–8, 292, 316
    definition of Skilled Health Personnel providing care during childbirth 2018 333
    Expert Committee on Midwifery Training 73–4, 81 n.14, 290–1
    Expert Committee on the Midwife in Maternity Care 291–3, 327
    Global Advisory Group on Nursing and Midwifery (GAGNM) 226, 235 n.17, 296, 319–20
    Global Strategy for Women's, Children's, and Adolescents' Health 326
    and the ICM 36, 75–6, 78–9, 81 n.16, 110, 120, 290–7, 348, 349–50
    Making Pregnancy Safer (MPS) 296, 328
    Midwifery Services Framework 190
    ongoing relationship 293
    Partnership for Safe Motherhood and Newborn Health (PSMNH) 323
    State of the World's Midwifery (SoWMy) reports 303
    Technical Liaison Officers 293–5
    use of 'midwife' 328–30
    workshops with ICM 169–70
    World Health Assembly 319–20, 349
World War I 34, 41
World War II 34, 43

Young Midwifery Leaders Programme (YML) 187–8, *189*, 240, 255

Zimbabwe 170–1